Ethics and Epidemiology

Ethics and Epidemiology

Edited by

Steven S. Coughlin
Tom L. Beauchamp

New York   Oxford
OXFORD UNIVERSITY PRESS
1996

Oxford University Press

Oxford   New York
Athens   Auckland   Bangkok   Bombay
Calcutta   Cape Town   Dar es Salaam   Delhi
Florence   Hong Kong   Istanbul   Karachi
Kuala Lumpur   Madras   Madrid   Melbourne
Mexico City   Nairobi   Paris   Singapore
Taipei   Tokyo   Toronto

and associated companies in
Berlin   Ibadan

Published by Oxford University Press, Inc.,
198 Madison Avenue, New York, New York 10016

Oxford is a registered trademark of Oxford University Press

Library of Congress Cataloging-in-Publication Data
Ethics and epidemiology /
edited by Steven S. Coughlin, Tom L. Beauchamp
p.   cm.   Includes index.
ISBN 0-19-510242-8
1. Epidemiology—Research—Moral and ethical aspects.
I. Coughlin, Steven S. (Steven Scott), 1957– .
II. Beauchamp, Tom L.
[DNLM: 1. Ethics, Medical.   2. Epidemiology.
3. Epidemiologic Methods.   4. Social Medicine.
W 50 E8423 1996]   RA652.E84   1996   174'.2—dc20
DNLM/DLC   for Library of Congress   95-4802

9 8 7 6 5 4 3 2

Printed in the United States of America
on acid-free paper

Preface

Epidemiologists, like other scientists, accept ideals of free inquiry and the pursuit of knowledge. The goal of science, after all, is to explain and to predict natural phenomena. But epidemiologists also cherish values of improving the public's health through the application of scientific knowledge. Epidemiologists have professional obligations both to advance scientific knowledge and to enhance, protect, and restore public health through the application of this knowledge.

These dual professional obligations sometimes give rise to moral problems. An example is found in the recent report of a dramatic increase over the past decade in the numbers of infants and toddlers living in poverty in the United States. Should epidemiologists knowledgeable about these findings be expected or encouraged to take public stands on policies that may protect the health of poor children, or is such advocacy by epidemiologists an inappropriate professional activity that causes scientific objectivity to suffer? As this and many other examples illustrate, epidemiologists are often confronted with moral problems that need careful analysis, and yet such questions cannot be adequately answered by reference to current ethics guidelines.

Epidemiologists need to be in a position to ensure that subjects are adequately informed and protected from undue risks, and that potential social benefits of epidemiology are maximized. The essays in this volume were undertaken with these challenges in mind, tempered by the knowledge that they present serious problems around which it may be difficult to build consensus.

The chapters are organized topically and divided into five parts. The first part is titled "Foundations" because the chapters introduce basic and recurring concepts and principles. The subsequent parts deal with "Informed Consent, Privacy, and Confidentiality," "Balancing Risks and Benefits," "The Study of Vulnerable Populations," and "The Regulatory Context and Professional Education." The latter subject includes discussion of the institutional review board (IRB) system and issues surrounding scientific misconduct in epidemiologic research. Each chapter is original, developed to fit into the structure of this volume.

The objective of this work is to make students, epidemiologists, and other health professionals aware of situations that require moral reflection, judgment, or decision, while pointing to ways in which justified moral conclusions can be reached. We hope the book will also be of use to persons interested more broadly in bioethics and health policy. The text is most suited to the situation in epidemiology in North America, whose history, institutions, and studies represent the bulk of the material covered. However, several chapters examine international issues, and much of the book's content can easily be construed beyond the North American context of epidemiology and bioethics.

We have received many helpful suggestions for improving this work. It is impossible to recognize them all, but we owe a major debt of gratitude to Kenrad Nelson, Kenneth Goodman, Douglas Weed, Rebecca Clark, Colin Soskolne, George Annas, and Virginia Ktsanes, and special thanks to Catherine Metayer, who has assisted us for two years in the collection of materials. Superb assistance was also provided through our university offices, where for several months drafts were faithfully prepared. Moheba Hanif and Miranda Kobritz deserve our special thanks.

We also thank Jeffrey House and Susan Hannan of Oxford University Press for their helpful editorial advice. We acknowledge with warm appreciation the assistance provided by the Tulane Medical Center Library and the Kennedy Institute's Bioethics Library and information retrieval project, which kept us in touch with the most important literature and reduced the burdens of library research.

New Orleans, La.   S.S.C.
Washington, D.C.   T.L.B.
April 1995

Contents

PART IV   The Study of Vulnerable Populations

PART V   The Regulatory Context and
Professional Education

Contributors

KAREN GLANZ
Professor
Cancer Research Center of Hawaii
University of Hawaii
Honolulu, HI

ELLEN B. GOLD
Associate Professor
Division of Occupational and
    Environmental Medicine
University of California at Davis
Davis, CA

KENNETH W. GOODMAN
Director
Forum for Bioethics and Philosophy
University of Miami
Miami, FL

JOHN LAST
Emeritus Professor of Epidemiology and
    Community Medicine
University of Ottawa
Ottawa, Ontario, Canada

SANFORD LEIKIN
Professor and Director
Office of Ethics
Children's National Medical Center
Washington, DC

CARYN LERMAN
Associate Professor
Cancer Prevention and Control
Georgetown University Medical Center
Washington, DC

CAROL LEVINE
Executive Director
The Orphan Project: The HIV Epidemic
    and New York City's Children
Fund for the City of New York
New York, NY

ROBERT J. LEVINE
Professor
Department of Medicine
Yale University School of Medicine
New Haven, CT

DOROTHY K. MACFARLANE
Division of Research Investigations
Office of Research Integrity
U.S. Department of Health and Human
    Services
Rockville, MD

JOANNE M. MCGLOIN
Associate Director
Program on Aging
Yale University School of Medicine
New Haven, CT

ADRIAN M. OSTFELD
Professor Emeritus
Department of Epidemiology and Public
  Health
Yale University School of Medicine
New Haven, CT

RONALD J. PRINEAS
Professor and Chair
Department of Epidemiology
University of Miami
Miami, FL

BARBARA K. RIMER
Director, Cancer Control Program
Duke University Comprehensive Cancer
  Center
Durham, NC

MARJORIE M. SHULTZ
Professor
Boalt Hall School of Law
University of California at Berkeley
Berkeley, CA

PAUL A. SCHULTE
Chief, Screening and Notification Section
Division of Surveillance, Hazard
  Evaluations and Field Studies
Industrywide Studies Branch
National Institute for Occupational
  Safety and Health
Cincinnati, OH

MITCHELL SINGAL
Screening and Notification Section
Division of Surveillance, Hazard
  Evaluations and Field Studies
Industrywide Studies Branch
National Institute for Occupational
  Safety and Health
Cincinnati, OH

COLIN L. SOSKOLNE
Professor and Director
Epidemiology Program
University of Alberta
Edmonton, Alberta, Canada

DOUGLAS L. WEED
Chief, Preventive Oncology Branch
Division of Cancer Prevention and
  Control
National Cancer Institute
Bethesda, MD

I

FOUNDATIONS

1

Historical Foundations

STEVEN S. COUGHLIN
TOM L. BEAUCHAMP

In this first chapter we consider the historical and ethical roots of epidemiology and the public health movement. This brief history includes major developments in the last half of the twentieth century in regulatory safeguards and professional epidemiologic ethics. Our goal is to explain how we got where we are today.

Early Developments in Public Health and Ethics

The major writings of prominent figures in ancient, medieval, and modern medicine contain a storehouse of information about professional commitments to patients. But this history is disappointing from the perspective of public health ethics because of the nearly complete absence of many themes now considered central to ethics in the health professions.

Beginning with the classic texts of ancient medicine, the Hippocratic corpus, the primary focus of medical ethics was assumed to be the obligation of physicians to provide medical benefits to patients and to protect them from harm. The purpose of medicine as expressed in the Hippocratic oath is to benefit the sick and keep them from harm and injustice. Information management in interactions with patients is portrayed as a matter of prudence and discretion. Although the Hippocratic writings mention the importance of a few moral requirements that are prominent today, such as confidentiality, these writings do not even hint at most of the obligations we now consider central to biomedical and public health ethics, among them respect for the autonomy of persons and social justice in promoting the public's health.

5

Rudiments of public health were themselves primitive in ancient, medieval, and early modern societies. They included little more than the segregation of persons with leprosy and religious requirements to avoid foods thought to be unclean. The ancient Greeks favored the miasmic theory of the origin of epidemics (the belief that epidemics are caused by "bad air" and the odors of putrefaction), but little evidence suggests that they regarded health and disease as the proper subjects of broad public action or moral responsibility.[1] Aristotle and Galen lived in societies in which hygienic measures and health education (to the extent they existed) were directed at the elite, rather than lower classes, foreigners, or slaves.[1]

During the Middle Ages societal values often did not favor the development of public health or the provision of health services, and authorities accepted no obligation to protect the public's health. Public health advanced little throughout the Middle Ages, except for the control of a very limited number of communicable diseases achieved through the segregation and quarantine of persons thought to be infectious.[2]

Around the sixteenth century in Europe, hypotheses began to emerge about the social genesis of disease and some proposals were advanced about the role of government in public health. At the outset these ideas had little practical meaning, but they ultimately contributed to the emerging realization that government has an obligation to correct unsanitary conditions that threaten the health of rich and poor alike.[1] The early writings relied on speculative hypotheses and came more from the humanities than the sciences. For example, Thomas More (1478–1535) wrote about a fictitious land in *Utopia* (1516) in which hygiene protected health and where there was insurance against sickness and unemployment, and Jean-Jacques Rousseau (1712–1778) speculated about the social origins of illness in his *Discourse on the Origin and Foundations of Inequality Among Men* (1755).[2-4] In the context of an angry criticism of all "civil society," Rousseau suggested that disease developed from social circumstances and that ill health resulted from many factors, most beyond the power of medicine to touch:

With regard to illnesses, [I note] the extreme inequality in our lifestyle: excessive idleness among some, excessive labor among others; the ease with which we arouse and satisfy our appetites and our sensuality; the overly refined foods of the wealthy, which nourish them with irritating juices and overwhelm them with indigestion; the bad food of the poor, who most of the time do not have even that, and who, for want of food, are inclined to stuff their stomachs greedily whenever possible; staying up until all hours, excesses of all kinds, immoderate outbursts of every passion, bouts of fatigue and mental exhaustion; countless sorrows and afflictions which are felt in all levels of society and which perpetually gnaw away at souls: these are the fatal proofs that most of our ills are of our own making, and that we could have avoided nearly all of them by preserving the simple, regular and solitary lifestyle prescribed to us by nature.[4]

Rousseau's ideas subsequently influenced some leading Enlightenment figures in ethics, as well as later public health writers such as the influential German physician Johann Peter Frank (1745–1821), who held high positions in government and academia (in Germany, Austria, Italy, and Russia) and was an early proponent of social medicine controlled by the state. Frank promoted the idea of "medical police," that is, physicians with a public health role of sufficient authority to protect people against the health consequences of squalid urban living conditions. He argued that the physician's primary obligations are not owed merely to patients or the local community, but to the state as a whole (and the monarch in particular). Public health responsibilities were thereby reconceived as primary physicians' responsibilities.[1,5]

However, pathogenic microorganisms were still unknown during the Enlightenment. With the exception of a few diseases such as smallpox, disease was explained in terms of unhealthy lifestyles and environments rather than of contagion. Poor air, water, and living conditions were thought to foster miasmas that caused illness. Hence, many Enlightenment physicians undertook public health campaigns emphasizing both personal hygiene and environmental hygiene. They appreciated that methods of prevention were more effective than those of cure, and saw it as a matter of personal responsibility to maintain one's health. The success of their efforts was not surprising because standard therapies such as laxatives, bloodletting, and vomits yielded less impressive results than did public health efforts.[6,7]

A small number of Enlightenment figures with these preoccupations also exhibited an interest in professional ethics. They were among the first in history to lecture on and publish extensive writings devoted to this subject. American Benjamin Rush (1745–1813) and Scottish physician John Gregory (1724–1773) have in recent years been recognized for their views on the moral obligations of physicians to educate the public and to make disclosures to patients. However, neither advocated moral obligations that we think of today on the model of informed consent. They wanted patients and the general public to be sufficiently educated so that they could understand physicians' recommendations and therefore be motivated to comply. But they were not optimistic that nonphysicians could form their own opinions and make appropriate medical choices. For example, Rush advised physicians to "yield to them [patients] in matters of little consequence, but maintain an inflexible authority over them in matters that are essential to life." Gregory was quick to underscore that the physician must be keenly aware of the harm untimely revelations might cause to private patients or to the public. There is no assertion by these or any other Enlightenment figures of the importance of respecting patient rights of self-determination, nor of obtaining consent for any purpose other than a medically good outcome. Gregory and Rush appreciated the value of information, but ideas of informed consent in health care did not originate in their writings. Indeed, the concept was not mentioned during the Enlightenment.[8,9]

An organized social system for the protection of public health did not appear

until the nineteenth century in England.[10] Before such protections were instituted, England had become the first country to experience the social costs of the
Industrial Revolution.[2] But due to the efforts of Sir Edwin Chadwick (1800–1890)
and other English reformers, laws were enacted that improved the method of providing relief to the poor, made it illegal to employ children under the age of nine
in factories, and advanced the health and welfare of industrial workers.[1,10]
Chadwick was largely responsible for the passage of the Public Health Act of
1848, for example, which created a Board of Health to oversee sanitary improvements at about the time that John Snow began his classic series of investigations on the occurrence of cholera in London.[1,3,10] Legislation of this type
quickly spread to other countries and had a substantial impact on public health
and life expectancy.[1] A Royal commission headed by Chadwick recommended
improvements in drainage systems in large towns, where a lack of sanitation had
resulted in the spread of typhoid, cholera, and other diseases.[1]

The primary motivation for reform was the realization that poverty and unsanitary conditions had adverse economic and social consequences.[1,10] Chadwick
maintained a close association with English philosopher Jeremy Bentham
(1748–1832), whose progressive social reforms to benefit children employed in
the factories, the poor, the protection of animals, and women's liberation had a
major impact in Victorian England and repercussions throughout Europe and
India. In early adulthood, Chadwick was assistant to Bentham, and later applied
Bentham's utilitarian theories[11] to practical problems of public health. Chadwick
came to see poverty as a major cause of ill health and he ultimately concluded
that poverty was often caused by disease.

Chadwick was a contemporary of John Stuart Mill (1806–1873), himself a
Benthamite and the foremost utilitarian writer of the nineteenth century (Chapter
2). Mill was elected to the British Parliament in 1865, but his causes were un-
popular with both major parties. These causes were similar to Chadwick's and
included increased protections for the more vulnerable members of society, especially women, poor people, and persons condemned to capital punishment. The
flavor of Mill's convictions and objectives is well captured in a passage in his
Utilitarianism, which remains the most widely read statement of utilitarian ethics:

Even that most intractable of enemies, disease, may be indefinitely reduced in dimensions
by good physical and moral education, and proper control of noxious influences; while
the progress of science holds out a promise for the future of still more direct conquests
over this detestable foe. And every advance in that direction relieves us from some, not
only of the chances which cut short our own lives, but, what concerns us still more, which
deprive us of those in whom our happiness is wrapt up.[12]

Many of the founders of the public health movement in nineteenth century
England were guided by a utilitarian moral theory—Bentham's, Mill's, or some
other. Whether or not their utilitarian foundations were adequate, the leaders of

the sanitary movement attempted to use epidemiologic methods of observation to prevent or control diseases that afflicted those who were less well off in society. For example, Chadwick organized an inquiry into the diseases and unsanitary living conditions that were prevalent among the impoverished working-class population of England. The resulting *General Report on the Sanitary Conditions of the Labouring Population of Great Britain* (1842) was a powerful indictment of the appalling living conditions of industrial workers and their families.[1,10,13]

A similar sanitary survey was undertaken subsequently by Lemuel Shattuck (1793–1859) in Massachusetts. Shattuck's influential report (1850) outlined the basis for an organized system of public health.[14] Industrialization in the United States had caught up with and surpassed that in England by the latter part of the nineteenth century. The arrival of large numbers of immigrants from Europe and rapid industrialization resulted in a number of social problems, including unplanned urban growth and the spread of urban slums. Voluntary societies and governmental agencies were formed to tackle public health problems such as poverty, malnutrition, and disease.[10]

During the closing decades of the nineteenth century, the germ theory of disease gained widespread acceptance because of important bacteriological discoveries by Koch, Pasteur, and others.[15,16] Microbiology and bacteriology became the most important of the medical sciences, and, in both the United States and Europe, the emphasis in public health and epidemiology was on the prevention of infectious diseases.[16,17] By the turn of the century, environmental health concerns began to be overtaken by a new approach to public health: meeting the needs of affected persons, particularly of vulnerable persons such as mothers and children. With major breakthroughs in bacteriology and immunology, disease prevention in the individual moved to the forefront.[10]

These developments occurred in conjunction with a broad philosophic and social revolution that was driven by a growing appreciation for the value and dignity of the person. Since the beginnings of the public health movement, the goal of public health and epidemiology has been the prevention of premature death and disease through the application of scientific and technical knowledge.[18] However, as some events now to be discussed indicate, the rights of individuals have not always been respected in pursuing these important societal objectives.

Twentieth-Century Developments in Public Health and Ethics

At the beginning of the twentieth century, epidemiology in the United States developed primarily as a function of federal, state, and local health departments. In 1891 the Hygienic Laboratory was organized by the Marine Hospital Service (later the United States Public Health Service), and became a major center for epidemiologic research in the United States. Investigators at the Hygienic

Laboratory, renamed the National Institute of Health in 1930, focused on both infectious diseases and deficiency diseases such as pellagra. The Hygienic Laboratory was a training ground for Joseph Goldberger, Wade Hampton Frost, and other prominent epidemiologists.[17]

Epidemiology developed separately in England, where leading practitioners in the 1930s, such as Major Greenwood of the London School of Hygiene, were concerned with both infectious and noninfectious epidemiology.[16,17] Greenwood was an active member of the Socialist Medical Association and an early advocate of socialized medicine. Like other British epidemiologists of that era, he was concerned with social causes of disease and the health of all groups in society.[10,16]

As John Last notes in Chapter 3, it is difficult to find any mention of ethical issues in the writings of the leading epidemiologists during this period. Moreover, medicine, public health, and moral philosophy also showed no deep interest in what we would consider today the major issues of biomedical ethics. A noteworthy exception is found in United States Army surgeon Walter Reed's yellow-fever experiments, which involved formal procedures for obtaining the consent of potential subjects using a written contract that set forth his understanding of the ethical duties of medical researchers.[19] Although deficient by contemporary standards of disclosure and consent, these procedures recognized the right of the individual to refuse or authorize participation in the research.

By the mid-twentieth century, the focus in epidemiology had shifted in both Europe and the United States in response to the increasing predominance of chronic diseases such as cardiovascular disease, cancer, and diabetes, which were seen as having multiple environmental and genetic etiologies. The period of the late 1940s was notable for both the start-up of the World Health Organization and the initiation of the Framingham Study (a well-known cohort study of heart disease, continuing since 1949).[20] The Nuremberg Code and the Declaration of Geneva were also developed during this period (as discussed below). In 1956, Doll and Hill released the results of their cohort study of cigarette smoking and lung cancer among British doctors.[21] A few years later, in 1960, Brian MacMahon and his colleagues published *Epidemiological Methods*, the first text to provide a clear description of case-control and cohort study designs.[20,22]

Throughout the early years of the post-World War II era, it is difficult to find any reference to ethical issues in the epidemiologic literature, outside of some narrowly focused discussions of the ethics of randomized controlled trials.[23,24] Epidemiologic researchers, primarily physicians, undertook studies with little or no public scrutiny of their methods or professional obligations, and unencumbered by what would later become regulatory safeguards for the protection of human subjects, such as the shift to committee review. Since that time, major regulatory changes have been made in the United States and many other countries, as discussed below and then more fully by Robert Levine in Chapter 13. These changes have resulted in substantially improved safeguards for protecting the welfare and rights of human research subjects, and were driven primarily by acceptance of the idea that individuals possess fundamental rights that should not be violated in the pursuit of scientific and medical progress.[25,26,27]

The Origins of Regulatory Safeguards for Human Subjects Research

In 1908 Sir William Osler appeared before the Royal Commission on Vivisection, and used the occasion to discuss the subject of Reed's research on yellow fever. When asked by the commission whether risky research on humans is morally permissible—a view Osler attributed to Reed—Osler answered: "It is always immoral without a definite, specific statement from the individual himself, with a *full knowledge* of the circumstances. Under these circumstances, any man, I think is *at liberty to submit himself to experiments*" (emphasis added). When then asked if "voluntary consent . . . entirely changes the question of morality," Osler replied, "Entirely."[28] Some writers on the history of this period describe his testimony as reflecting the usual and customary ethics of research at the turn of the century,[29] but this sweeping historical claim needs more supporting evidence than is now available. The extent to which any principle of scrutiny of research obligations and any requirement of consent was then ingrained in the ethics of research, or would become ingrained in the next half century, is still today a matter of historical controversy.

One reason for the relatively late emergence of interest in research ethics is that scientifically rigorous research involving human subjects did not become common in the United States and Europe until the middle of the twentieth century. Only shortly before the outbreak of World War II had research evolved into an established and thriving concern.[30,31,32] Not surprisingly, then, research ethics prior to World War II were no more influential on research practices than the parallel history of clinical ethics were on clinical practices.[33]

The major events that pushed the ethics of research to the forefront occurred at the Nuremberg trials. The Nuremberg Military Tribunals unambiguously condemned the sinister political motivation of Nazi experiments in the tribunals' review of "crimes against humanity." A list of ten principles constitutes the Nuremberg Code, whose famous Principle 1 states, without qualification, that the primary consideration in research is the subject's voluntary consent, which is "absolutely essential."[34]

The Nuremberg Code was not an attempt to formulate new rules of professional conduct.[35] Rather, it delineated certain principles of medical and research ethics in the context of a trial for war crimes. Although it had little immediate impact on the conduct of biomedical research, the Nuremberg Code served as a model for many professional and governmental codes formulated in the 1950s and 1960s, and its provision requiring *voluntary* consent was a forerunner of practices of informed consent in biomedical research.[33,36]

The gross violations investigated at Nuremberg were gradually perceived by the medical community as a threat to the reputation and integrity of biomedical research. Partially in response to this perceived threat, the General Assembly of the World Medical Association (WMA) drafted the less impressive Declaration of Geneva in 1948.[35] Eventually the WMA began to formulate a more suitable code to distinguish ethical from unethical clinical research. A draft was produced in 1961, but the code was not adopted until a WMA meeting at Helsinki in 1964.[37] This three-year delay was not caused by vacillation or indifference, but was the result of international political processes and a determination to produce a universally applicable and useful document.[38]

The Declaration of Helsinki made consent a central requirement of ethical research and introduced an important distinction between therapeutic and nontherapeutic research. The former is defined in the declaration as research "combined with patient care," and is permitted as a means of acquiring new medical knowledge only insofar as it "is justified by its potential diagnostic or therapeutic value for the patient." The latter is defined as purely scientific research without therapeutic value or purpose for the specific subjects studied. The declaration requires consent for all instances of nontherapeutic research, unless a subject is incompetent, in which case guardian consent is necessary. Paragraph I.9 of the declaration reads: "In any research on human beings, each potential subject must be adequately informed of the aims, methods, anticipated benefits and potential hazards of the study and the discomfort it may entail [and] that he is at liberty to abstain. . . . The doctor should then obtain the subject's freely given informed consent."[25,35]

The American Medical Association (AMA), the American Society for Clinical Investigation, the American Federation for Clinical Research, and many other medical groups either endorsed the Declaration of Helsinki or established ethical requirements consonant with its provisions.[39] Officials at federal agencies in the United States also looked to Helsinki before developing their provisions, some of which were close-to-verbatim reformulations of the declaration. Whatever its shortcomings, the Helsinki code will be remembered as a foundational document in the history of research ethics and the first significant attempt at self-regulation internal to medical research itself. It can be said that Nuremberg was the first code prescribed for medicine externally by a court system, and Helsinki the first code prescribed internally by a professional body in medicine.

More comprehensive guidelines formulated in 1982 by the World Health Organization (WHO) and the Council of International Organizations of Medical Sciences (CIOMS) took Helsinki (1975 revision) as a starting point.[25,35] Both Helsinki and the WHO/CIOMS guidelines (revised in 1993) state that all human-subjects research should be reviewed by an independent committee.[35] The latter guidelines contain special provisions for protecting vulnerable persons included in medical experiments, such as pregnant women, children, the mentally ill, and individuals in developing countries.[35] Many of these aspects are discussed by John Last in Chapter 3 and Robert Levine in Chapter 13.

In the United States, Congress passed the Drug Amendments of 1962 with the intent of making fundamental changes in federal regulation of the drug industry.[40] Public concern over the thalidomide disaster in the early 1960s (when the drug was approved for use in Europe but still considered experimental in the United States) was a strong incentive for regulatory action. This gripping example of the effects of a drug that was harmless to the pregnant woman but devastating to the fetus was presented to a congressional subcommittee headed by Senator Hubert Humphrey.[41] Humphrey, Senator Estes Kefauver, and other senators argued vigorously that loopholes in testing and warning requirements existed at the Food and Drug Administration (FDA), and procedures for monitoring research protocols and consent procedures were discussed at the hearings.[42,43] In its deliberations on the amendments, the Senate focused on problems of cost, competition, safety, and efficacy. A so-called consent requirement was added at the last moment by Senator Jacob Javits during committee and floor debate.

This provision required—for the first time in U.S. legislative history—that researchers inform subjects of a drug's experimental nature and receive their consent before starting an investigation, except under circumstances in which researchers "deem it not feasible or, in their professional judgment, contrary to the best interests of such human beings."[44] This exception proved troublesome, and is an outstanding example of the way confusion arose in the early days of attempts to change practices of biomedical ethics in the United States. Frances Kelsey—Chief of the Investigational Drug Branch, Division of New Drugs, FDA—argued that the best-interests exception could not be validly invoked merely because an investigator believed informed consent would negatively affect the research design or would disturb the patient-physician relationship. Kelsey held that the exception could be legitimate in only a few extreme cases, usually with special classes of subjects such as children, or in emergency contexts. However, the matter went unclarified at FDA for the next two years. In 1965, FDA Commissioner George P. Larrick obstinately refused to offer an interpretation of the consent provisions beyond the literal letter of the law as enacted. This refusal compounded the vagueness surrounding the policy at FDA, and critics pointed to the objectionable implication that research on the seriously ill and unconscious patient would be permissible, without consent, under these guidelines.[43]

On January 17, 1966, James Lee Goddard succeeded Larrick as FDA Commissioner. Beset by numerous reports of experimentation without consent, as well as by the swirl of controversy caused by the major case of the Jewish Chronic Disease Hospital, Goddard determined to resolve the ambiguities surrounding informed consent. He appointed several FDA officials to study the matter and make recommendations. In August 1966, new provisions were published as "Consent for Use of Investigational New Drugs on Humans: Statement of Policy."[42,43]

This development took place two months after the appearance of an influential 1966 article by Henry Beecher in the *New England Journal of Medicine*. Beecher charged that many patients included in clinical research experiments never had the risks satisfactorily explained to them or were unaware they were the subjects of an experiment.[45] Beecher's pioneering article spawned a great deal of interest in the ethics of research and was noticed by high officials at the National Institutes of Health (NIH).

James Shannon, Director of NIH from 1955 to 1968, was deeply impressed by Beecher's article and was at the time of its publication troubled by dramatic and morally unacceptable events. He and other officials at NIH had concluded that federally funded research could be ethically insensitive and politically explosive, and could be initiated without adequate peer review or consent by patients and subjects. In late 1963, Shannon asked the NIH division that supported research centers to investigate these problems and make recommendations. An Associate Chief for Program Development, Robert B. Livingston, was selected to chair this study.[46] His report, in November 1964, warned of "possible repercussions of untoward events which are increasingly likely to occur" in "unfavorable" circumstances, including events that could "rudely shake" the NIH. It noted the absence of an applicable code of conduct for research, as well as an uncertain legal context.[47,48] Problems of risk, liability, and the inhibition of research dominated this report.

The Livingston report argued that it would be difficult for NIH to assume responsibility for ethics and research practices without striking an unduly authoritarian posture on requirements for research. The report also noted that there were ethical problems raised by policies "inhibiting the pursuit of research on man," and added that "NIH is not in a position to shape the educational foundations of medical ethics, or even the clinical indoctrination of young investigators."[46] Shannon was disappointed with this part of the report because he believed that NIH should command a position of increased responsibility. However, he accepted the report and regarded some of its recommendations as urgent. In early 1965 he asked the U.S. Surgeon General to give "highest priority" to "rapid accomplishment of the objectives" of the basic recommendations. He suggested broad consultation with members of the legal profession and the clergy as well as the medical profession, and endorsed the idea of "review by the investigator's peers."[49]

Shannon and Surgeon General Luther Terry then reached a joint decision to present problems raised by the report to the National Advisory Health Council (NAHC) in September 1965. At this decisive meeting, Shannon argued that the agency should assume responsibility for placing formal controls on the independent judgment of investigators, in order to remove conflict of interest and bias.

Specifically, he argued for subjecting research protocols to impartial, peer review of the risks of the research and of the adequacy of protections of subjects' rights.[50] Shannon knew that "consent" could easily be manipulated through the authority of physicians, and he prompted a discussion of how impartiality could be introduced into the consent process as well. The members of NAHC accepted all of these concerns as valid, but they doubted that the many fields encompassed by government-supported research—which included epidemiology and the social sciences—could be governed by a single set of procedures or regulations. Nevertheless, within three months, at its meeting on December 3, 1965, NAHC supported a resolution that followed the broad outlines of Shannon's recommendations and proposed guidelines for federal research ethics.[51]

The resolution was accepted by newly installed Surgeon General William H. Stewart, who issued a policy statement in February 1966 that would become a landmark in the history of research ethics in the United States—as historically important as any comparable event in clinical ethics. This policy statement on "Clinical Investigations Using Human Subjects" compelled institutions receiving federal grant support from the Public Health Service to provide prior review by a committee for proposed research with human subjects. The subjective judgment of a principal investigator or program director was no longer sufficient. The three areas requiring review were (1) the rights and welfare of subjects, (2) the appropriateness of methods used to obtain informed consent, and (3) the balance of risks and benefits.[52]

A memorandum that explained this policy and made it effective immediately was sent the same day to the heads of all institutions receiving grant support. The Surgeon General said simply that "the wisdom and sound professional judgment of you and your staff will determine what constitutes the rights and welfare of human subjects in research, what constitutes informed consent, and what constitutes the risks and potential medical benefits of a particular investigation."[53] Tough questions about research ethics were thus being afforded a *procedural* answer only: Committees would make the final substantive determinations.

These developments formed the genesis of what has been called the "movement to ethics committees."[54] Peer review was destined to serve as the basis of a string of federal policies governing research ethics. The federal initiatives gained endorsement by much of the biomedical community,[55] and were adopted in modified form by the Association of American Medical Colleges as one requirement for the accreditation of medical schools.[56] Over a period of a decade they served as a crude model, which gradually was refined and finally became an accepted part of institutional practices for the protection of human research subjects throughout the United States.

Shortly after these developments, the Department of Health, Education, and Welfare issued a series of guidebooks and regulations for the protection of human research subjects. The National Research Act of 1974 then established the

National Commission for the Protection of Human Subjects of Biomedical and Behavioral Research, which by 1978 made a number of important recommendations, many having the effect of federal law.[25,33,57] Subsequent federal regulations for the protection of human research subjects in the United States, including those of the FDA and the Department of Health and Human Services, have resulted in a complex institutional review board system (IRB) and other regulatory safeguards.[25,26,33] The purpose of the IRB is to ensure the rights and welfare of research subjects as well as justice in the selection of subjects. Many of these developments and their importance are discussed by Robert Levine in Chapter 13.

The Origins of Contemporary Epidemiologic Ethics

By the early 1970s, the Tuskegee Syphilis Study, the Jewish Chronic Disease Hospital case, and Beecher's article had fostered a growing awareness of the potential for ethical problems and dilemmas in epidemiology and clinical research.[25,33,58,59,60] Some ethical issues in epidemiologic research and practice drew widespread attention in the 1970s when U.S. legislators responded to public concern and began drafting stringent laws to protect the privacy and confidentiality of medical records.[61] (Privacy and confidentiality are discussed by Ellen Gold in Chapter 6.) The Privacy Act of 1974 soon became law. Similar data protection legislation had been enacted in the Federal Republic of Germany in 1970, and Great Britain would follow suit in 1984. Because of this legislative trend, some forms of epidemiologic research and routine surveillance activities—including study designs that had provided important insights into environmental causes of disease—were at risk of becoming unjustifiably restricted. Leading epidemiologists responded to the threat of growing limitations on the use of routinely collected medical records by explaining the utility of the endangered research to society and future patients, and by outlining the confidentiality safeguards that ought to be employed by epidemiologists.[62] An influential article by Leon Gordis, Ellen Gold, and Raymond Seltser on privacy protection in epidemiologic research appeared in the *American Journal of Epidemiology* in 1977, the same year that the Privacy Protection Study Commission report was released in the United States.[62,63]

A year later, Mervyn Susser, Zena Stein, and Jennie Kline published a far-ranging paper on ethical issues in epidemiology.[64] At the time, epidemiologists had no ethics guidelines or professional codes of conduct and, unlike many other professional groups, had no acknowledged means of self-regulation.[61] In part because of the growth of epidemiology graduate programs for non-physicians, epidemiologists were being trained without direct exposure to the ethical traditions of medicine.[20,61] Soon new public health problems, such as the global spread of the acquired immunodeficiency syndrome (AIDS), brought new ethical questions, as discussed by Carol Levine in Chapter 12. In the mid-1980s, Colin Soskolne and others proposed the development of ethics guidelines for epidemiologists.[65,66] In a paper published in the *American Journal of Epidemiology* in 1989, "Epidemiology: Questions of Science, Ethics, Morality, and Law," Soskolne argued that ethics guidelines could be useful for teaching purposes and as a framework for the debate of ethical issues.[61] Other epidemiologists at the time were beginning to discuss and develop ethical guidelines, as John Last covers in Chapter 3.

The American College of Epidemiology approved the establishment of an ethics committee in 1985, and a Committee on Ethics and Standards of Practice was in place by 1991.[61] By 1987, the Society for Epidemiologic Research had instituted committees to examine ethical problems of conflict of interest and access to data by third parties. The International Epidemiological Association held a major session on ethics the same year in Helsinki, Finland, and the Industrial Epidemiology Forum conducted a conference on Ethics in Epidemiology in Birmingham, Alabama, in 1989, in conjunction with the annual meeting of the Society for Epidemiologic Research. The papers presented at this conference were published in 1991, together with proposed ethics guidelines for epidemiologists.[67,68]

In 1990 the International Epidemiological Association held an ethics workshop in Los Angeles that circulated draft ethics guidelines for epidemiologists,[69] and the International Society of Pharmacoepidemiology established an Ethics Committee the same year. The next development came in 1991, when the Council of International Organizations of Medical Sciences published the CIOMS International Guidelines for Ethical Review of Epidemiological Studies.[70] By this time ethical interests had developed among most major groups of epidemiologists. For example, a symposium on Ethics and Law in Environmental Epidemiology was held in Mexico in 1992 in conjunction with the annual meeting of the International Society for Environmental Epidemiology (ISEE),[71] and an International Workshop on Ethical and Philosophical Issues in Environmental Epidemiology was convened jointly by WHO and ISEE in North Carolina in 1994.[72] Findings of an international ethics survey carried out that year by ISEE and the Global Environmental Epidemiology Network were presented at the latter meeting.[73] The International Clinical Epidemiology Network Ethics Group also met during 1994 to discuss the recently published CIOMS ethics guidelines and to determine what participating clinical epidemiology units around the world were doing to protect human subjects.

Other contemporaneous developments included the incorporation of ethics curriculum into epidemiology graduate programs,[74] as discussed by Kenneth Goodman and Ronald Prineas in Chapter 15, and the inclusion of ethics workshops at annual meetings of the Society for Epidemiologic Research, the American College of Epidemiology, and other professional organizations for epidemiologists internationally. The Society for Epidemiologic Research, for instance, held a workshop titled "Symposium on Ethics: A Guiding Force in the Practice of Epidemiology" at the annual meeting in Keystone, Colorado, in 1993. Chapter 7 in this volume is an expanded version of a paper presented at that workshop. By July 1994, membership in the American Public Health Association (APHA) Forum on Bioethics—which hosts sessions on bioethics and public health in conjunction with the APHA annual meeting—had risen to 145 interested bioethicists, legal experts, epidemiologists, and other public health professionals. The *Epidemiology Monitor* had also featured a spirited series of articles and letters on ethical topics of interest to epidemiologists.

These developments in professional ethics in epidemiology occurred against a background of social and political movements in the early 1990s that included vigorous efforts to ensure that women and minorities are adequately represented in research projects funded by the National Institutes of Health.[75,76] The Womens' Health Initiative was launched in the United States during this period, along with other epidemiologic investigations of understudied womens' health problems.[77] Womens' health advocates testified on Capitol Hill on behalf of increased federal spending in breast cancer research and for improved procedures for recruiting and obtaining the informed consent of patients in breast cancer chemoprevention trials. Legislators and regulatory agencies also responded to increasing public concern about the integrity of scientific research, as discussed by Colin Soskolne and Dorothy MacFarlane in Chapter 14.

Another recent development, with important implications for epidemiologists in Europe and North America, has been renewed concern among legislators, data-protection advocates, and members of the general public over the privacy and confidentiality of information contained in health information systems. These issues are discussed by Marjorie Schultz in Chapter 5 and by Ellen Gold in Chapter 6. In light of pending legislation in the European Community that would severely restrict the use of routinely collected medical data for epidemiologic research,[78] both the International Society of Pharmacoepidemiology Ethics Committee and the joint WHO-ISEE International Workshop on Ethical and Philosophical Issues in Environmental Epidemiology have made recommendations to policy makers and legislative bodies that underscore the societal value of epidemiologic research.[72]

Summary and Conclusions

The upsurge of interest in the ethics of epidemiologic research and practice in the late 1980s and early 1990s could be interpreted as a sign of both the maturation of epidemiology as a profession and the important role that epidemiology plays in contemporary society. In the spirit of William Farr and other founders of the public health movement, today's epidemiologists are addressing a wide range of public health problems, such as environmental injustices experienced by migrant farm workers, malnutrition and diarrheal diseases in the developing world, osteoporosis in elderly women, Kaposi's sarcoma in homosexual men, and the plight of minority children and adolescents living and dying in inner cities in the United States. It seems certain that such studies will give rise to new ethical problems, many of which are anticipated in the remaining chapters in this volume.

References

1. Brockington, C. F. "The History of Public Health." In *The Theory and Practice of Public Health*, ed. W. Hobson. London: Oxford University Press, 1971: 1–7.
2. Kerkhoff, A. H. M. "Origin of Modern Public Health and Preventive Medicine." In *Ethical Dilemmas in Health Promotion*, ed. S. Doxiadis. New York: John Wiley & Sons, 1987: 35–45.
3. Lilienfeld, A. M. and Lilienfeld, D. E. "Threads of Epidemiologic History." In *Foundations of Epidemiology*. New York: Oxford University Press, 1980: 23–45.
4. Rousseau, Jean-Jacques. *The Basic Political Writings*, trans. and ed. Donald A. Cress. Indianapolis: Hackett Publishing Co., 1987.
5. Frank, Johann Peter. *A System of Complete Medical Police*, trans. Erna Lesky. Baltimore: Johns Hopkins University Press, 1976.
6. Porter, R. *Disease, Medicine and Society in England, 1550–1860.* London: Macmillan, 1987.
7. Temkin, O. "Health and Disease." In *The Double Face of Janus*. Baltimore: Johns Hopkins University Press, 1977.
8. Gregory, J. *Lectures on the Duties and Qualifications of a Physician*. London: W. Strahan and T. Cadell, 1772.
9. Rush, B. *Medical Inquiries and Observations*. Vol. 2, ch. 1. Published as a single essay titled *An Oration . . . An Enquiry into the Influence of Physical Causes upon the Moral Faculty*. Philadelphia: Charles Cist, 1786.
10. Chave, S. P. W. "The Origins and Development of Public Health." In *Oxford Textbook of Public Health*, ed. W. W. Holland, R. Detels, and G. Knox. New York: Oxford University Press, 1984: 3–19.
11. Bentham, J. *An Introduction to the Principles of Morals and Legislation*, ed. Burns & Hart. Oxford: Clarendon Press, 1970.
12. Mill, J. S. *Utilitarianism*. In vol. 10 of the *Collected Works of John Stuart Mill*. Toronto: University of Toronto Press, 1969.
13. Flinn, M. W., ed. *Report on the Sanitary Condition of the Labouring Population of Great Britain, Chadwick, E. (1842)*. Edinburgh: University Press, 1964.
14. Shattuck, L. *Report of the Sanitary Commission of Massachusetts, 1850*, Cambridge, MA, 1948.
15. Geison, G. L. "Pasteur's Work on Rabies: Reexamining the Ethical Issues," *Hastings Center Report* 8 (1978): 26–33.
16. Terris, M. "The Changing Relationships of Epidemiology and Society: The Robert Cruikshank Lecture," *Journal of Public Health Policy* 6 (1985): 15–36.

17. Terris, M. "Epidemiology and the Public Health Movement," *Journal of Public Health Policy* 8 (1987): 315–29.
18. Hanlon, J. J. and Pickett, G. E. "Philosophy and Purpose of Public Health." In *Public Health Administration and Practice*. 7th ed. St. Louis: C.V. Mosby Co., 1979: 2–12.
19. Bean, W. B. "Walter Reed and the Ordeal of Human Experiments," *Bulletin of the History of Medicine* 51 (1977): 75–92.
20. Susser, M. "Epidemiology in the United States After World War II: The Evolution of Technique," *Epidemiologic Reviews* 7 (1985): 147–77.
21. Doll, R. and Hill, A. B. "Lung Cancer and Other Causes of Death in Relation to Smoking," *British Medical Journal* 2 (1956): 1071–81.
22. MacMahon, B., Pugh, T. G., and Ipsen, J. *Epidemiological Methods*. Boston: Little, Brown & Co., 1960.
23. Hill, A. B. "The Clinical Trial," *British Medical Bulletin* (1951) 7: 278–82.
24. Mainland, D. "The Clinical Trial. Some Difficulties and Suggestions," *Journal of Chronic Diseases* 11 (1959): 484–96.
25. Levine, R. J. *Ethics and Regulation of Clinical Research*. 2d ed. New Haven: Yale University Press, 1986.
26. Katz, J. "The Regulation of Human Experimentation in the United States—A Personal Odyssey," *IRB: A Review of Human Subjects Research* 9 (1987): 1–6.
27. Katz, J. "Ethics and Clinical Research Revisited. A Tribute to Henry K. Beecher," *Hastings Center Report* 23 (1993): 31–9.
28. Cushing, H. *The Life of Sir William Osler*. London: Oxford University Press, 1940.
29. Brady J. V. and Jonsen, A. R. "The Evolution of Regulatory Influences on Research with Human Subjects." In *Human Subjects Research*, ed. R. Greenwald, M. K. Ryan, and J. E. Mulvihill. New York: Plenum Press, 1982.
30. Ivy, A. C. "The History and Ethics of the Use of Human Subjects in Medical Experiments," *Science* 108 (July 2, 1948): 1–5.
31. Beecher, H. *Experimentation in Man*. Springfield: Charles C. Thomas, 1959.
32. Brieger, G. H. "Human Experimentation: History." In *Encyclopedia of Bioethics*, ed. W. T. Reich. 4 vols. New York: Free Press, 1978: 684–92.
33. Faden, R. R. and Beauchamp, T. L. *A History and Theory of Informed Consent*. Ch. 3–6. New York: Oxford University Press, 1986.
34. *United States v. Karl Brandt, Trials of War Criminals Before the Nuremberg Military Tribunals under Control Council Law No. 10*. Vols. 1 and 2. "The Medical Case" (Military Tribunal I, 1947). Washington, DC: U.S. Government Printing Office, 1948–49.
35. Howard–Jones, N. "Human Experimentation in Historical and Ethical Perspectives," *Social Sciences and Medicine* 16 (1982): 1429–48.
36. Katz, J. *The Silent World of Doctor and Patient*. New York: Free Press, 1984.
37. "Declaration of Helsinki: Recommendations Guiding Medical Doctors in Biomedical Research Involving Human Subjects." Adopted by the 18th World Medical Assembly, Helsinki, Finland, 1964. *New England Journal of Medicine* 271 (1964): 473.
38. Winton, R. R. "The Significance of the Declaration of Helsinki: An Interpretative Documentary," *World Medical Journal* 25 (July-August 1978): 58–59.
39. World Medical Association. "Human Experimentation: Declaration of Helsinki," *Annals of Internal Medicine* 65 (1966): 367–68.
40. Public Law 87–781, 21 U.S.C. 355, 76 Stat. 780; amending Federal Food, Drug, and Cosmetic Act.

41. Temin, P. *Taking Your Medicine: Drug Regulation in the United States*. Cambridge, MA: Harvard University Press, 1980.
42. Curran, W. J. "Governmental Regulation of the Use of Human Subjects in Medical Research: The Approach of Two Federal Agencies," *Daedalus* 98 (spring 1969).
43. Curran, W. J. "1938–1968: The FDA, the Drug Industry, the Medical Profession, and the Public." In *Safeguarding the Public: Historical Aspects of Medicinal Drug Control*, ed. J. Blake. Baltimore: The Johns Hopkins University Press, 1970.
44. Federal Food, Drug, and Cosmetics Act, Sec. 505(i), 21 U.S.C. 355(i).
45. Beecher, H. K. "Ethics and Clinical Research," *New England Journal of Medicine* 274 (1966): 1355–60.
46. Livingston, R. B. Memorandum to Director J. A. Shannon on "Moral and Ethical Aspects of Clinical Investigation" (February 20, 1964).
47. Memorandum from Clinical Director, NCI (Nathaniel I. Berlin) to Director of Laboratories and Clinics, OD-DIR, on "Comments on Memorandum of November 4, 1964 from the Associate Chief of Program Development DRFR, to the Director, NIH" (August 30, 1965).
48. Livingston, R. B. Memorandum to Director J. A. Shannon on "Progress Report on Survey of Moral and Ethical Aspects of Clinical Investigation" (November 4, 1964).
49. Shannon, J. A. Memorandum and Transmittal Letter to the U.S. Surgeon General on "Moral and Ethical Aspects of Clinical Investigations" (January 7, 1965).
50. Transcript of the NAHC meeting. Washington, DC, September 28, 1965.
51. "Resolution Concerning Clinical Research on Humans" (December 3, 1965), transmitted in a Memorandum from Dr. S. John Reisman, Executive Secretary, NAHC, to Dr. J. A. Shannon ("Resolution of Council") on December 6, 1965. Reported in a Draft Statement of Policy on January 20, 1966.
52. U.S. Public Health Service, Division of Research Grants, Policy and Procedure Order (PPO) 129, February 8, 1966, "Clinical Investigations Using Human Subjects," signed by Ernest M. Allen, Grants Policy Officer.
53. Memorandum from Surgeon General William H. Stewart on "Clinical Research and Investigation Involving Human Beings" (February 8, 1966).
54. Curran, W. "Evolution of Formal Mechanisms for Ethical Review of Clinical Research." In *Medical Experimentation and the Protection of Human Rights*, ed. N. Howard–Jones and Z. Bankowski. Geneva: Council for International Organizations of Medical Sciences, 1978.
55. Editorial. "Friendly Adversaries and Human Experimentation," *New England Journal of Medicine* 275 (1966): 786.
56. Marston, R. Q., Director, NIH. "Medical Science, the Clinical Trial, and Society," a speech delivered at the University of Virginia on November 10, 1972 (typescript).
57. National Commission for the Protection of Human Subjects of Biomedical and Behavioral Research. *The Belmont Report: Ethical Principles and Guidelines for the Protection of Human Subjects of Research*. Washington, DC: U.S. Government Printing Office, 1978.
58. Brandt, A. M. "Racism and Research: The Case of the Tuskegee Syphilis Study," *Hastings Center Report* 8 (1978): 21–29.
59. *Final Report of the Tuskegee Syphilis Study Ad Hoc Panel*. Public Health Service, April 28, 1973.
60. Hearings before the Subcommittee on Health of the Committee on Labor and Public Welfare, U.S. Senate. "Quality of Health Care—Human Experimentation" (1973).

61. Soskolne, C. L. "Epidemiology: Questions of Science, Ethics, Morality, and Law," *American Journal of Epidemiology* 129 (1989): 1–18.
62. Gordis, L., Gold, E., and Seltser, R. "Privacy Protection in Epidemiologic and Medical Research: A Challenge and a Responsibility," *American Journal of Epidemiology* 105 (1977): 163–68.
63. Privacy Protection Study Commission. *Personal Privacy in an Information Society.* Washington, DC: U.S. Government Printing Office, 1977.
64. Susser, M., Stein, Z., and Kline, J. "Ethics in Epidemiology," *Annals of the American Academy of Political and Social Sciences* 437 (1978): 128–41.
65. Soskolne, C. L. and Zeighami, E. A. "Research, Interest Groups, and the Review Process." Paper presented at the 10th Scientific Meeting of the International Epidemiological Association, Vancouver, British Columbia, Canada, August 19–25, 1984.
66. Soskolne, C. L. "Epidemiological Research, Interest Groups and the Review Process," *Journal of Public Health Policy* 7 (1985): 173–84.
67. Fayerweather, W. E., Higginson, J., Beauchamp, T. L., eds. Industrial Epidemiology Forum's Conference on Ethics in Epidemiology. *Journal of Clinical Epidemiology* 44 (suppl. I) (1991).
68. Beauchamp, T. L., Cook, R. R., Fayerweather, W. E., et al. "Ethical Guidelines for Epidemiologists," *Journal of Clinical Epidemiology* 44 (1991): 151S–69S.
69. American Public Health Association. 1991 Section Newsletter—Epidemiology. Winter (1990).
70. Council for International Organizations of Medical Sciences. "International Guidelines for Ethical Review of Epidemiological Studies," *Law, Medicine and Health Care* 19 (1991): 247–58.
71. Soskolne, C. L., ed. Proceedings of the Symposium on Ethics and Law in Environmental Epidemiology. *Journal of Exposure Analysis and Environmental Epidemiology* 3 (suppl. 1) (1993).
72. World Health Organization Meeting Report. Joint WHO-ISEE International Workshop on Ethical and Philosophical Issues in Environmental Epidemiology, Research Triangle Park, North Carolina, U.S.A., September 16–18, 1994.
73. Soskolne, C. L., Jhangri, G. S., Hunter, B., and Close, M. "Interim Report on the International Society for Environmental Epidemiology/Global Environmental Epidemiology Network Ethics Survey." Working paper presented at the joint WHO-ISEE International Workshop on Ethical and Philosophical Issues in Environmental Epidemiology, Research Triangle Park, North Carolina, U.S.A., September 16–18, 1994.
74. Coughlin, S. S., Etheredge, G. D., Metayer, C., and Martin, S. A., Jr. "Curriculum Development in Epidemiology and Ethics at the Tulane School of Public Health and Tropical Medicine. Results of a Needs Assessment and Plans for the Future." Paper presented to the Association of Schools of Public Health Council on Epidemiology, Washington, DC, October 30, 1994.
75. Coughlin, S. S. and Beauchamp, T. L. "Ethics, Scientific Validity, and the Design of Epidemiologic Studies," *Epidemiology* 3 (1992): 343–47.
76. U.S. House of Representatives, Committee on Energy and Commerce. National Institutes of Health Revitalization Amendments of 1990 (report 101-869). Washington, DC: U.S. Government Printing Office, 1990.
77. Cummings, N. B. "Women's Health and Nutrition Research: U.S. Governmental Concerns," *Journal of the American College of Nutrition 12* (1993): 329–36.

78. James, R. C. "Consent and the Electronic Person." Working paper contributed at the joint WHO-ISEE International Workshop on Ethical and Philosophical Issues in Environmental Epidemiology, Research Triangle Park, North Carolina, U.S.A., September 16–18, 1994.

2

Moral Foundations

TOM L. BEAUCHAMP

The issues discussed in this book have emerged from professional practice in epidemiology. In later chapters, we consider specific moral problems that confront epidemiologists. The goal of this chapter is to provide a framework for epidemiologic ethics and to explain some central concepts and methods of biomedical ethics and moral philosophy needed for reading and interpreting subsequent chapters.

The terms *ethical* and *moral* are treated in this introduction as identical in meaning, but *morality* and *moral philosophy* (as well as *ethical theory*) have very different meanings. The general term *morality* refers to social conventions about right and wrong human conduct that are so widely shared that they form a stable (although incomplete) communal consensus. *Moral philosophy, ethical theory*, and *philosophical ethics* are reserved for philosophical theories.

In section I of this chapter, several questions about the nature of morality and moral responsibility are discussed, including, "What morality is already embedded in epidemiologic practice?" In section II, problems and methods in moral philosophy are addressed, and in section III, some ethical theories of importance to biomedical ethics are investigated.

I. Social Morality and Professional Morality

The term *morality* refers to a social institution with a code of learnable norms. Morality comprehends many forms of social protection that we acknowledge through language such as "moral rules" and "human rights." Like natural languages and political constitutions, morality exists before we are instructed in its

demands. As we grow up, we learn moral responsibilities along with other social responsibilities, such as those imposed by laws. Eventually we learn to distinguish general social rules of both law and morals from particular social rules
fashioned for and binding on the members of special groups, such as the members of a profession. Hence, we learn to distinguish general or social morality
from professional morality. But how sharp is this distinction?

Morality

The morality that is shared by all morally committed persons in all societies is
not one morality among others; it is simply morality, or what is sometimes called
"the common morality." This morality is universal because it contains a body of
fundamental ethical precepts constituting morality wherever it is found. I will
call this body of norms "morality in the *narrow* sense." There are no distinctive
moralities in this narrow sense, but, as will be discussed later, there are distinctive moralities in a "*broad* sense of morality" that recognizes divergent moral
norms and positions springing from cultural, philosophical, religious, and other
differences.

Not everyone in every society accepts or lives up to the demands of morality
in the narrow sense, but this failure is not because they have a different morality. Such persons are simply not moral; they are either amoral or immoral.
Morality, so understood, is not a philosophical theory about morality, but a core
of unphilosophical precepts most often categorized as principles, rules, rights,
and the like. In recent years the favored category in international discourse has
been universal or basic human rights,[1,2] but we can also capture large parts of
our common morality through the language of obligations and virtues.

Many attempts have been made in the history of philosophy, political theory,
and law to formulate the precepts of morality (in the narrow sense) in order to
show that these precepts do not depend, as do mere customs and positive law,
on local codifications. As the Dutch jurisprudential thinker Hugo Grotius put it,
basic moral rules are obligatory and binding on everyone, kings not excepted.[3]
However, many problems are present in the particular formulations of the basic
demands of morality found in these writings, in part because such formulations
presuppose controversial ethical theories (this chapter, section III).

These longstanding controversies in ethical theory cannot be considered here,
but I can provide some examples of universal morality. All moral persons in all
moral traditions accept the following universal precepts (stated in the form of
obligations):

1. Tell the truth.
2. Respect the privacy of others.
3. Protect confidential information.

4. Obtain consent before invading another person's body.
5. Be loyal to friends who return the loyalty.
6. Do not kill.
7. Do not cause pain.
8. Do not incapacitate.
9. Do not cause offense.
10. Do not deprive of goods.
11. Protect and defend the rights of others.
12. Prevent harm from occurring to others.
13. Remove conditions that will cause harm to others.
14. Help persons with disabilities.
15. Rescue persons in danger.

No rule in this list is absolute and some are limited in scope; all can in some circumstances be validly overridden by rules with which they come into conflict. Which rule overrides in a case of conflict will depend on the particular context and the way specific societies deal with that context. These rules are wholly binding *unless* they conflict with another moral rule, making some balancing of the two necessary. The list is not exhaustive. It could easily be supplemented by precepts of loyalty, obligations of reparation for wrongful interventions, obligations of gratitude for the generous services or gifts of others, and the like.

Professional Morality

Just as there is a common morality with shared principles and rules, so most professions have, at least implicitly, an indigenous morality whose precepts are widely shared in the field. Some measure of professional morality is transmitted in informal ways, but formal instruction and attempts at the codification of professional morality have increasingly appeared in recent years. We have seen many new formal codes of medical, behavioral, nursing, and research ethics, reports by government-sponsored commissions, and courses in professional schools.

Specific codes written for groups such as physicians, nurses, and psychologists are sometimes explicitly defended by appeal to general norms in the common morality, such as the fifteen rules listed above. Usually, however, professional codes are attempts to discover, formulate, and develop an inchoate morality widely accepted by practitioners in a given field. Professions often control entry into occupational roles by formally certifying that candidates have acquired the necessary knowledge and skills. Authorities may require some forms of instruction in ethics, or at least some evidence verifying good moral character. Professions typically specify and enforce responsibilities, seeking to ensure that persons who enter into relationships with their members will find them competent and of good moral character. Many of these responsibilities are role obligations that are correlative with the rights of persons served. A professional code commonly emphasizes role obligations, but it may also be broader in scope.

Professional Morality in Epidemiologic Research and Practice

In recent years, codes of ethics for epidemiologists have been the subject of numerous meetings and commentaries,[4,5,6,7] as discussed in Chapters 1 and 3. Attempts to devise codes have been difficult because of the diversity of professional backgrounds found in epidemiology, which draws its practitioners and consultants from a number of different disciplines including medicine, statistics, public health, demography, sociology, genetics, anthropology, psychology, and industrial hygiene. Ethics for epidemiologists involves an interplay between the model of public health (protecting the public welfare) and the model of medicine (protecting the welfare of the individual), and must also take into account ethical issues arising from the social sciences.

Despite the diversity of training brought into epidemiologic practice and its continuing evolution and change, we can meaningfully speak of a morality internal to epidemiologic practice and research.[8,9,10] The remainder of this section will be devoted to explaining these professional moral commitments. That is, I will attempt to formulate a framework of rules that draws primarily on the internal morality already accepted by epidemiologists. However, I do not assume that acceptable moral standards for epidemiologists are entirely a matter of rules and beliefs that already have an embedded and well-articulated position in epidemiologic practice. The formulations provided here occasionally develop and extend the professional morality in epidemiology, but remain faithful to its fundamental moral commitments.

The following types of responsibilities, with their major components, constitute the basic professional moral commitments in epidemiology:*

> *Responsibilities to Research Subjects*
> Welfare Protection
> Informed Consent
> Privacy
> Confidentiality
> Committee Review
>
> *Responsibilities to Society*
> Providing Benefits
> Public Trust

---

*This analysis is heavily indebted to T. L. Beauchamp, R. R. Cook, W. E. Fayerweather, et al. "Ethical guidelines for epidemiologists." *Journal of Clinical Epidemiology* 44 (1991): 151S–69S. I thank Ralph Cook and Bill Fayerweather for many stimulating conversations and suggestions.

Avoiding Conflict of Interest
Impartiality

Responsibilities to Employers and Funding Sources
Formulating Responsibilities
Protecting Privileged Information

Responsibilities to Professional Colleagues
Reporting Methods and Results
Reporting Unacceptable Behavior and Conditions

The remainder of section I will focus on the topics listed above, which will be developed as rules that specify responsibilities (or obligations). These rules are not mechanical or definitive procedures for decisionmaking; experience and sound judgment are indispensable allies for any system of rules. I will now develop this framework by explaining its basic commitments.

Responsibilities to Research Subjects

Research involving human subjects is an ancient practice, but serious concern about its consequences and about the protection of human subjects emerged relatively recently. Mechanisms of control such as the Declaration of Helsinki, government commissions, regulatory agencies, and professional societies have become prominent parts of the historical landscape of research ethics (see Chapter 1). However, epidemiology needs more specific and detailed guidelines.

PROTECTING THE WELFARE OF SUBJECTS. The mid-twentieth-century developments in protecting human subjects were primarily directed at eliminating dangerous research that exploited subjects' confidence in a physician-patient therapeutic relationship.[11] Although risks are usually lower in epidemiology than in most other areas of biomedicine, epidemiologists should always strive to minimize discomfort, disturbances, inconveniences, and risks caused to subjects, and they should be aware of any intrusive or harmful potential present in their investigations. A fundamental responsibility exists to avoid harming subjects and, insofar as conditions permit, to prevent or remove anything potentially harmful.

The idea that professionals are obligated to avoid inflicting injury has been associated for centuries with the maxim *primum non nocere*—"above all [or first] do no harm." This obligation is a complex responsibility not to cause harm, to prevent harm, and to remove harm.[12] In epidemiology, risks of harm presented by studies must constantly be weighed against possible benefits for patients, subjects, or the public. The epidemiologist who professes to "do no harm" is not pledging never to cause harm, but only to strive to create a positive balance of good over inflicted harms. Whenever risk of harm is imposed on subjects, law and morality alike recognize a standard of "due care." Negligence is a departure from the standard of due care owed to others and includes not only deliberately imposed risks that are unreasonable but also carelessly imposed risks.

The epidemiologist should gather, store, and use data in a fashion that minimizes risk to subjects. Even in situations in which the data have been gathered for purposes other than epidemiologic research (personnel records, death certificates, tax rolls, and the like), epidemiologists should recognize that with these data goes a trust to protect persons from harm. Failure to disclose hazards in work environments or risks in medical procedures are examples of violations of this trust. In some cases harm can be caused by overemphasizing a risk or by suggesting a risk where none truly exists. The epidemiologist should also guard against circumstances in which information gathered for health research might be used for unjustifiable purposes such as determining employability, promotion, or insurability.

Finally, epidemiologic research may inadvertently pose potential risks to groups of individuals and communities. For example, populations defined by race, ethnicity, or lifestyle may suffer stigmatization or lowered self-esteem following the publication and dissemination of research findings that create or reinforce negative cultural stereotypes, as Steven Coughlin discusses in Chapter 7. Disparaging information about a group can result in harms such as discrimination in employment, housing, or insurance, and injured racial or cultural pride.[13,14,15]

OBTAINING INFORMED CONSENT. As concerns about subjects' rights to autonomy gradually grew more insistent in twentieth-century research, the idea of respect for autonomy gained recognition equal to that of protection against risk. At this point informed consent began to play a central role in research ethics. The justification of requirements of informed consent is the principle of respect for autonomy. However, the goal of enabling an "autonomous choice" is difficult to articulate with precision.

In studies requiring the active participation of human subjects, explicit informed consent must be obtained. Disclosures should be made regarding the aims, methods, anticipated benefits and risks of the research, any inconvenience or discomfort that may be involved, and the right to withdraw from the research. If participation in the study is voluntary, subjects should understand that they may refuse to cooperate initially or at any stage in the research.[16,17]

An informed consent is, by definition, an *autonomous authorization* given by individual patients or subjects. Thus, a patient or subject must understand the relevant circumstances, make a decision in substantial absence of control by others, and intentionally authorize a professional to proceed with a medical or research intervention. The person does more than merely acquiesce in or comply with a proposal; he or she actively consents. A truthful disclosure therefore does not by itself constitute a morally acceptable consent solicitation or practice, because it says nothing about the basis on which the subject consented.[18]

It is neither feasible nor necessary to obtain informed consent in certain types of research. For example, some research in epidemiology could not be conducted if consent were needed in order to obtain access to records. Use of data without consent is not necessarily an ethical violation. Research may be the first stage of an investigation to determine whether one needs to trace particular individuals to obtain their permission for further participation. In other cases, third-party consent is sometimes acceptable when access to a subject is impractical or the subject is incompetent.[19,20]

Epidemiologists often analyze data initially gathered by others for purposes beyond health research. Application of informed consent requirements under these conditions may be overly burdensome, and in some cases subjects of research do not need to be contacted at all. In other cases it suffices to notify persons in advance of how data will be used and give them the opportunity to decline participation. Thus, disclosures and warnings may sometimes be substituted for informed consents. (Further qualifications and examples are given in Chapter 5.)

Finally, significant issues arise in epidemiology regarding surveillance activities, cohort studies, and sequential study designs. In some cases, the processes of data collection and analyses are continuous, and some analyses that might take place in the future cannot be anticipated. The investigator should periodically consider whether informed consent is needed and should place any judgments about bypassing informed consent before a review panel. In some circumstances written informed consent is needed, whereas in others ongoing communication of study results and continuing review may be the best policy.

PROTECTING PRIVACY. Privacy, the condition of limited access to a person, should be aggressively protected by epidemiologists. Research requiring massive bodies of data involves the disclosure of medical and other confidential records to third parties, creating a threat to privacy and a special concern for epidemiologists. Here questions can be raised about to whom the disclosures may be made, whether the entire record should be open to inspection (including, for example, a psychiatric record), whether the subject is to be informed of the disclosure, and whether the subject must authorize the disclosure.[21,22,23,24]

Infringements of privacy are at times justified, but only under exceptional circumstances such as contact tracing for sexually transmitted diseases, as mandated by law. An epidemiologist should carefully weigh legal obligations to make disclosures against the moral importance of preserving the privacy of subjects. Breaking the law or ignoring a court order may be required in rare cases. If an epidemiologist must infringe on privacy, those involved should be informed of the reasons and of their rights in the circumstances. For epidemiologic research that invades privacy to be justified, several conditions must be satisfied. First, the infringement must be necessary for the conduct of the research. Second, there must be no reason to believe that substantial risks of harm to subjects are created, (for example, the possibility that a person might be fired or divorced by a spouse). Third, the research must show promise of societal benefit by contributing to the protection of health or survival.

Those zealous in the defense of medical and other stored records have sometimes argued that a further condition must be present: that these records cannot be examined without the authorization of the patient.[25,26,27,28] Requirements for such permission would, however, threaten epidemiologic and other legitimate forms of medical and social research, which often depend on unauthorized disclosure to third parties. Moreover, the condition would be overprotective of persons' interests and inconsistent with the objectives of public health.

MAINTAINING CONFIDENTIALITY. Privacy and confidentiality are often blended in professional guidelines on ethics, as if protecting a person's privacy is essentially a matter of protecting confidential information about the person. However, privacy and confidentiality are distinct concepts. An infringement of confidentiality occurs only if a person to whom information was disclosed *in confidence* fails to protect that information. Confidentiality can be violated or infringed in several ways, including deliberate and accidental disclosure.

As discussed elsewhere in this volume, measures that may and should be taken to protect the confidentiality of health information include securing records with personal identifiers, limiting access to records to a small set of members of the research team, eliminating personal identifiers whenever possible, emphasizing the importance of confidentiality at training sessions for study personnel, and preventing release of information in a form that would enable identifications.[29,30]

A breach of confidentiality cannot be justified unless it is necessary to meet a strong conflicting obligation, such as a court order, but this rule does not restrain epidemiologists from obtaining and using confidential information. The obligation to protect confidential information does not mean it cannot be collected or shared with appropriate parties (assuming adequate safeguards). Indeed, confidential medical and other vital records that identify individuals are essential to epidemiologic research in order to prevent those individuals or others associated with them from developing disease, or to identify the disease at an early stage. Although confidential data may be passed between responsible professionals, just as clinical data are passed between physicians, care must be exercised as to how and under what protections the information is transmitted (see Chapter 6).

Whenever an epidemiologist publicly disseminates information collected from confidential data, anything that might point to individuals should be removed. Under unusual circumstances, such as a threat to the public health or to the safety of other persons, the epidemiologist may be justified in infringing confidentiality by communicating personally identifying information to public health officials, family members, or other involved parties. Nevertheless, in almost all cases the individuals identified should be notified of the action taken.[31,32,33,34,35,36]

Epidemiologists often obtain access to medical records, school records, social agency records, employment records, and some federal records. Credit, census, and Internal Revenue records are far less accessible. These restraints are socially important, but from a moral perspective the type of record is usually irrelevant.

REVIEWING RESEARCH PROTOCOLS. A massive, increasingly international system of prior review of research involving human subjects has developed since the late 1960s and early 1970s. Epidemiologists are obligated to submit their research protocols for approval and to provide justification of their procedures. Review committees and (if appropriate) administrative review are often structured so that officials work closely with investigators to improve the ethical quality of the research. However, investigators have a personal responsibility to evaluate and maintain a study's ethical adequacy; this duty cannot be justifiably transferred to the review committee or to administrative review.

In order for epidemiologic research with human subjects to be approved, the following minimum conditions should be satisfied: (1) consent procedures are adequate for obtaining permission from each individual subject; (2) the privacy of subjects and the confidentiality of information have been adequately protected; (3) risks to subjects have been minimized and shown to be justifiable by anticipated benefits of the research; (4) subjects especially vulnerable to influence or harm have been protected by stringent measures; (5) selection of subjects is fair and the research does not place an undue burden on a particular class of subjects; (6) provisions have been made to monitor the research as it continues in order to deepen the protection of human subjects; (7) plans have been included for the communication of study results.

Occasionally, research conducted by epidemiologists need not meet these conditions because some research is legitimately exempted from ethical review or handled through an expedited review process. But regardless of the judgments and demands of particular committees, every study in epidemiology involving human subjects should have an approved, written protocol.

Responsibilities to Society

The main argument justifying epidemiologic research is that its societal benefits are substantial and that various risks are reduced or eliminated. Because of the commitment to better the public's health and improve survival rates, epidemiologists often have dual professional obligations to advance scientific knowledge and to enhance, protect, and restore public health through the application of this knowledge.[37,38] The freedom to perform epidemiologic research also entails a correlative responsibility to perform it with due care, competence, and objectivity.

PROVIDING BENEFITS. Obligations to confer benefits, to prevent and remove harm, and to weigh and balance an action's possible good against its possible harm are central to the health professions. By the very nature of epidemiology and its implicit contract with the members of society, risks to rights or welfare must be justified by potential benefits. The advantages of epidemiologic research can be substantial in providing knowledge about areas such as cancer, cardiovascular disease, infectious disease, psychiatric disorders, injuries, and child health.[39] Consequently, epidemiologists have role obligations to provide such benefits when the opportunity arises—and obligations to advance the profession as well.

Epidemiologists should employ the means available to them to enlarge the reach of sound epidemiologic inquiry and to disseminate their findings, so that the widest possible community benefits from the research. When properly carried out, the review of protocols also requires a justification of the research through an honest and comprehensive comparison of anticipated benefits and anticipated risks.

SUSTAINING PUBLIC TRUST. Epidemiologists should attempt to promote and preserve public confidence by properly presenting the methods, results, and public health significance of their inquiries. All information vital to public health should be communicated in a timely, comprehensive, understandable, and responsible manner.

Difficult judgments sometimes have to be made about whether issues involving security, confidentiality, or trade secrets justify withholding information, and, if so, whether restricted dissemination of findings might outweigh any larger need for the information. Withholding of information can be justified in unusual cases. However, to do so for personal or institutional reasons is almost always a violation of the epidemiologist's responsibility. Failure to provide full information (except in highly unusual situations) is morally no better than failure to provide any information at all, and may be worse if the presentation is distorted in the interests of a party at risk.

AVOIDING CONFLICT OF INTEREST. A conflict of interest occurs when an investigator's personal goal or role obligation conflicts with an obligation to uphold another party's interest, thereby compromising normal expectations of objectivity and impartiality. Conflicts of interest typically arise when a person must make a judgment in a context free of interests or influences that jeopardize objectivity and professionalism.

An epidemiologist on the payroll of a corporation, a university, or a government does not encounter a conflict of interest simply by the condition of em-

ployment. However, a conflict exists whenever an epidemiologist's role obligation or personal interest in accommodating the institution, such as job security,
compromises responsibilities to others who have a right to expect impartial treatment.

The "conflict" in conflict of interest is a confrontation between professional
judgment and an influence that potentially could impair that judgment. Some influences clearly distort judgment, others have a reasonable probability of doing
so, and still others hold only a distant possibility. Thus, a difference exists between a conflict of interest and a potential conflict of interest. There is also a difference between a real conflict of interest and a perceived conflict of interest.
Perceived conflicts can erode trust, even though such perceptions may be little
more than unfounded suspicions. Moreover, potential conflicts of interest cannot
always be foreseen. Obviously it is best to avoid such circumstances if possible,
but, when conflicts arise, there is no reason to assume that loyalty to an employer, agency, or academic institution is always the foremost consideration.
Personal integrity, moral responsibilities to other parties, or responsibilities to
professional colleagues may turn out to be more weighty motivations.

Epidemiologists can and have confronted many forms of conflict of interest
involving sources of support (including grants and contracts) and in their work
as consultants, witnesses, and the like. Widely discussed problems of conflict of
interest concern gifts, favors, potential gains from products with commercial
value, and lucrative side contracts.[40,41,42]

MAINTAINING IMPARTIALITY. Closely related to issues of conflict of interest are
failures of impartiality, which occur when a value-directed departure from accuracy, objectivity, and balance takes place. Partiality can be a factor in research
design, critical analysis, the publication of results, and peer review. It is a reasonable presumption that the deeper the commitment to sound principles of scientific method, the lower the risk that partiality will threaten results and conclusions. There is no reason to assume, however, that epidemiologists who employ
observational study designs are more susceptible to partiality than experimental
scientists. Perhaps most importantly, the presence of a value judgment does not
entail that partiality taints the judgment. Epidemiologists are often called upon
to reach legitimate value judgments about the conclusions and implications of
their research. Epidemiologic research and the reporting of its results also necessarily involve selection among facts for emphasis and the taking of points of
view, which often are openly stated in the study conclusions. We therefore should
distinguish partiality from legitimate forms of opinion and appraisal.

Failures of impartiality do not occur unless there is a *value-directed* departure
from accuracy, objectivity, and balance. If, for example, an epidemiologist fails
to notice that an accidental omission has distorted a crucial part of a study, the
distortion results from error, not from partiality. Failures of impartiality in sci-

entific research may have many specific motivations, such as an ideology, an employer-controlled framework of beliefs, affiliation with special-interest groups, career ambition, irrationality, prejudice, greed, and even religious fervor.

In scientific research, charges of partiality often stem from the belief that an epidemiologist has adopted an inappropriate advocacy role, or has been hired as a consultant or employee to represent narrow institutional views or special interests—for example, to take public stands on policies to protect the health of vulnerable children the epidemiologist has studied. The concern is that this relationship may lead an investigator to report results in a fragmentary or imbalanced fashion that promotes the desired values and conclusions (or at least to report conclusions in a way that limits dangers to those values), causing a loss of scientific objectivity.[43,44] However, value-directed roles do not themselves produce partiality. A partisan or institutionally loyal epidemiologist may restrain or even completely eliminate his or her beliefs when conducting a study or reporting its findings.

Responsibilities to Employers and Funding Sources

Valid interests and rights are held by funders and employers. The epidemiologist's responsibilities to them sometimes conflict with responsibilities to subjects, society, or colleagues.[45,46]

FORMULATING RESPONSIBILITIES. Epidemiologists should inform employers and funders, preferably in contractual form, how research is to be conducted and how it might involve moral and legal obligations. The respective responsibilities of employer, funder, and epidemiologist, including responsibilities to report findings, should be clearly articulated in documents such as program manuals or protocols. All parties should be aware of any moral or other professional codes to which an epidemiologist should adhere. No valid agreement exists unless the arrangements have been thoroughly disclosed and all parties understand their specific duties. Epidemiologists should not accept any contractual responsibilities if particular conclusions must be reached from a proposed study or if one must refrain from publishing conclusions.

PROTECTING PRIVILEGED INFORMATION. Epidemiologists may use privileged information furnished by a funder or employer under a requirement that the information remain confidential. An example of such information is intellectual property, such as trade secrets. However, epidemiologic methods, procedures, and results should not be treated as confidential and should be included in any final report(s). Conflicts between the various parties sometimes arise over proprietary or other privileged information. An epidemiologist who possesses confidential information that could damage the economic interests of an employer or the privacy interests of a subject is under an obligation of confidentiality that should not be broken except in highly unusual circumstances when a more demanding moral obligation requires it. This responsibility remains in force when the epidemiologist leaves a firm or completes a project.

Responsibilities to Professional Colleagues

Codes of professional ethics typically assert that colleagues should be dealt with honestly and should be criticized when deficient in character, competence, or action. These demands are sensitive in professional practice, and codes and guidelines usually say little about how to handle such responsibilities. Less problematic, but no less important, are professional obligations to report methods and results publicly and to communicate ethical requirements to colleagues and associates in institutions.

REPORTING METHODS AND RESULTS. Upon completion of their studies, epidemiologists should provide adequate information to colleagues in order to permit the methods, procedures, techniques, and findings of their research to be critically assessed. The communication should occur within a reasonable period after research is finished (that is, within the standard amount of time it takes to write, critique, and polish such work) and should address all results, including those that do not fit investigators' preferences or preconceptions. It is unacceptable to withhold the results of a study because they turned out differently than expected.

Epidemiologists should also avoid being placed in a situation in which their results might be suppressed or edited by others. For example, academic epidemiologists and their universities should not accept grants or contracts in which a funding source retains the right to edit or hold back results; government and corporate epidemiologists should avoid circumstances in which their superiors can unduly edit, suppress, or delay publication; and epidemiologic reviewers should only attempt to deter publication of work by other epidemiologists for reasons of inferior science.

Quality assurance and internal review procedures may legitimately delay publication. Some responsible institutions and departments believe that the reputation of the institution, the development of younger colleagues, and related considerations justify manuscript-clearance procedures prior to submission for publication. There may be sound informational and educational reasons for such policies, resulting in constructive critique of studies and manuscripts. However, the constructive side of the process can be subverted, which suggests the need for oversight of these review procedures.

REPORTING UNACCEPTABLE BEHAVIOR AND CONDITIONS. Epidemiologists at times encounter fraud, illegal behavior, unethical conduct, and incompetence. When such behavior is discovered in colleagues or in other associates, an epidemiologist has a responsibility to confront the problem and to encourage the repudiation of improper activities. Some cases may require that specific action be taken to correct the behavior, though protection against unjust accusations should also be maintained. Fraud and misrepresentation in research are instructive examples. Even a single act of misrepresentation or tampering with data is a morally serious matter.

Disclosures about colleagues and others found to be engaging in unacceptable conduct are essential in order to preserve trust with the public, an employing institution, and professional colleagues. In exposing unacceptable behavior or conditions, the epidemiologist sometimes must assume the role of advocate for the public, colleagues, and perhaps the institution at which the research is conducted—although institutions often have a vested interest in not having such problems brought to light.

These observations conclude the overview of professional morality. Several issues deriving from this morality are discussed in subsequent chapters, and we now move to a study of some problems and methods in moral philosophy.

II. Problems and Methods in Moral Philosophy

Professionals are typically not trained in or exposed to moral philosophy even when they receive formal instruction in professional ethics. Moral philosophy involves disciplined reflection on the nature, function, and justification of moral beliefs. The purpose is to confront fundamental problems and to introduce clarity, substance, and precision of argument into moral thinking. Section II is devoted to a few questions and methods in moral philosophy that should improve the quality of moral thinking in epidemiology.

The Moral Basis of Professional Ethics

Many scholars of professional ethics believe that morality should be grounded in or justified in terms of fundamental norms or principles. This idea was alluded to in section I, where it was proposed that the justification of requirements of informed consent is the *principle* of respect for autonomy. We also noted that many codes have traditionally relied on the implications of the general principle "do no harm." Ideally, a set of general principles, such as the two just mentioned, could be developed as an analytical framework that expresses the values underlying specific guidelines, including rules of confidentiality, disclosure, impartiality, and conflict of interest. I have defended the view that four clusters of moral principles can serve this function by mapping our most general values.[12] These clusters are:

1. Respect for autonomy (respecting the decisionmaking capacities of autonomous persons);
2. Nonmaleficence (avoiding the causation of harm);
3. Beneficence (providing benefits and balancing benefits against risks);
4. Justice (fairness in the distribution of benefits and risks).

I will not attempt to show how these four groups of principles are related to particular rules, such as the rules of professional ethics found in section I. Instead, I will focus on a related problem that is pertinent to constructing practical moral guidelines: Principles (and all general moral norms) are abstract instruments that dispense vague, nonspecific advice open to competing interpretations. Morality in the narrow sense is composed entirely of general precepts, and has little power to demand particular actions until the precepts are given content that will render them suitable for specific contexts. Over time, the basic precepts of morality become implemented in many different ways in cultures, groups, and even by individual decision makers—thereby creating morality in the broad sense. To see how this process of growth in moral belief occurs and how it should occur, I begin with the need for specification.

Specification and Reform

Practical moral problems typically require that we make our general norms specific (whether principles, rules, or more particular maxims).[47] General precepts have insufficient resources to resolve deep or complex moral problems, and even specific norms are often indeterminate. Progressive specification is needed on an ongoing basis, especially as new problems arise. Such specification in biomedical ethics is the means to the formulation of institutional and public policy. None of this should be surprising. There is no way we can anticipate the range of commitments that must be made in the process of accepting a moral precept, such as a rule of confidentiality, and we are unable in advance to specify a precept to the unique circumstances of concrete cases.

In managing difficult cases, the first line of attack should be to specify general norms and thereby reduce or eradicate conflicts. The following is a typical example of the kind of problem an epidemiologist might confront, together with a possible solution: Research data and conclusions generated by private corporations that produce commercial health care products and services are often valuable to the health community at large. Yet the information is proprietary to the corporation, and the interests of stockholders must be protected. Publishing research that is valuable to the public's health is a moral responsibility, but so is protecting the stockholder's interests. Corporate officers therefore must carefully balance duties to stockholders with duties to society and professional colleagues. A corporation attempting to devise an adequate set of guidelines to govern these responsibilities must state the conditions under which the methods, techniques, and findings of its research and product development will be shared and the conditions under which the data will remain confidential. In so acting, corporate officers will be engaged in a process of specifying abstract norms and rendering them coherent.

For instance, the corporate officers in this health information example might specify as follows: (1) Disclose *all* available information about (a) *epidemiologic research* regarding workplace safety and (b) *research on product risks and safety*; disseminate all findings, so that the widest possible community benefits from the research. (2) Disseminate *no* findings of research pertaining to (a) product development and (b) consumer preferences.

Although contingent conflicts are still possible even among these rules (for example, between rule 1b and rule 2a), opportunities for incoherence, contingent conflict, and subjective balancing are reduced by these specifications of general norms. In the process, the corporation has developed a policy to handle contingent conflicts.

Because we inventively create rather than simply discover these more specific rules and policies, John Mackie argues that ethics is "invented."[48] Mackie does not mean that individuals create personal moral policies, but that specific standards are built up over time through communal agreements and decision making. What is morally demanded, enforced, and condemned is not merely what we discover in already available basic precepts, but what we decide in the development of those precepts. We constantly invent rules and policies that clarify and specify both the commitments of morality in the narrow sense and our previous specifications. For example, since about 1966 we have been inventing many of the rules and policies that protect human subjects of biomedical and behavioral research in the United States. These rules extend well beyond the content of any pre-1966 guidelines and practices relevant to their development (Chapter 1).

We cannot reasonably expect that these strategies of specification will function as cure-alls for our deepest problems of moral conflict. Specification will not always eliminate competing proposals for the resolution of contingent conflicts, but specification is often of assistance in professional ethics.

Moral Dilemmas and the Resolution of Moral Disagreements

Many situations in professional practice present moral dilemmas in which strong moral reasons support the rival conclusions of at least two well-supported points of view. If any one set of reasons is acted upon, events will result that are desirable in some respects but undesirable in others. Here an agent morally ought to do one thing and also morally ought to do another thing, but the agent is precluded by circumstances from doing both. Parties on both sides of dilemmatic disagreements can correctly present good moral reasons in support of their competing conclusions. Most moral dilemmas therefore present a need to balance alternative claims.

However, some dilemmas and disputes can be mitigated or even eliminated. The following six methods for dealing constructively with moral disagreements have been employed in the past, and each deserves recognition as a method of addressing dilemmas and controversies.

1. *Specification.* The most important method is specification, discussed previously in this section. The need for specification is often particularly evident when dilemmas arise.

2. *Adopting a code or policy.* Resolution of moral problems can be facilitated if disputing parties agree on a common set of moral guidelines. Of course, agreement will rarely be achieved if this method requires a complete shift from one starkly different moral point of view to another, but discussion and negotiation often can lead to the adoption of a new or modified moral framework. Specification will likely play a critical role in this process, which frequently eventuates in a code of ethics or institutional policy.

3. *Obtaining information.* Many moral disagreements can be resolved by gathering facts about matters central to the moral controversy. For example, debates about the fairness of allocating health dollars to preventive programs have often bogged down over issues of whether these strategies actually do function to prevent illness and promote health. New information often facilitates negotiation and compromise. For instance, additional epidemiologic information about the alleged dangers created by certain industries has often affected controversies over risks in science. Debates about sweetening agents for drinks, toxic substances in the workplace, pesticides in agriculture, and radiation therapies, among others, have all involved issues of both values and facts. Current controversies over compulsory versus voluntary screening for HIV often turn critically on factual claims about how the virus is transmitted, which benefits can be gained by screening, how many persons are threatened and the magnitude of their risks, whether testing and counseling reduces HIV risk, and the like.[49,50,51,52,53]

4. *Providing definitional clarity.* Controversies have been settled by reaching agreement on the meaning of the language used by disputing parties. In some cases stipulation of a definition or a clear explanation of a term may prove sufficient, but in others agreement will involve negotiation. Debates over the ethics of obtaining informed consent, for example, are often needlessly entangled because disputing parties use different senses of the term *informed consent* and have invested heavily in their particular definitions. One party may equate informed consent with *disclosure* by a physician or investigator, while another equates it with *mutual decision making* between patient and physician or investigator. Any resulting moral controversy over obligations of informed consent

will be ensnared in terminology, rendering it doubtful that disputants are discussing the same problem.

5. *Using examples and counter examples.* Resolution of moral controversies can be aided by constructive use of an example and a counterexample. Cases or examples favorable to one point of view are brought forward, and counterexamples are proposed to refute them. This form of debate was employed when a national bioethics commission considered the level of risk that can justifiably be permitted in scientific research involving children as subjects, where no therapeutic benefit is offered to the child. Commissioners were at first inclined to accept the view that only "minimal" risk procedures could be justified for children (where "minimal risk" refers to the level of risk present in standard medical examinations of patients). Many examples were put forth of unnecessary risk that had been presented to children in research. Instances from the history of medicine were then cited that revealed how significant diagnostic, therapeutic, and preventive advances in medicine would have been retarded or prevented unless procedures that posed a higher level of risk had been employed. Counterexamples of overzealous researchers who placed children at too much risk were then thrown up against these examples, and the debate continued in this way for several months.[54] Eventually a majority of commissioners abandoned their original view that nontherapeutic research involving more than minimal risk was unjustified. Instead, most accepted the position that a higher level of risk can be justified by the potential benefits provided to other children, as when a group of terminally ill youngsters is studied in the hope that something will be learned about their disease that can be applied to help other children. Resolution was thereby achieved on the primary moral controversy.

6. *Analyzing arguments.* One of the most important methods of philosophical inquiry—that of exposing the inadequacies, gaps, and fallacies in an argument—can also be brought to bear on moral disagreements. For example, if an argument rests on two incompatible positions, then pointing out the incoherence will require a change in the argument. If a moral argument leads to conclusions that a proponent is not prepared to defend and did not anticipate, part of the argument will have to be reconsidered, and this process may reduce the distance between the parties who disagree. The method of analyzing arguments is often supplemented by one or more of the above five ways of addressing moral disagreement.

Much of the work published in journals of ethics takes the form of attacking arguments, using counterexamples, and proposing alternatives. To use these methods is not to assume, of course, that conflicts can always be eliminated. The moral life will always be plagued by some conflict or ambiguity that cannot easily be eradicated without producing another problem. Our pragmatic goal should be a method that helps push the discussion forward through refinements, not a method that will always resolve the problems.

Relativism and Objectivity in Ethics

Problems of moral disagreement raise questions about whether there can be correct or objective moral judgments. Discrepancies between the belief that morality is purely personal or a matter of social convention and the belief that it has an objective grounding lead to issues of relativism in morals. Cultural differences raise these questions in profound ways.

A widespread view challenges the validity of moral precepts that are accepted in one culture when these precepts are applied to a different culture. Some figures in contemporary biomedical ethics cite "American values" such as requiring informed consent as a representative example of the problem. Because they fear "medical-ethical imperialism," they defend notions such as "culturally sensitive" standards, thereby rejecting a transcultural applicability for standards of informed consent, confidentiality, peer review, and the like.[55,56,57]

The most obvious thesis to counter this relativist position is one presented at the beginning of this chapter: Obligations such as those of obtaining informed consent express universally applicable moral values that cannot be compromised without compromising morality itself.[58] Morality *in the narrow sense* is not relative to cultures or individuals, and any norms closely associated with these fundamental moral values can never be validly compromised. At the same time, morality *in the broad sense* does show considerable diversity, and we can expect many well-grounded cultural and philosophical differences to appear. For roughly this reason, other writers have proposed a partial relativism (of morality in the broad sense) that retains a core of universal components.[59,60,61,62]

Relativism can also be criticized by showing the *inapplicability* of leading relativistic views on factual grounds, without showing their *unjustifiability* on moral grounds.[63] Relativists often start with and defend their position by appealing to anthropological data indicating that moral rightness and wrongness vary from place to place and that no absolute or universal moral standards apply to all persons at all times. They add that rightness is contingent on cultural beliefs and that rightness and wrongness are meaningless apart from the specific contexts in which they arise.

Relativist arguments pertaining to epidemiology have been used largely when researchers from developed countries are engaged in research in developing countries. Informed consent has been a particularly important topic. Relativists who challenge the importation of informed consent from one culture to another question the appropriateness of first-person informed consent in nations with no history of its use, on three grounds. They argue (1) that informed consent is culturally insensitive, (2) that potential patients and subjects are of questionable competence, and (3) that the critical importance of clinical interventions or research investigations renders informed consent requirements dangerous for certain cultures. The first argument is the most important of the three.

In many countries, relativists say, persons view their social roles in terms of close relationships rather than in terms of individual rights or personal ambitions. Culture is multiform, and every culture contains values, beliefs, and rituals that are of overriding importance. Relativists further maintain that these should not be nullified by values imported from external cultures, such as informed consent. But how adequate are the data on which relativist claims rest? In many societies it is easy to misrepresent or overstate widespread beliefs, social structures, and changing circumstances. There is often a time lag in our evidence about many cultures, and before we can claim a lack of interest in (or preparation for) informed consent in a given culture we have a responsibility to obtain solid and recent evidence. In many societies we know that major groups have diverse moral and political commitments, which necessitate a threshold line of guaranteed international rights (drawn from morality in the narrow sense) that cannot be overturned even by the most culturally sensitive analysis.

Relativists also sometimes point to a lack of competence to consent in many cultures. This proposal is difficult to assess, because such claims sometimes rely for their credibility on inadequate resources for obtaining valid consent from persons in developing countries. But questions about *resources* should be kept separate from questions of *competence*. The idea that normal patients and research subjects in countries other than one's own are psychologically incompetent to give an informed consent is likely to be offensive, and perhaps abusive. It can demean people and fail to respect them in ways persons in one's own culture are respected.[64]

Finally, relativists have argued that the need for interventions or data is so critical in many countries that the time required to obtain bona fide informed consent should not be taken. Everyone can, of course, agree that interventions without consent are permissible under emergency circumstances. The crisis situation is a long-established exception to many moral requirements, including informed consent. But is there any justification for the claim that the gravity of medical, public health, or research interventions *generally* warrants an exception to informed consent?

No one would deny that we should be "culturally sensitive" in exporting moral requirements to other cultures, but whether we can validly dispense with the responsibility to obtain first-person informed consent or with any other norm required by morality in the narrow sense is a difficult claim to sustain. Except in the aberrant case, such acts may simply be failures to treat one human being as he or she ought to be treated. At the same time, we can recall the distinction between morality in the narrow sense and morality in the broad sense and put it to a new use by distinguishing between a *relativism of judgments* and a *relativism of standards*. A relativism of judgment (involving morality in the broad sense) is so pervasive in human social life that it would be foolish to deny it. For example, when individuals and committees differ about whether one policy for keeping health information confidential is more acceptable than another, they differ in their moral judgments about alternative policies, but it does not follow that they have different moral standards of confidentiality. Many divergent *particular* judgments can call upon the same *general* standards (those of morality in the narrow sense) for their justification.

III. Ethical Theories

Many figures in the history of philosophical ethics have attempted more than an examination of problems and methods of the sort addressed in section II. They have undertaken to develop general, systematically organized ethical theories. These theories are complicated and only the most general features of a few influential types of ethical theory will be examined here: utilitarian theories, Kantian theories, and virtue theories. Casuistry, which is not an ethical theory in the usual sense, will also be discussed. Some knowledge of these theories is indispensable for reflective study in biomedical ethics, because a sizable part of the field's literature draws on their terminology, arguments, methods, and conclusions.

Utilitarian Theories

Utilitarianism is rooted in the thesis that an action or practice is right (when compared with any alternative action or practice) if it leads to the greatest possible balance of good consequences or to the least possible balance of bad consequences. Utilitarians defend only one basic principle of ethics: the principle of utility. This principle asserts that we ought always to produce the maximal balance of positive value over disvalue (or the least possible disvalue, if only undesirable results can be achieved). To utilitarians, the larger objective or function of morality is to promote human welfare by minimizing harms and maximizing benefits: Utilitarians see moral rules as the means to the fulfillment of individual needs as well as to the achievement of broad social goals.

The most influential exposition of utilitarianism is John Stuart Mill's book *Utilitarianism*.[65] In this work Mill refers to the principle of utility as the Greatest Happiness Principle: "Actions are right in proportion as they tend to promote happiness, wrong as they tend to produce the reverse of happiness, i.e., pleasure or absence of pain." Four essential features of utilitarianism may be extracted from the reasoning of Mill and other utilitarians.

The principle of utility: maximize the good. First, as noted above, actors are obliged to maximize the good: We ought always to produce the greatest possible balance of value over disvalue (or the least possible balance of disvalue). But what is the interpretation of "good" or "valuable"? This question takes us to the second feature of utilitarianism.

The standard of goodness. The goodness or badness of consequences is to be measured by items that count as the primary goods or utilities. Many utilitarians agree that ultimately goodness should be analyzed in terms of values that do not vary from person to person. But many other utilitarians interpret the good as that which is subjectively desired or wanted, and in this account the satisfaction of desires or wants is the goal of our moral actions.

Consequentialism. All utilitarian theories decide which actions are recommended entirely by reference to the consequences of the actions, rather than by virtue of any intrinsic moral features they may have, such as truthfulness or fidelity. The utilitarian does not demand that all future consequences be anticipated, but only that we take account of what can reasonably be expected to produce the greatest balance of good or least balance of harm.[66]

Impartiality (universalism). In utilitarian theory all parties affected must receive equal and impartial consideration. Utilitarianism stands in sharp contrast to egoism, which proposes maximizing consequences for the actor rather than for the other parties affected. Utilitarianism thus aligns good and mature moral judgment with personal distance from the choices to be made.

Kantian Theories

Another type of theory departs significantly from utilitarianism. Sometimes called *deontological*, it is now increasingly called *Kantian* because of its origins in the theory of Immanuel Kant (1734–1804).

Duty from rules of reason. Kant believed that an act is morally praiseworthy only if done neither for self-interested reasons nor as the result of a natural disposition; the person's motive for acting must be a recognition of the act as resting on duty. It is not good enough that one performs the morally correct action, because one could act for self-interested reasons having nothing to do with morality. For example, if an employer discloses a health hazard to an employee only because he or she fears a lawsuit, and not because of a belief in the importance of truth telling, then the employer acts rightly but deserves no moral credit for the action.

Kant regarded all considerations of utility and self-interest as secondary, because the moral worth of an agent's action depends exclusively on the moral acceptability of the rule on which the person is acting. An action has moral worth only when performed by an agent who possesses a good will, and a person has a good will only if moral duty based on a universally valid rule is the sole motive for the action. Morality, then, provides a rational framework of universal principles and rules that constrain and guide everyone.

Kant's supreme principle, called "the moral law" and "the categorical imper-

ative," is expressed in several ways in his writings. In what appears to be his favored formulation, the principle is stated as follows: "I ought never to act except
in such a way that I can also will that my maxim should become a universal
law."[67] This moral law offers worthwhile lessons for biomedical ethics. Many
clear cases of immoral behavior involve a person trying to make a unique exception of himself or herself for personal reasons. This conduct could not be
made universal, or else the moral rules presupposed by the idea of "being an exception" would be destroyed.

The Kantian view is that wrongful practices, including invasion of privacy,
theft, cheating, and bribes, are "contradictory"; that is, they are not consistent
with what they presuppose. Consider cases of lying. The universalization of rules
that allow lying would entitle everyone to lie to you, just as you could lie to
them. One could never tell if a person were telling the truth or lying. The rule
acted upon would be inconsistent with the practice of truth telling that it pre-
supposes. Similarly, fraud in research is inconsistent with the practice of publishing honestly gathered scientific evidence. All such wrongdoings are inconsistent with a rule or practice that they presuppose.

The requirement to never treat persons as means. Kant stated his categorical
imperative in another and distinctly different formulation (which many inter-
preters take to be a wholly different principle). This form is probably more widely
quoted and endorsed in contemporary philosophy than the first form, and certainly it is more frequently invoked in biomedical ethics. The formulation stip-
ulates that "one must act to treat every person as an end and never as a means
only."[69] Thus, one must treat persons as having their own autonomously established goals.

It has been widely reported in contemporary textbooks that Kant was arguing
categorically that we can never treat another as a means to our ends. This interpretation, however, misrepresents his views. He argued only that we must not treat
another *exclusively* as a means to our own ends. When adult human research subjects are asked to volunteer to test new drugs, for example, they are treated as a
means to a researcher's ends (and perhaps society's ends). However, they are not
exclusively used for others' purposes, because they do not become mere servants
or objects. Their consent justifies using them as means to the ends of research.
Kant's imperative demands only that persons in such situations be treated with the
respect and moral dignity to which all persons are always entitled.

Virtue Ethics

In discussing utilitarian and Kantian theories, we have looked chiefly at theories
erected on obligations and rights, but we often reflect on the *agents* who perform
actions, have motives, and follow principles. In recent years, several philoso-

phers have proposed that ethics should redirect its preoccupation with principles of obligation and look to decisionmaking by persons of good character, that is, virtuous persons.

Virtue ethics descends from the classical Greek tradition of ethics represented by Plato and Aristotle. Here the cultivation of virtuous traits of character is viewed as morality's primary function. Aristotle held that virtue is neither a feeling nor an innate capacity, but a disposition bred from a properly trained innate capacity. For example, epidemiology students acquire virtues much as they do skills such as learning to develop a questionnaire or perform statistical tests. They become just by performing just actions and become temperate by performing temperate actions.[68]

This approach relies on the importance of a person's characteristic motivational structure. A just person, for example, not only has a disposition to act fairly, but a morally appropriate desire to do so. The person characteristically has a moral concern and reservation about acting in a way that would be unfair. Having only the motive to act in accordance with a rule of obligation, as Kantian theory demands, is not morally sufficient for virtue.

Imagine someone who always performs his or her obligation because it is an obligation, but intensely dislikes having to allow the interests of others to be taken into account. Such a person does not cherish, feel congenial toward, or think fondly of others, and respects them only because obligation requires it. Suppose this person is a physician who always meets his moral responsibilities, but his underlying motives and desires are morally inappropriate. This physician detests his job and hates having to spend time with every patient who comes through the door. He cares not at all about being of service to people or creating a better environment in the office. All he wants to do is make money and avoid malpractice suits. Although this man meets his moral responsibilities, something in his character is defective morally. The admirable compassion guiding the lives of many dedicated health professionals is absent in this person, who merely engages in rule-following behavior.

Virtue ethics has practical value for biomedical ethics because a morally good person with right desires or motives is more likely to understand what should be done, more likely to perform required acts, and more likely to form and act on moral ideals than a morally bad person. A person who is ordinarily trusted is one who has an ingrained motivation and desire to perform right actions, and who characteristically cares about morally appropriate responses. Someone who simply follows rules of obligation and who otherwise exhibits no special moral character may not be trustworthy. A proponent of virtue ethics need not claim that analysis of the virtues subverts or discredits ethical principles and rules. It is enough to argue that ethical theory is more complete if the virtues are included and that moral motives deserve to be at center stage.[69,70]

Casuistry

An alternative to traditional theories is the recent revival of an approach that was influential during the medieval and early modern periods. Casuistry focuses on practical decisionmaking based on the experience of previous cases, and holds that judgments cannot be reached by using general norms such as principles and rules. Casuists are skeptical of principles, rules, rights, and theory divorced from history, experience, and circumstance. One can make successful moral judgments of agents, actions, and policies, casuists say, only when one has an intimate understanding of particular situations and an appreciation of treating similar cases similarly.

How exactly is a moral judgment made? The casuist believes it cannot come through traditional appeals to general principles and rules, because many forms of moral thinking and judgment do not derive from rules, rights, or virtues. The casuist holds that we sometimes appeal to narratives or paradigm cases, to classification schemes, and to the precedents established by previous cases.[71,72]

An analogy to law is helpful in understanding the casuist's point. In case law, the normative judgments of courts of law become authoritative. That is, they form the primary normative grounds for later judges who assess other cases—even though the particular features of each new case will be different. Matters are similar in ethics: Normative judgments about certain cases emerge through consensus in society and in institutions. That consensus then becomes authoritative and is extended to similar cases.[73]

At first sight, casuistry seems strongly opposed to the frameworks of principles and rules at work in traditional moral theory. However, closer inspection of casuistry shows that its primary concern is with an *excessive* reliance in recent philosophy on impartial, universal action-guides. Some proponents hold that casuistry often applies well-understood general principles to particular cases. Acceptance of general rules is therefore not necessarily incompatible with casuistry. The casuist can consistently hold that as a history of similar cases and similar judgments mounts, we legitimately become confident in our general judgments. As confidence in these generalizations increases, they can be accepted less tentatively and moral knowledge develops. Just as case law (legal rules) develops incrementally from legal decisions in actual cases, so the moral law (moral rules) develops incrementally.[74]

From the casuists' perspective, moral reasoning is also similar to that of a physician in clinical diagnosis: Paradigms of proper treatment function as sources of comparison when new problem-cases arise. Recommendations are made by analogy to the paradigm. If the analogy is proper, a resolution of the problem and a recommendation will be achieved; but uncertainty may remain if there is no close analogy. Casuists thus remind us of the importance of analogical reasoning, paradigm cases, and practical judgment. They also emphasize that generalizations and new knowledge are often learned, accommodated, and implemented by using case discussion and methods of case analysis.

Conclusion

Some perspective is needed on the limitations of moral philosophy and ethical theory as sources for our judgments in practical ethics. Philosophical theory is abstract and contains within its fabric a sustained body of controversies that render it unsuitable for generating specific, applied rules for practical ethics. Just as theoretical epidemiology concentrates on mathematical-statistical models to explain disease occurrences, so ethical theory concentrates on abstract models that attempt to explain and justify general principles and features of the moral life. These fields serve us well, but usually cannot be directly applied in our thinking about particular cases and policies.

In Chapter 3, John Last analyzes several of the themes of professional morality mentioned in section I above. In Chapter 4, Douglas Weed treats some of the problems of method and theory raised in section III of this chapter.

References

1. Macklin, R. "Universality of the Nuremberg Code." In *The Nazi Doctors and the Nuremberg Code*, ed. G. J. Annas and M. Grodin. New York: Oxford University Press, 1992: 240–257.
2. Gostin, L. "Human Rights in Mental Health: A Proposal for Five International Standards Based upon the Japanese Experience," *International Journal of Law and Psychiatry* 10 (1987): 353–68.
3. Grotius, H. *De jure belli ac pacis*, ed. J. B. Scott, trans. Francis W. Kelsey. Oxford: Clarendon Press, 1925.
4. Last, J. M. Association News. "Guidelines on Ethics for Epidemiologists," *International Journal of Epidemiology* 19 (1990): 226–29.
5. Fayerweather, W., Beauchamp, T. L., and Higginson, W., eds. *Ethics and Epidemiology*. Oxford: Pergamon Press, 1991.
6. Beauchamp, T. L., Cook, R. R., Fayerweather, W. E., et al. "Ethical Guidelines for Epidemiologists," *Journal of Clinical Epidemiology* 44 (1991): 151S–69S.
7. Bankowski, Z., Bryant, J. H., and Last, J. M., eds. *Ethics and Epidemiology: International Guidelines*. Proceedings of the XXVth Council for International Organizations of Medical Sciences Conference, November 7–9, 1990 (Summary of Discussions). Geneva: CIOMS, 1991.
8. Susser, M., Stein, Z., and Kline, J. "Ethics in Epidemiology," *Annals of the American Academy of Political and Social Science* 437 (1978): 128–41.
9. Gordis, L. "Ethical and Professional Issues in the Changing Practice of Epidemiology," *Journal of Clinical Epidemiology* 44 (1991): 9S–13S.
10. Capron, A. M. "Protection of Research Subjects: Do Special Rules Apply in Epidemiology?" *Law, Medicine and Health Care* 19, no. 3–4 (fall-winter 1991): 184–90.
11. National Commission for the Protection of Human Subjects of Biomedical and Behavioral Research. *The Belmont Report: Ethical Principles and Guidelines for the Protection of Human Subjects of Research*. Washington, DC: U.S. Government Printing Office, 1978.

12. Beauchamp, T. L. and Childress, J. F. *Principles of Biomedical Ethics*. 4th ed. New York: Oxford University Press, 1994.

13. Gostin, L. "Ethical Principles for the Conduct of Human Subject Research: Population-Based Research and Ethics," *Law, Medicine and Health Care* 19 (1991): 191–201.

14. Dickens, B. M. "Issues in Preparing Ethical Guidelines for Epidemiological Studies," *Law, Medicine and Health Care* 19 (1991): 175–83.

15. Dickens, B. M., Gostin, L., and Levine, R. J. "Research on Human Populations: National and International Ethical Guidelines," *Law, Medicine and Health Care* 19 (1991): 157–61.

16. Levine, R. J. *Ethics and Regulation of Clinical Research*. 2d ed. New Haven: Yale University Press, 1988.

17. President's Commission for the Study of Ethical Problems in Medicine and Biomedical and Behavioral Research. *Making Health Care Decisions*. Vols. 1–3. Washington, D.C.: Government Printing Office, 1982.

18. Faden, R. R., and Beauchamp, T. L. *A History and Theory of Informed Consent*. New York: Oxford University Press, 1986.

19. Meisel, A. "The 'Exceptions' to the Informed Consent Doctrine: Striking a Balance Between Competing Values in Medical Decisionmaking," *Wisconsin Law Review* 1979 (1979): 413–88.

20. Buchanan, A. E. and Brock, D. W. *Deciding for Others: The Ethics of Surrogate Decision Making*. Cambridge: Cambridge University Press, 1989.

21. Gordis, L., Gold, E., and Seltser, R. "Privacy Protection in Epidemiologic and Medical Research: A Challenge and a Responsibility," *American Journal of Epidemiology* 105 (1977): 163–68.

22. Last, J. M. "Individual Privacy and Health Information: An Ethical Dilemma?" *Canadian Journal of Public Health* 77 (1986): 168–70.

23. Privacy Protection Study Commission. *Personal Privacy in an Information Society*. Washington, D.C.: Government Printing Office, 1977.

24. Schoeman, F. D., ed. *Philosophical Dimensions of Privacy: An Anthology*. New York: Cambridge University Press, 1984.

25. Kelsey, J. L. "Privacy and Confidentiality in Epidemiological Research Involving Patients," *IRB* 3 (1981): 1–4.

26. Kmentt, K. A. "Private Medical Records: Are They Public Property? A Survey of Privacy, Confidentiality and Privilege," *Medical Trial Technique Quarterly* 33, no. 3 (1987): 274–307.

27. Cleaver, C. M. "Privacy Rights in Medical Records," *Fordham Urban Law Journal* 13, no. 1 (1984–1985): 165–204.

28. Parmet, W. "Public Health Protection and The Privacy of Medical Records," *Harvard Civil Rights–Civil Liberties Law Review* 16 (1981): 265–304.

29. NCHS Staff Manual on Confidentiality. Hyattsville, MD: National Center for Health Statistics, 1984. DHHS Publ. No. (PHS) 84–1244.

30. McCarthy, C. R. and Porter, J. P. "Confidentiality: The Protection of Personal Data in Epidemiological and Clinical Research Trials," *Law, Medicine and Health Care* 19 (1991): 238–41.

31. Rennert, S. American Bar Association. Commission on the Mentally Disabled [and] Center on Children and the Law. *AIDS/HIV and Confidentiality: Model Policy and Procedures*. Washington: American Bar Association, 1991.

32. Maney, A. and Wells, S., eds. *Professional Responsibilities in Protecting Children: A Public Health Approach to Child Sexual Abuse*. New York: Praeger, 1988.

33. Lako, C. J. and Lindenthal, J. J. "The Management of Confidentiality in General Medical Practice: A Comparative Study in The U.S.A. and The Netherlands," *Social Science and Medicine* 32, no. 2 (1991): 153–57.

34. Appelbaum, P. S. and Rosenbaum, A. "Tarasoff and The Researcher: Does The Duty to Protect Apply in The Research Setting?" *American Psychologist* 44, no. 6 (June 1989): 885–94.

35. Price, D. P. T. "Between Scylla and Charybdis: Charting a Course to Reconcile The Duty of Confidentiality and The Duty to Warn in The AIDS Context," *Dickinson Law Review* 94 (1990): 435–87.

36. Marshall, S. E. "Doctors' Rights and Patients' Obligations," *Bioethics* 4, no. 4 (October 1990): 292–310.

37. Lappé, M. "Ethics and Public Health." In *Public Health and Preventive Medicine*, ed. J. M. Last. 12th ed. Norwalk: Appleton-Century-Crofts, 1986: 1867–77.

38. Armenian, H. K. "In Wartime: Options for Epidemiology," *American Journal of Epidemiology* 124 (1989): 28–32.

39. Gordis, L. and Gold, E. "Privacy, Confidentiality, and the Use of Medical Records in Research," *Science* 207 (January 11, 1980): 153–56.

40. American Medical Association. Council on Scientific Affairs and Council on Ethical and Judicial Affairs. "Conflicts of Interest in Medical Center/Industry Research Relationships," *Journal of the American Medical Association* 23 (May 23/30, 1990): 2790–93.

41. Kenney, M. *Biotechnology: The University-Industrial Complex*. New Haven: Yale University Press, 1986.

42. Healy, B. et al. "Conflict-of-Interest Guidelines for a Multicenter Clinical Trial of Treatment After Coronary-Artery Bypass-Graft Surgery," *New England Journal of Medicine* 320 (April 6, 1989): 949–51.

43. Rothman, K. J. and Poole, C. "Science and Policy Making," *American Journal of Public Health* 75 (1985): 340–41.

44. Weed, D. L. "Science, Ethics Guidelines, and Advocacy in Epidemiology," *Annals of Epidemiology* 4 (1994): 166–71.

45. Blumenthal, D. et al. "University-Industry Research Relationships in Biotechnology: Implications for the University," *Science* 232 (June 13, 1986): 1361–66.

46. Relman, A. S. "Economic Incentives in Clinical Investigation" (Editorial), *New England Journal of Medicine* 320 (April 6, 1989): 933–34.

47. Richardson, H. S. "Specifying Norms as a Way to Resolve Concrete Ethical Problems," *Philosophy and Public Affairs* 19 (Fall 1990): 279–310.

48. Mackie, J. L. *Ethics: Inventing Right and Wrong*. New York: Penguin Books, 1977.

49. Mayer, K. H. "The Epidemiological Investigation of AIDS," *Hastings Center Report* 15, no. 4 (August 1985): S12–S15.

50. Dickens, B. M. "Legal Rights and Duties in the AIDS Epidemic," *Science* 239 no. 4840 (February 1988): 580–86.

51. Faden, R. R., Geller, G., and Powers, M., eds. *AIDS, Women and the Next Generation*. New York: Oxford University Press, 1991.

52. Fox, D. M. "From TB to AIDS: Value Conflicts in Reporting Disease," *Hastings Center Report* 16, no. 6 (December 1986): S11–S16.

53. Walters, L. "Ethical Issues in the Prevention and Treatment of HIV Infection and AIDS," *Science* 239, no. 4840 (February 5, 1988): 597–603.

54. The National Commission for the Protection of Human Subjects of Biomedical and Behavioral Research. *Research Involving Children*. Washington, D.C.: U.S. Government Printing Office, DHEW Publication, 1977.

55. Christakis, N. A. "Ethics are Local: Engaging Cross-Cultural Variation in the Ethics for Clinical Research," *Social Science and Medicine* 35 (1992): 1079–91.

56. Christakis, N. A., Fox, R. C., Faden, R. R., IJsselmuiden, C. B., et al. "Informed Consent in Africa" (letters and replies), *New England Journal of Medicine* 327 (October 8, 1992): 1101–02.

57. Christakis, N. A. "The Ethical Design of an AIDS Vaccine Trial in Africa," *Hastings Center Report* 8 (June/July 1988): 31–37EM.

58. Angell, M. "Ethical Imperialism? Ethics in International Collaborative Clinical Research" (Editorial), *New England Journal of Medicine* 319 (1988): 1081–83.

59. Barry, M. "Ethical Considerations of Human Investigations in Developing Countries: The AIDS Dilemma," *New England Journal of Medicine* 319 (1988): 1083–86.

60. Levine, R. J. "Informed Consent: Some Challenges to the Universal Validity of the Western Model," *Law, Medicine and Health Care* 19 (Fall-Winter 1991): 207–213.

61. De Craemer, W. "A Cross-Cultural Perspective on Personhood," *Milbank Memorial Fund Quarterly* 61 (1983): 19–34.

62. Council for International Organizations of Medical Sciences. "International Guidelines for Ethical Review of Epidemiological Studies," *Law, Medicine and Health Care* 19 (1991): 247–58; and *International Ethical Guidelines for Biomedical Research*. Geneva: CIOMS, 1993.

63. IJsselmuiden, C. B. and Faden, R. R. "Research and Informed Consent in Africa—Another Look," *New England Journal of Medicine* 326 (1992): 830–34.

64. Ekunwe, E. O. and Kessel, R. "Informed Consent in the Developing World," *Hastings Center Report* 14 (1984): 22–24.

65. Mill, J. S. "Utilitarianism." In *Collected Works of John Stuart Mill*, vol. 10. Toronto: University of Toronto Press, 1969.

66. Scheffler, S. ed. *Consequentialism and its Critics*. Oxford: Clarendon Press, 1988.

67. Kant, I. *Foundations of the Metaphysics of Morals*, trans. Lewis White Beck. Indianapolis: Bobbs-Merrill Co., 1959.

68. Aristotle. *Nicomachean Ethics*, trans. T. Irwin. Indianapolis: Hackett, 1985.

69. Foot, P. *Virtues and Vices*. Oxford: Basil Blackwell, 1978.

70. Pence, G. *Ethical Options in Medicine*. Oradell: Medical Economics Co., 1980.

71. Jonsen, A. R. and Toulmin, S. *Abuse of Casuistry*. Berkeley: University of California Press, 1988.

72. Jonsen, A. R. "Casuistry as Methodology in Clinical Ethics," *Theoretical Medicine* 12 (December 1991): 295–307.

73. Arras, J. D. "Getting Down to Cases: The Revival of Casuistry in Bioethics," *Journal of Medicine and Philosophy* 16 (1991): 29–51.

74. Jonsen, A. R. "Casuistry and Clinical Ethics," *Theoretical Medicine* 7 (1986): 67, 71.

3

Professional Standards of Conduct for Epidemiologists

JOHN LAST

Members of a wide diversity of the health professions follow the calling of epidemiology. Many work in national agencies like the U.S. Centers for Disease Control and Prevention, in regional cancer registries, in local health departments, or as hospital infection-control officers. They do the routine work of epidemiology, but the boundary between research and practice is ill-defined. Others are primary health care providers and clinicians: family doctors like the British rural general practitioner Wilfred Pickles,[1] public health nurses such as those who monitor sexually transmitted diseases in Uganda,[2] and specialists in all clinical fields who have embraced the analytic approaches and methods of clinical epidemiology.[3] Still others participate on research teams that conduct hypothesis-testing studies aimed at identifying causes or assessing risk factors for public health problems such as cancer, heart disease and the dementias associated with aging. Members of these teams may be professionally trained in medicine, nursing, social or behavioral science, or biostatistics; they may be technically qualified in computing, coding and editing data; or they may be interviewers, secretaries, or filing clerks. Although those in the last three staff categories are not epidemiologists, they often work with sensitive confidential material and therefore require some understanding of the concepts of privacy and confidentiality discussed in this chapter.

Another variety of epidemiologists are theoreticians, refining the scientific basis of epidemiology by enhancing methodologic rigor or by making conceptual breakthroughs. As epidemiology expands into new territory such as clinical decision analysis and molecular biology, new kinds of biomedical scientists are using epidemiologic methods. The techniques of molecular epidemiology[4] have considerable value. For instance, we can now identify precisely who is the source of an epidemic due to a particular strain of microorganism; and distinguish between persons who may safely be exposed to chemicals in an occupational setting and those who may not (raising ethical questions about disclosure and discriminatory hiring practices respectively).

Epidemiologists usually work on salary at an institution such as a university or health department, or they are supported by research funds rather than fees for services. They are accountable to the organization or institution that provides their financial support. As members of a team they also have obligations to colleagues.

Professional Education of Epidemiologists

Until the 1960s, many who practiced or did research in epidemiology had little or no formal training in this science, but used their professional skills in settings that gave them opportunities to study populations rather than (or as well as) individuals. They acquired these skills in service or by happenstance, sometimes learning just enough to work on a specific research problem. Most were competent clinicians who were self-selected by their interest in a population-based approach to medical practice. Typically they were individuals with a desire to generalize on the basis of experience, reinforced by analytic examination of numbers of cases, events, procedures, outcomes, and the like.

The mid twentieth century was in some respects a golden age of epidemiology in which new methods were being developed to solve difficult problems. But the classic papers from that era sometimes contain methodologic inadequacies that would lead, if the same work were being peer reviewed in the 1990s, to insistence on revision if not outright rejection of research proposals and reports of results.* In short, the science was sometimes flawed. Those epidemiologists were steeped in the traditions of the healing professions (medicine, nursing, dentistry). As part of these traditions they usually had become aware of and adhered to a code of conduct such as a modern variation of the Hippocratic oath; but this did not ensure that their ethical standards were impeccable. Some of the methods of those we recognize as founders of modern epidemiology, including some studies that led to important advances in our understanding of disease, would be looked on askance by an institutional review board of the 1990s. For example,

---

*For example, papers by Kennaway and by Wynder et al. on cancer of the cervix, reprinted in *The Challenge of Epidemiology*, an anthology of classic papers published by the Pan American Health Organization in 1988, report the association of incidence rates with ethnic origin and socioeconomic status; both fail to note the confounding factors and effect modifiers that might render the associations spurious and the conclusions flawed. There are many other examples of what would now be regarded as shortcomings of methodology in the same volume.

several of Joseph Goldberger's studies of pellagra[5] would not survive modern ethical review (as they were done in prisons, orphanages, and insane asylums, apparently without informed consent).[6] Other deplorable episodes of professional misconduct occurred then just as they do today, regardless of ancient traditions dating from the time of Hippocrates.

Formal education in epidemiology has proliferated in North America. All schools of public health and most medical schools now offer graduate programs at least to master's level, and many to doctoral level. Although less widespread, the same trends can be observed in Europe and the rest of the world, including a number of developing countries.

Increasingly in the past twenty-five years, epidemiology has attracted recruits with no prior training or experience in a setting of patient care or service to the general public. Instead, they may have professional education in biology, statistics or computing. These epidemiologists, lacking acquaintance with professional codes of conduct such as those encountered by medical and nursing students during their educational programs, may not always appreciate the subtle interactions that occur among members of the health professions, patients and their families, and the general public. Their previous education may also have failed to acquaint them with other aspects of professional conduct such as how to relate to colleagues, employers, and the media. Research assistants, interviewers, and data processors may be quite unfamiliar with these aspects of their work. The impetus to develop guidelines or codes of conduct has come at least in part from epidemiologists with such backgrounds.[7]

Master's level programs in epidemiology at universities or schools of public health offer formal courses in epidemiology, statistics, behavioral sciences, environmental sciences, and related fields such as toxicology. There are often vocational courses in survey methods, health services research, and, for students without previous education or experience in a health discipline or a health care setting, introductory courses in human biology and pathology, concepts of health and sickness, and organization of the health care system. Education in biomedical ethics is not required for completion of a master's or doctoral degree, although ethical topics may be discussed in seminars, perhaps at the request of students. Ethical dilemmas arise often enough in both epidemiologic research and practice to have become a popular topic at scientific meetings of epidemiologists, which has helped heighten awareness.[†] Examinations to verify professional competence may or may not include questions aimed at assessing whether candidates are acquainted with ethics, or appreciate the moral nuances of their role,

---

†Since the late 1980s, there has been at least one session dedicated to ethical topics or issues at every annual meeting of the Society for Epidemiologic Research. Ethical issues and case studies have been published frequently in *Epidemiology Monitor*, which offers a more convenient forum for exchange of ideas than peer-reviewed journals of epidemiology.

duties, and responsibilities in relation to research subjects, colleagues, and the general public. Some students do not understand, for instance, that they may be held accountable not only for their own actions but for those of staff under their supervision.

Obligations and Responsibilities of Epidemiologists

Whether engaged in routine practice or research, epidemiologists have obligations and responsibilities to the human subjects of our studies, to the organizations and institutions at which we work, to employers and granting agencies, to our colleagues, to students, to our science, and to society at large. We should understand the basic principles of biomedical ethics. We should be familiar with the Nuremberg Code and the Helsinki Declaration (see Chapter 1), and be aware of the relevance of these documents to our work. In our practice and research we must recognize the four basic principles developed by Beauchamp and Childress in *Principles of Biomedical Ethics*:[8] respect for autonomy, beneficence, nonmaleficence, and justice (fairness in the distribution of benefits and risks).

These codes and principles express our belief systems, or values. We should ask ourselves what additional values we have in common as epidemiologists, and we should consider how these values relate to our professional behavior. We must be conscious of the moral climate in which we work, that is, of the values and belief systems of an increasingly complex, multicultural society. Moreover, sometimes we have a fiduciary responsibility to the subjects of our studies. An understanding of the *virtues*[9] is also desirable in epidemiology; we should uphold the virtues of trust, compassion, prudence, and integrity.

Respect for Autonomy: Informed Consent

Respect for autonomy requires that we do not carry out any biomedical or social research without the informed consent of the subjects or their proxies. Informed consent is an integral part of medical practice and of research involving human subjects.[10] Subjects must not only be informed, they must understand what is asked of them; they must be advised of their right to withdraw their consent at any time; there must be no coercion or undue influence, or inappropriate inducements to participate in a research study. These and other requirements for informed consent are specified in the revised *International Ethical Guidelines for Biomedical Research Involving Human Subjects*,[11] drafted by a working group of the Council for International Organizations of the Medical Sciences (CIOMS) and approved by the World Health Assembly in 1993. These guidelines should be observed in epidemiologic studies. The valid, although rare, exceptions are specified in the 1991 CIOMS *International Guidelines for Ethical Review of*

Epidemiological Studies.[12] The subject is further discussed later in this chapter and elsewhere in this book.

Privacy and Confidentiality

We have a duty to protect the privacy of individuals and to preserve the confidentiality of information about them. Privacy is the state of being undisturbed or free of public attention; confidentiality is the right of a person to withhold information from others and the obligation not to disclose private information. Privacy and confidentiality can conflict with the imperative societal need for access to and perhaps disclosure of information in the public interest. The clash between the privacy rights of persons and the need for access to and disclosure of personal health-related information is the most frequent ethical dilemma to confront epidemiologists. As this chapter will discuss, in some nations the right to privacy has so much higher priority than the socially important need for access to information that the public interest can be undermined.

Avoiding Harms and Wrongs

Stigmatizing and Segregating the Sick

The oldest task of the epidemiologist is to investigate and control epidemics in order to protect the public against the threat to health and life from contagious diseases. Two ancient customs associated with this task are older than the field of epidemiology. In biblical times, victims of leprosy (and often any other disfiguring conditions believed to be contagious) were required in some societies to carry a bell and wear distinctive clothing so others would recognize and avoid them. Thereby the victims often were stigmatized. In some communities such persons were also required to be segregated in leper houses or lazarettos, and in the fourteenth century the Venetians added the practice of quarantine for healthy contacts. Thus stigmatization and restriction of freedom have long been associated with infection control. These practices were codified by Johann Peter Frank[13] in *System einer vollständigen medicinischen Polizey* (1779), which contributed to the concept of the police function of public health.

During World War I, public health authorities in the United States, Australia, and other countries regarded prostitutes, who might transmit what were then called venereal diseases, as war criminals sabotaging the war effort. They were rounded up and incarcerated.[14] In the severe polio epidemic of 1916, public health authorities in New York searched private homes to detect and remove children who had been in contact with cases of polio.[15] Thereafter, the unhappy image of "medical police" almost vanished from modern public health practice until it was reinvigorated by some of the measures thought necessary to control the HIV epidemic.[16] In many communities, public health authorities, sometimes in collaboration with local police forces, have taken punitive action against persons thought to be responsible for knowingly engaging in sexual practices that might contribute to the spread of HIV infection. The confidentiality of medical records has been violated, for instance by physicians' receptionists, and the HIV status of patients revealed to unauthorized persons. Medical records must be kept secure so that intimate personal information cannot be disclosed to the media, the police, or the general public.[17] There are legal exceptions, however. In many jurisdictions, for example, physicians must report suspected child abuse to law-enforcement authorities.

Avoiding Harmful Disclosures

Epidemiologists must be aware of and sensitive to the feelings of individuals and identifiable groups, and must avoid actions that can needlessly cause harm by invading privacy and violating confidentiality. We often believe that everything we do is in the public interest, but at times this may lead us to disclose information in ways that can be harmful to individuals or social groups. One of our obligations is the need to consider carefully the potential harm that may follow invasion of privacy and violation of confidentiality.

There have been many recent examples in the context of the HIV epidemic, but we need not enter this emotionally charged arena to encounter damaging disclosures. Consider the commonplace incident that is the basis for an exercise in almost every elementary course in epidemiology, an epidemic of staphylococcal food poisoning with explosive vomiting and diarrhea a few hours after a supper in the church basement on a Sunday evening. If investigation reveals that the incriminated food was prepared by a prominent member of the congregation, tact is required in reporting to prevent needless feelings of guilt or shame and acrimony among parishioners. The same tact is necessary in all communicable disease reporting.

Insensitive or inaccurate disclosure can harm communities or social groups. A *Mortality Atlas*[18] identified the "unhealthiest town in Canada," leading to media publicity that embarrassed and angered the residents, partly because the accompanying commentary implied that alcohol and other substance abuse were responsible for many deaths. To remedy the situation, an expensive study was conducted. This showed that the death rates were inflated by nonresidents who died in the local hospital.[19] Epidemiologists and vital statisticians have an obligation to present findings in a manner that does not stigmatize communities or identifiable social groups.

Epidemiologic studies often define risks to the health of an identifiable group. Smokers or people who are overweight or sedentary, for example, may be stigmatized as individuals or as groups by the image of poor health. Such labeling of persons for their characteristics or occupations (such as those employed in the alcohol or gambling industries) can cause them to experience victim-blaming at the hands of their health care providers, or make them feel guilty about their high-risk characteristic. Even more emotionally loaded are studies that identify members of a particular race or ethnic group as having a high risk of certain diseases. African American men are prone to hypertension and cancer of the prostate, native Americans have a high incidence of alcohol-related disorders and diabetes associated with obesity, and members of certain Jewish sects have a high risk of hereditary transmission of Tay-Sachs disease. In the reverse of this situation, the low risk of cancer and heart disease and "health consciousness" among Mormons and Seventh Day Adventists, for example, is sometimes equated with elitism and may be resented or envied ("Members of our sect live longer").

Tactlessly disclosed epidemiologic findings can cause harm by stigmatizing a group and in other ways as well—for instance, by aggravating the adversarial relationship between a labor union and management.

Interactions with Others

Relationships with Colleagues

As in other fields of science, epidemiologists have obligations to colleagues and to science itself. With the exception of work that involves national security or trade secrets, we must be open in our dealings and be prepared to share our methods and results with others. Failure to disclose our methods can raise suspicions about scientific misconduct. Indeed, it is often regarded as prima-facie evidence of wrongdoing. We must respect our duty to students under our supervision, teach them honestly, and demonstrate exemplary conduct in all scientific respects.

Epidemiologists and Society

We relate directly to society or the community in several ways. Increasingly our research results are making headlines. But epidemiologic findings are sometimes open to misinterpretation if presented carelessly or without caveat. In our dealings with the media, we must not sensationalize: we should make conscious efforts to present the facts objectively and with sufficient explanation to ensure that the news reaching the general public does not mislead either by unnecessarily arousing alarm or by falsely reassuring people that their way of life is conducive to longevity. We should inform the media about errors that can be made when population-based findings are used to infer risks to individuals. For instance, smokers are at higher risk than nonsmokers from life-shortening diseases such as lung cancer and coronary atherosclerosis, but this does not mean that non-smokers never have heart attacks or get lung cancer.

Impartiality and Advocacy

The aim of epidemiology and public health is to enhance the human condition by identifying causes of premature death and disability and finding ways to control or eliminate these causes. Often epidemiologists who have identified sources of prominent life-threatening conditions become advocates, taking public positions in debates about control measures. But advocacy is incompatible with scientific objectivity and impartiality. It is difficult, but particularly important, to preserve scientific objectivity when we are employed by a special-interest group such as an industrial management, a labor union, or a lobbying organization. In such situations we need to be aware of the potential for conflict of interest.

Unbecoming Professional Conduct

Epidemiologists are sometimes disturbed by what they consider wrongful conduct of their peers. There have been disputes over the nature and quality of epidemiologic evidence, and the interpretation of data and conclusions that may be derived from studies. Such controversies are often related to the methods and procedures used to demonstrate "statistically significant" associations (presumed cause-effect relationships) between exposure to a risk factor and the occurrence of serious disease such as cancer. One hallmark of professional competence is the ability to decide on the appropriate methods and procedures to yield valid results in particular circumstances. The choice of inappropriate methods and procedures can indicate shoddy science or impaired scientific objectivity. Our impartiality can be compromised when we have a vested interest in the outcome of a study—when there is a conflict of interest. This is a disservice to science and to society, and an egregious departure from ethical conduct. The subjects of scientific integrity and responsible conduct of science have been discussed in the United States by the National Science Foundation,[20] the Institute of Medicine of the National Academy of Science,[21] the American Association for the Advancement of Science,[22] and by similar groups in other nations.[23]

Toward a Code of Conduct for Epidemiologists

The preceding discussion has dealt with several problems that can arise in epidemiologic practice and research. It suggests that we should be able to formulate some guidelines on the ethical conduct of epidemiology.

Leaders of epidemiologic thought in the late nineteenth and early twentieth centuries—Hamer, Stallybrass, Frost, Greenwood, Goldberger, Maxcy, and many others—were untroubled by ethical issues and concerns. It is hard to find even indirect allusions to medical ethics anywhere in their writings. If they professed ethical beliefs, they would most likely have embraced utilitarianism, a philosophical theory pervasive in public health literature of the 1800s and early 1900s. Indeed, public health practice is based largely on a belief in the greatest good for the greatest number, with the understanding that sometimes individuals must suffer harm in order that the community as a whole will benefit. As mentioned above, Goldberger's studies of pellagra were done without informed consent. Greenwood's views were paternalistic, even authoritarian (epitomized in the title of his collection of essays on men he admired, *The Medical Dictator*[24]). Some epidemiologic studies of that and later eras, notably the Tuskegee Syphilis Experiment, an observational study of the natural history of untreated syphilis,[25] display an insensitivity to human rights that horrifies us today. The early studies of fluoridation of drinking water in New York State and Ontario, Canada, did not observe the niceties of informed consent.[26] In research sponsored by the United States Atomic Energy Agency in the 1950s to test the effects of exposure to ionizing radiation, mentally retarded adolescents were given food contaminated by radioactive substances and pregnant women received doses of radioactive iron. The consent procedures in these studies were seriously flawed, because information about the experiments was not provided to the subjects or their proxies.[27,28]

After the trials of Nazi war criminals at Nuremberg in the late 1940s, formal consent procedures became increasingly common and ultimately mandatory in randomized controlled trials and other experiments on human subjects. In the early 1960s, however, only two (E. M. Glaser and J. Knowelden) of eighteen contributors to an anthology of papers on medical surveys and clinical trials mentioned the importance of informed consent.[29] Even now, some clinical researchers rationalize that informed consent is not always necessary or even desirable,[30] although most realize that with rare exceptions, discussed below, it is mandatory.[31]

Recognition of the potential for ethical problems and dilemmas has led epidemiologists to discuss and develop ethical guidelines and codes of conduct. These initiatives have come from different directions and have originated in several nations. Codes of conduct have an ancient tradition in the medical profession, and have been developed for other health-related professions and human service activities such as the work of official statisticians[32] (who are responsible for compiling statistics based on registrations of births, marriages, deaths, and other officially collected information). The existence of a code of conduct is sometimes seen as a hallmark of professional maturity. Thus epidemiologists, seeking to enhance the stature of their calling, have been motivated to compose a formal statement setting out criteria of desirable, acceptable, and unacceptable conduct.

The Nuremberg Code

Some of the major concerns of biomedical scientists—including epidemiologists—date from the Nuremberg trials, when Nazi atrocities came to light. Revelations about "experiments" in which people were regarded as expendable animals outraged civilized people everywhere. The Nuremberg Code[33] was an outcome of these trials. It states that ten basic principles must be observed in order to satisfy moral, ethical, and legal concepts. The first principle begins, "The voluntary consent of the human subject is absolutely essential." (Table 3–1.)

Principle One is usually conceded to have certain exceptions, but it has been interpreted literally in Germany; the same will be true throughout Europe if European Community directives are fully implemented. The consequences will be detrimental to epidemiology and other kinds of research that require access to medical and other records for purposes beyond the intent of those who originally compiled them, as discussed below.

The Declaration of Helsinki

The World Medical Association refined and expanded on the ideas in the Nuremberg Code at its 1964 meeting in Finland, where the Declaration of

---

Table 3–1. Summary of the Nuremberg Code

1. Voluntary consent of the human subject is absolutely essential
   Legal capacity to give consent
   Free power of choice
   No force, fraud, deceit, duress or other constraint or coercion
   Sufficient knowledge and comprehension for an enlightened decision
   Personal duty and responsibility of researcher to obtain consent

2. Experiment should yield fruitful results for good of society
   Unprocurable by other means
   Not random or unnecessary

3. Experiment should be designed and based on animal experiment, knowledge of natural history of disease or other problem under study
   Anticipated results will justify the experiment

4. Avoid unnecessary physical and mental suffering and injury

5. No experiment when *a priori* reason to believe death or disabling injury will occur

6. Degree of risk should never exceed that determined by the humanitarian importance of the problem to be solved

7. Adequate facilities to protect study subjects

8. Conducted only by scientifically qualified persons

9. Subject has right to withdraw at any time

10. Scientist must be prepared to terminate experiment if continuation likely to cause injury, disability or death

---

Helsinki was drafted to address research on human subjects. This has been revised and embellished with more specific statements about patient care and aspects of medical research several times since 1964, most recently in Hong Kong in 1989[34] (Table 3–2).

Recognition that research on human subjects should comply with the conditions set out in the Declaration of Helsinki has had a pervasive influence on many forms of such research, including even observational epidemiologic studies that do not require intervention or any alteration in the status of study subjects.

Epidemiology differs from other branches of biomedical science in several ways, such as the ill-defined distinction between observational research and routine surveillance (the latter is the everyday practice of epidemiology). Furthermore, situations arise in epidemiologic studies when it makes no sense to adhere to the "human subjects" provisions of the Helsinki declaration. For instance, if the study requires no intervention and the subjects are deceased, it is not practicable to insist on informed consent. If the study involves huge numbers, perhaps millions as in record-linkage studies, it is not feasible to obtain informed consent from everybody. These exceptions to the rules about informed consent are sanctioned in the 1991 CIOMS *International Guidelines for Ethical Review of Epidemiological Studies*, described and discussed below.

Codes of Conduct and HIV Infection

Surveillance and control of HIV infection require recognition of unprecedented ethical and moral dilemmas, and have prompted many statements about "correct" conduct of health workers, including epidemiologists. It may be impossible, however, to establish codes of conduct that apply universally to aspects of surveillance, control, and research on HIV disease. Some examples make this point. To monitor the changing prevalence of HIV infection in the population, the World Health Organization (WHO) Global Programme on AIDS has recommended the use of anonymous, unlinked HIV tests.[35] Blood drawn from neonates is a useful source. After testing for inherited metabolic defects, which is routine in many jurisdictions, the specimens are stripped of personal identifiers and used to test for the presence of HIV. This can yield prevalence estimates for a large, representative population of the live offspring of sexually active young women, and is regarded as a reasonably valid surrogate for general population prevalence.

However, such tests can give rise to several ethical problems. One is that specimens of blood are used for a purpose other than that for which parents or others may have given consent. In some jurisdictions, including the European Community (EC), this is now illegal. Another ethical problem arises if the specimen tests positive: there is no way to identify infected individuals for counseling, case, and contact tracing. Nevertheless, public health authorities in most nations have agreed that the public interest is best served by using this method to

Table 3–2. Summary of the Declaration of Helsinki

Drafted by World Medical Association, intended for medical doctors, but applicable to all working in the medical field

Introduction

"The health of my patient will be my first consideration"

"The purpose of biomedical research involving human subjects must be to improve diagnostic, therapeutic and prophylactic procedures and understanding of the aetiology and pathogenesis of disease"

I. Basic principles

1. Research must conform to accepted scientific principles, be based on laboratory and animal experiments and thorough knowledge of the scientific literature

2. Design and performance of experiment clearly formulated in an independently reviewed experimental protocol

3. Conducted only by scientifically qualified persons under supervision of a clinically competent medical person
   Responsibility for human subjects rests with medical person, not with subjects of research

4. Importance of objectives is in proportion to inherent risk

5. Experiment must be preceded by assessment of predictable risk in comparison to expected benefits
   Concern for the interests of the subject must prevail over the interests of science or society

6. Rights of subjects to safeguard their integrity, and to privacy, must be respected

7. No experiment unless hazards predictable
   Terminate experiment if hazards outweigh potential benefits

8. Publish results accurately

9. Informed consent is mandatory; subjects should understand aims, methods, benefits, hazards; should know they have the right to withdraw from the study

10. When subject is in a dependent relationship to the investigator, consent must be obtained by third party

11. Informed consent should be provided by a proxy when subject is legally incompetent

12. Research protocol should contain statement about compliance with the above ethical considerations

II. Medical research combined with professional care (Clinical research)

1. Doctor must be free to use new diagnostic and therapeutic measures according to best judgement

2. Benefits, hazards, discomforts of new measures should be weighed against advantages of best current methods

3. Every patient should be assured of the best proven diagnostic and therapeutic method

4. Refusal of a patient to participate in a study must never interfere with the doctor-patient relationship

5. If the doctor considers it essential not to obtain informed consent, the specific reason should be stated in the protocol that is to be submitted for independent review

6. Medical research can be combined with professional care with the objective of acquiring new knowledge only to the extent that research is justified by its potential value to the patient

Table 3–2. (*continued*)

III. Non-therapeutic biomedical research involving human subjects
(Non-clinical biomedical research)

1. It is the duty of the doctor to remain the protector of life and health of persons on whom research is being conducted

2. The subjects should be volunteers

3. Investigators should discontinue research if in their judgment its continuation might be harmful to the subjects

4. The interests of science and society should never take precedence over the well-being of the subjects

estimate the prevalence of HIV infection. Different conclusions have been reached in some countries, including the Netherlands. If EC directives are enforced, anonymous, unlinked HIV tests based on samples of neonates' blood will be illegal and unethical in all EC nations.

Another example of the difficulty in establishing universal ethical codes in HIV surveillance is more controversial. Common ways for HIV infection to spread are sharing of needles for intravenous drug abuse, and unprotected receptive anal sexual intercourse. Both of these dangerous and often illegal practices are prevalent among prison inmates, despite the efforts of prison staff to eliminate them. The risk of HIV transmission among convicts can be reduced by providing "no-questions-asked" circumstances for sterile needle exchange and condom distribution. Yet to take these actions would violate legal, ethical, and moral standards that prison wardens are expected to honor, and pose other potential dangers such as use of needles to make weapons and condoms to smuggle drugs. The approach to this problem varies greatly from one jurisdiction to another. No code of conduct or guidelines could state universally applicable rules to cope with this situation; it has to be decided by prevailing circumstances and moral values in each setting where the problem arises.

Guidelines for Ethical Review of Epidemiologic Studies

Research grant review committees and national research funding agencies, such as the United States National Institutes of Health,[36] the United Kingdom Medical Research Council,[37] the Canadian Medical Research Council,[38] the Australian National Health and Medical Research Council (NHMRC),[39] and the Swedish[40] and other European medical research councils,[41] have been concerned for many years about the need for standards for ethical review of medical research. Some have recognized that standards in epidemiologic studies may differ from those applied to other aspects of research involving human subjects.[42]

Many research funding agencies have prepared statements about ethics for the benefit of both applicants for research support and members of research grant review committees. These documents deal with ethical issues that can arise in research involving human subjects. A report by the NHMRC in Australia[43] and a book on ethical issues in psychiatric epidemiology[44] directly address ethical issues in epidemiologic research, such as the unique problem of access to personal medical records.

These initiatives attracted the attention of the Council for International Organizations of the Medical Sciences (CIOMS). In 1989, CIOMS established a working group to develop guidelines for ethical review of epidemiologic research. The group recognized the ill-defined boundary between research and routine practice, such as investigating outbreaks of contagious disease, and the need to draft guidelines that might be used to govern both. The document that ultimately emerged, however, did not specify the need for routine epidemic investigation to adhere to ethical standards comparable to those that apply in epidemiologic research. During the XXV CIOMS International Conference, at which the draft guidelines were the principal topic of discussion, practicing epidemiologists insisted that it was not feasible to require ethical review of procedures to be followed in routine epidemic investigation.[45] In fact this was never intended, but members of the working group hoped that discussing the issue might lead public health authorities at national, regional, and local levels to develop greater ethical sensitivity and awareness than they had sometimes hitherto shown in their approach to surveillance and control of diseases of public health importance.

The CIOMS *International Guidelines for Ethical Review of Epidemiological Studies* include discussion of the unique problems associated with informed consent in epidemiologic studies: it is not always feasible or desirable to apply the same procedures for consent as in clinical research. For example, if subjects receive detailed information about the aims of a health promotion research project, their behavior may change in ways that would invalidate the research. The principle of "conscientious nondisclosure" was suggested to cope with this circumstance. Issues relating to maximizing benefit and minimizing harm, to confidentiality, and to conflict of interest are also discussed in the CIOMS Guidelines. Ethical review procedures are addressed and responsibilities of members of ethics review committees are delineated, including respect for privileged information. It is pointed out that ethical review should assess scientific soundness—unsound research is unethical. The ethics of randomization and the status of control groups are discussed. Randomization is described not as a discriminatory procedure but as a necessary step in ensuring scientific validity.

The CIOMS guidelines were approved by the World Health Assembly in 1991. The working group that drafted the document hoped it would become a model for guidelines subsequently to be developed by member nations of WHO. Indeed, the CIOMS guidelines help to ensure sound ethical review of epidemiologic studies, and they could be adopted by national and local ethical review committees such as institutional review boards in the United States.

Initiatives of Professional Associations

Associations and societies of epidemiologists, along with eminent practitioners, have held discussions and debates on ethical aspects of the profession. In the early 1970s, the Society for Epidemiologic Research (SER) became concerned about the rising tension between guardians of privacy and those who need access to information in personal files in order to conduct analytic studies. Several presentations and published papers at that time expressed concern about the rising tide of opinion in favor of protecting privacy at the expense of access to information that it would be in the public interest to analyze in depth.[46,47,48] Later discussions at meetings of SER turned to other topics such as conflicts of interest and scientific misconduct,[49,50] and then to questions related to data sharing.[51] SER has produced several short statements about these ethical issues, but has not developed a formal set of guidelines or a code of conduct.

The International Epidemiological Association (IEA) resolved at its meeting in Helsinki in 1987 to begin developing ethical guidelines. Drafts of the IEA guidelines were circulated late in 1987 and subsequently to progressively widening circles of correspondents worldwide over the next two to three years, and were periodically revised several times to reflect feedback received.[52] These guidelines were the principal topic of discussion at an international workshop attended by IEA delegates from about twenty-five nations in the industrial and developing world preceding the 1990 IEA meeting in Los Angeles.[53] The IEA guidelines comprise a preamble, a statement about values, a summary of ethical principles, and sections or clauses dealing with the duties or obligations of epidemiologists to individuals, communities, colleagues, students, employers and granting agencies, and the science itself (Table 3–3).

The IEA guidelines state that the same rules apply in routine practice as in epidemiologic research. After the change in membership of the IEA Council in 1990, this initiative was suspended, for two reasons. First, the CIOMS working group had taken over all essential aspects of the task; and second, as an international organization, the IEA had no mandate to prescribe ethical rules for its members in any given country. That function, it was felt by the new Council, was best performed by national associations of epidemiologists.

The initiative to compose a Code of Conduct for Epidemiology was taken up in the late 1980s by the Industrial Epidemiology Forum (IEF), an American society of epidemiologists employed in industrial settings. The group engaged in these deliberations included an ethicist as well as epidemiologists. Drafts of the IEF "code" were discussed at several meetings, including a conference convened specifically for that purpose preceding the SER annual meeting in Birmingham,

Table 3–3. Summary of IEA Ethics Guidelines

1. Definition and purpose of epidemiology
    Research and practice—guidelines apply to both, and to all who do any kind of epidemiology

2. Values of epidemiology—concerned with health of population
    • aim to identify interventions that will restore, maintain, improve health
    • aim to improve state of knowledge
    • obligation to communities rather than individuals
    • distinguish science from advocacy

3. Basic principles of biomedical ethics
    Autonomy, beneficence, nonmaleficence, justice

4. Obligations to individuals
    Informed consent
    Respect privacy, preserve confidentiality
    Obtain consent when privacy must be invaded, e.g., when notifying infectious diseases
    Weigh benefits and risks, harms

5. Obligations to communities
    Communicate with community representatives
    Ensure provision of adequate care
    Avoid discrimination

6. Access to information
    Use personal information responsibly
    Share and disseminate findings and data

7. Scientific integrity
    Honesty and impartiality are essential
    Declare conflicts of interest
    Distinguish objectivity and advocacy

8. Professional standards
    Interactions with colleagues, students, others
    Exemplary conduct with students

9. Cultural variations in values
    Respect variations in moral values
    May have difficulty when culturally determined behavior harms health

10. Conclusions
    These are guidelines, not a formal code of conduct

Alabama, in 1989. The document that ultimately emerged from these discussions was published in 1991 as *Ethical Guidelines for Epidemiologists*.[54] This carefully composed statement is a model for anyone who seeks to draft guidelines for a professional group. It focuses on the epidemiologist's obligations to subjects of study, society, research funding agencies, employers, and colleagues (Table 3–4). The commentary accompanying the IEF guidelines is especially useful.

The Chemical Manufacturers' Association (CMA) set up an Epidemiology Task Group to produce *Guidelines for Good Epidemiology Practices for Occupational and Environmental Epidemiologic Research*. Its report,[55] published in 1991 after circulation of preliminary drafts, spells out ethical rules and describes and discusses aspects of research design, methods, procedures, staffing, facilities, resources, and other important topics (Table 3–5).

In discussing the organization and conduct of studies, the CMA guidelines advance the notion that epidemiologists working for the chemical industry have a primary duty of loyalty to their employers: they may not publish or otherwise distribute results of their studies without prior clearance from their companies. While this restriction may be desirable when trade secrets are at stake, it poses a disturbing potential threat of censorship of findings that it may be in the public interest to disclose.[56]

European Initiatives

The emphasis of discussions and actions regarding ethics at national and regional levels in Europe has varied according to locally perceived problems. For example, the Swedish Society for Public Health Research and several other European associations have been preoccupied mainly with problems and issues relating to access to health-related information.[57] In Sweden and other European nations, public sentiment has swung sharply toward protection of privacy, and guardians

---

Table 3–4. Summary of IEF Guidelines

Part I

   I. Obligations to subjects of research
       Protect welfare
       Obtain informed consent
       Protect privacy
       Maintain confidentiality

  II. Obligations to society
       Avoid conflicts of interest
       Avoid partiality
       Widen scope of epidemiology
       Pursue responsibilities diligently
       Maintain public confidence

 III. Obligations to funders and employers
       Specify obligations
       Protect privileged information

 IV. Obligations to colleagues
       Report methods and results
       Confront unacceptable conduct
       Communicate ethical requirements

Part II

Commentary

This sets out the ethical framework of the guidelines and discusses each of the clauses in detail

Table 3–5. Summary of the Chemical Manufacturers Association Guidelines for Good Epidemiology Practices for Occupational and Environmental Epidemiologic Research

Goals
- Provide a framework for researchers
- Promote sound epidemiologic research
- Facilitate continued improvement of research methods
- Provide a framework for evaluating research
- Improve acceptance of sound scientific methods
- Improve utility of epidemiologic studies in health policy
- Improve public confidence in epidemiology
- Facilitate conservation of resources

   I. Organization and personnel
      Delineate roles, responsibilities
      Appropriate education and training

  II. Facilities and resources
      Ensure adequacy

 III. Components of research protocol

 IV. Procedures for review and approval of research protocols, (including ethical review)

  V. Conduct of a study
      Protection of human subjects; data collection and verification; analysis; reporting

 VI. Communication
      With sponsors, government agencies, scientific peers, study subjects

VII. Archiving
      Specifications for secure storage of data and findings

VIII. Quality assurance
      Appointment of an independent quality assurance auditor

of privacy have erected increasingly intimidating barriers that impede or completely block access to sources of health-related information that are a sine qua non of epidemiologic studies. The barriers often are reinforced by regulations or laws. In Sweden this came about as a backlash against the "big brother" paternalism that long prevailed. Everyone has a personal identifying number that is used in all publicly compiled documents—school performance, tax records, police reports, and other official records as well as health information. However, recently the regulators have recognized the value of analyzed records and have loosened the restrictions.[58]

Restrictions on access to information are more stringent in the Netherlands. Privacy is considered by the Dutch to be so sacred that for more than thirty years they have not had a census with enumeration and recording of basic household information such as the presence of a flush toilet and hot-water services. It is very difficult to carry out population-based epidemiologic studies in the Netherlands for this reason. In the former West Germany, in reaction against the intrusive activities of the Nazis before and during World War II, the collection and storage of personal information were made illegal. After the unification of Germany, the same rules were applied; consequently, in the former East Germany previously compiled and very useful records of, for example, occupational diseases were destroyed—an act of scientific vandalism. In the United Kingdom, it is necessary to obtain informed consent before entering information about individuals in cancer registries, thus defeating their purpose of comprehensiveness and making them almost useless as an epidemiologic tool for investigation, especially of rare malignancies. For several years, officials of the European Community have been debating the application of regulations throughout the EC that would make data access for epidemiologic and other socially useful research purposes illegal and virtually impossible.[59] European epidemiologic societies have been much preoccupied with countermeasures that might ensure continuing access at least to health information.

Current Concerns of American Epidemiologists

The American College of Epidemiology (ACE) established a committee on Ethics and Standards of Practice (ESOP) in 1991. The ACE/ESOP committee includes representatives of SER, IEA, the Epidemiology Section of the American Public Health Association, and fields of occupational and industrial epidemiology. Committee members have discussed a wide range of issues, including aspects of scientific misconduct; interactions with colleages; the relationship between epidemiologists, the general public, and other health professionals; and the perennial problems of access to information. In order to engage epidemiologists at the grassroots level, questionnaires have been developed and circulated to samples of practitioners, both at national meetings and in random postal surveys. The ultimate aim is to develop a set of guidelines with input from a broadly representative sample of epidemiologists. To an outsider, Americans sometimes appear excessively preoccupied with respect for autonomy at the expense of the other three basic principles of biomedical ethics—justice, beneficence, and nonmaleficence. Perhaps this reflects the importance to Americans of "life, liberty, and the pursuit of happiness" (in contrast to the Canadian emphasis on "peace, order, and good government"). Statements on ethics display a concern for autonomy not only of subjects of research, but also of epidemiologists. There is a need to discuss the image of epidemiologists, both as perceived by the general public and as perceived by other health professions.[60] Guidelines and codes of conduct have not addressed this question.

Strengths and Weaknesses of Codes of Conduct

The process of developing codes and guidelines is a valuable exercise for all who participate: it educates, enlightens, and heightens awareness. Perhaps the process is more important than the outcome. One problem with codes of conduct and guidelines is that they may impose an implied rigidity where there is a need for flexibility.[61] There are so many variations among the innumerable situations in which ethical problems can arise that it is unwise to set strict rules: every situation is to some extent unique and requires moral reasoning. What ought to happen when an ethical problem arises is open discussion, then application of procedures for alleviating or resolving the problem. First, identify and characterize the problem and all affected by it, then consider the potential impact of possible solutions, choose one, act on it, and evaluate the consequences.

On the other hand, codes of conduct and guidelines have the advantage of offering moral support when individual professionals or organizations encounter situations that present ethical or moral dilemmas. Even though every situation is unique, general statements about appropriate actions can often be very helpful. Sometimes a code of conduct is used to reinforce decisions about violation of acceptable standards. For example, physicians can be punished by having their licence to practice revoked if they act in a manner that is regarded as infamous or heinous professional conduct. Epidemiologists do not require a licence to practice, so this severe sanction is not possible. Perhaps the worst penalty that could be imposed for violation of the standards set out in a code of conduct might be expulsion from a professional college or association, which might at some future time carry a threat of loss of employment. It is hoped that such potential sanctions remain theoretical, and that by discussion and debate whenever ethical problems arise, the high professional standards of epidemiologists will be maintained and will rise even higher in the future.

Conclusion

In this review, I have described various types of ethical issues that can arise in epidemiology and the increasing attention that epidemiologists are paying to these issues. Ethical problems are now frequent topics of discussion at formal and informal gatherings of epidemiologists. Whether such discussions lead to explicit guidelines or codes of conduct may be less important than the fact that the discussions are occurring, and thereby are heightening awareness of ethical issues among epidemiologists everywhere.

References

1. Pickles, W. *Epidemiology in Country Practice*. Bristol: John Wright & Sons, 1939.
2. Agyei, W. K. A., Epema, E. J., and Lubenga, M. "Contraception and Prevalence of Sexually Transmitted Diseases Among Adolescents and Young Adults in Uganda," *International Journal of Epidemiology* 21 (1992): 981–988.

3. Sackett, D. L., Haynes, R. B., Guyatt, G. H., and Tugwell, P. *Clinical Epidemiology: A Basic Science for Clinical Medicine.* Boston: Little, Brown, 1991.

4. Schulte, P. A., and Perera, F. P. *Molecular Epidemiology: Principles and Practices.* Orlando: Academic Press, 1993.

5. Terris, M., ed. *Goldberger on Pellagra.* Baton Rouge: Louisiana State University Press, 1964. Especially Part II on Human Experiments.

6. Susser, M., Stein, Z., and Kline, J. "Ethics in Epidemiology," *Annals of the American Academy of Political and Social Science* 437 (1978): 128–141. This paper discusses, among others, Goldberger's pellagra studies, drawing attention to the absence of ethical review.

7. Soskolne, C. L. "Epidemiology: Questions of Science, Ethics, Morality and Law," *American Journal of Epidemiology* 129 (1989): 1–18.

8. Beauchamp, T. L., and Childress, J. F. *Principles of Biomedical Ethics.* 4th ed. New York: Oxford University Press, 1994.

9. Pellegrino, E. D. and Thomasma, D. C. *The Virtues in Medical Practice.* New York: Oxford University Press, 1993.

10. Faden, R. R., and Beauchamp, T. L. *A History and Theory of Informed Consent.* New York: Oxford University Press, 1986.

11. *International Ethical Guidelines for Biomedical Research Involving Human Subjects.* Geneva: CIOMS and WHO, 1993.

12. *International Guidelines for Ethical Review of Epidemiological Studies.* Geneva: CIOMS and WHO, 1991.

13. Frank, J. P. "System Einer Vollständigen Medicinischen Polizey," *Mannheim, Tübingen, Wein,* 9 vols. (1779–1827). English translation, "A System of Complete Medical Police," selections by Erna Lesky. Baltimore: Johns Hopkins Press, 1976.

14. Brandt, A. M. *No Magic Bullet: A Social History of Venereal Disease in the United States Since 1880.* New York: Oxford University Press, 1987.

15. Paul, J. R. *A History of Poliomyelitis.* New Haven: Yale University Press, 1971: 148–52.

16. Shilts, R. *And the Band Played On.* New York: Penguin, 1987.

17. Last, J. M. "Medical Records, 2: Security and Confidentiality," *Annals of the Royal College of Physicians and Surgeons of Canada* 27 (1994): 8–9.

18. *Statistics Canada: Mortality Atlas of Canada,* vol. 2, General Mortality. Ottawa: Supply and Services Canada (cat. H49-6/2-1980).

19. Mao, Y., McCourt, C., Morrison, H., et al. "Community-based Mortality Surveillance; the Maniwaki Experience: Investigation of Excess Mortality in a Community," *Canadian Journal of Public Health* 75 (1984): 429–33.

20. U.S. National Science Foundation. "Misconduct in Science and Engineering: Final Rule," *Federal Register* 56 (1991): 22287–290.

21. Institute of Medicine, National Academy of Sciences. *Report of a Study on the Responsible Conduct of Research in the Health Sciences.* Washington: National Academy of Sciences, 1989.

22. Teich, A. H. and Frankel, M. S. *Good Science and Responsible Scientists: Meeting the Challenge of Fraud and Misconduct in Science.* Washington, D.C.: AAAS, 1992.

23. Royal College of Physicians of London. *Fraud and Misconduct in Medical Research.* London: Royal College of Physicians, 1989.

24. Greenwood, M. *The Medical Dictator.* London: Williams and Norgate, 1936.

25. Jones, J. H. *Bad Blood: The Tuskegee Syphilis Experiment: A Tragedy of Race and Medicine.* New York: Collier, Macmillan, Free Press, 1981.

26. Knutson, J. W. "Water Fluoridation After 25 Years," *Journal of the American Dental Association* 80 (1970): 765.

27. "When U.S. Risked Lives for Sake of Experiments," *Manchester Guardian Weekly*, January 9, 1994: 18.

28. McCally, M., Cassel, C., and Kimball, D. G. "U.S. Government-Sponsored Radiation Research on Humans 1945–1975," *Medicine & Global Survival* 1 (1994): 4–17.

29. Witts, L. J., ed. *Medical Surveys and Clinical Trials.* London: Oxford University Press, 1964.

30. "Correspondence on Informed Consent in Clinical Trials," *British Medical Journal* 307, (December 4, 1992): 1494–97.

31. Wald, N. "Ethical Issues in Randomized Prevention Trials," *British Medical Journal* 306 (1993): 563–65.

32. International Statistical Institute. "Declaration on Professional Ethics," *International Statistical Review* 54 (1986): 227–42.

33. The Nuremberg Code. *Trials of War Criminals Before the Nuremberg Military Tribunals under Control Council Law,* vol. 12, no. 10. Washington, D.Ç.: Government Printing Office, 1949: 81–82. (Reprinted many times.)

34. World Medical Association. "Declaration of Helsinki (1964)," *World Medical Journal* 19 (1972): 29. Revised 1975, 1982, 1989.

35. WHO Global Programme on AIDS. "Monitoring of National AIDS Prevention and Control Programmes: Guiding Principles," *WHO AIDS Series*, no. 4. Geneva: WHO, 1989.

36. Office of Technology Policy of the Executive Office of the President. *Federal Policy for the Protection of Human Subjects* (model policy). Washington, D.C.: U.S. Government Printing Office, 1991.

37. Medical Research Council. *Responsibility in Investigations on Human Subjects.* London: HMSO, 1986.

38. Medical Research Council. *Guidelines for Research Involving Human Subjects.* Ottawa: Medical Research Council, 1987.

39. Commonwealth of Australia, National Health & Medical Research Council. *Statement on Human Experimentation.* Canberra: Commonwealth Printer, 1983. [Supplementary statements on Gene Therapy (1987), Privacy (1988) and Genetic Registers (1991).]

40. Swedish Society for Public Health. *Statement on Ethical Considerations in Medical Research,* trans. C. G. Westrin. Personal communication, 1989.

41. Kelly, R. J., Fluss, S. S., and Gutteridge F. "The Regulation of Research on Human Subjects: A Decade of Progress." In *Ethics and Research on Human Subjects; International Guidelines,* ed. Z. Bankowski and R. J. Levine. Proceedings of the XXVIth CIOMS Conference, Geneva, February 5–7, 1992. Geneva: CIOMS/ WHO 1993: 127–66.

42. Fluss, S. S., Simon, F., and Gutteridge, F. "Development of International Ethical Guidelines for Epidemiological Research and Practice; a Survey of Policies and Laws." In *Ethics and Epidemiology: International Guidelines,* ed. Z. Bankowski, J. H. Bryant, and J. M. Last. Proceedings of the XXVth CIOMS Conference, Geneva, Switzerland, November 7–9, 1990. Geneva: CIOMS, 1991: 76–91.

43. Commonwealth of Australia, National Health and Medical Research Council, Medical Research Ethics Committee. *Report on Ethics in Epidemiological Research.* Canberra: Government Printing Office, 1985.

44. Tancredi, L., ed. "Ethical Issues in Epidemiologic Research," *Series in Psychosocial Epidemiology*, no. 7. New Brunswick, NJ: Rutgers University Press, 1986.

45. Bankowski, Z., Bryant, J. H., and Last, J. M., eds. *Ethics and Epidemiology: International Guidelines*. Proceedings of the XXVth CIOMS Conference. Summary of discussions. Geneva: CIOMS 1991: 137–142.
46. Gordis, L., Gold, E., and Seltser, R. "Privacy Protection in Epidemiologic and Medical Research: a Challenge and a Responsibility," *American Journal of Epidemiology* 105 (1977): 163–68.
47. Gordis, L., and Gold, E. "Privacy, Confidentiality and the Use of Medical Records in Research," *Science* 207 (1980): 153–56.
48. Rothman, K. "The Rise and Fall of Epidemiology, 1950–2000 AD," *New England Journal of Medicine* 304 (1981): 600–02.
49. *Report of the Society for Epidemiologic Research Committee on Ethical Guidelines*, ed. P. Stolley, K. Rothman, S. Shapiro, Z. Stein, M. Szklo. Society for Epidemiologic Research, May 12, 1989. Mimeographed.
50. Soskolne, C. L. "Epidemiological Research, Interest Groups and the Review Process," *Journal of Public Health Policy* 7 (1985): 173–84.
51. "Society for Epidemiologic Research: Statement on Data Sharing," *Epidemiology Monitor* 13, no. 6 (June 1992).
52. Last, J. M. "Guidelines on Ethics for Epidemiologists," *International Journal of Epidemiology* 19 (1990): 226–29. (Later version: *Newsletter of the Epidemiology Section*, American Public Health Association, winter 1991–92).
53. Last, J. M. "Workshop: Epidemiology and Ethics," *Lancet* 336 (1990): 497.
54. Beauchamp, T. L., Cook, R. R., Fayerweather, W. E., et al. "Ethical Guidelines for Epidemiologists," *Journal of Clinical Epidemiology* 44 (1991): 151S–69S.
55. Epidemiology Task Group, Chemical Manufacturers Association. "Guidelines for Good Epidemiology Practices," *Journal of Occupational Medicine* 33 (1991): 1221–29.
56. Soskolne, C. L., and Last, J. M. "CMA Epidemiology Guidelines" (letter to editor), *Journal of Occupational Medicine* 35 (1993): 97–98.
57. Westrin, C. G., Nilstun, T., Smedby, B., and Haglund, B. "Epidemiology and Moral Philosophy," *Journal of Medical Ethics* 18 (1992): 193–96.
58. Allebeck, P. "New Regulations on Databases," *Epidemiology Monitor* (November 1993): 6.
59. Knox, E. G. "Confidential Medical Records and Epidemiological Research" (editorial), *British Medical Journal* 304 (1992): 727–28.
60. Last, J. M. "New Pathways in an Age of Ecological and Ethical Concerns," *International Journal of Epidemiology* 23, no. 1 (1993): 1–4.
61. Last, J. M. "An Ethical Framework for Epidemiology." In *Ethics in Medicine*, ed. P. Allebeck and B. Janssen. New York: Raven, 1990: 125–136.

4

Epistemology and Ethics in Epidemiology

DOUGLAS L. WEED

Bertrand Russell wrote that the two great engines of progress in human society are a desire to *understand* the world and a desire to *improve* it.[1] Although penned over a half century ago, his thoughts seem ready-made for today's epidemiologists. As scientists we seek to understand the determinants and distribution of diseases, and as applied scientists we evaluate technologies and use those found effective to improve the health of the world's populations. Put another way, epidemiology contributes to progress through the coupled engines of science and technology.[2]

A primary thesis of this book is that the acquisition and use of epidemiologic knowledge should be guided by the theories, principles, case studies, and methods of bioethics. In the ensuing chapters, many practical implications of this thesis are developed, but in this chapter issues important to its philosophical foundations are examined. These issues, central to epidemiology, involve how *knowledge is acquired* and how *moral judgments are made* regarding the acquisition and use of knowledge. Such issues reside within the domain of two philosophical disciplines: epistemology and ethics (the latter including moral epistemology).

Epistemology is the branch of philosophy concerned with the nature, scope, and acquisition of knowledge. As an intellectual endeavor, it began as early as ancient Greek philosophy with writers such as Plato and the Sophists.[3] Ethics involves inquiries into the nature of rightness and the appropriateness of human conduct, and it too can be traced to ancient Greek sources, especially the Homeric code in its early, rudimentary stages and later in the works of Plato's predecessor, Socrates.[4] From those early days of inquiry to the present, a vast body of literature developed in both disciplines, documenting the philosophical discourse of two millennia.

Many parallels and frank overlaps exist between epistemology and ethics,[5] and some have argued that it is not always easy nor wise to ignore such connections.[6,7] In order to make epistemology and ethics (and their connections) meaningful and useful to the practicing epidemiologist without embarking on a protracted conceptual journey, this chapter focuses on methods, an important and popular concern among epidemiologists.

The specific emphasis is on methods of scientific and ethical reasoning; this focus is consistent with current thinking in epidemiology and bioethics. Since the mid-1970s, epidemiologists have been engaged in a debate regarding methods of scientific reasoning, primarily as they relate to the logic of causal inference. Bioethics is also currently involved in a methodological debate. It has centered on methods for making moral decisions, but it has also included such epistemological concerns as the logical relationships among theories, principles, and cases, as well as how moral knowledge is acquired. These debates are described separately, to provide background and context for the final section of this chapter. There, methods of scientific reasoning and ethical reasoning are shown to be jointly relevant to an issue of central importance to epidemiologists: making public health recommendations.

Public health recommendations emerge in the process of determining whether exposure factors can be considered causal. Epidemiologists and philosophers both term this process *causal inference*, and it requires criteria of evidence. The public health recommendations that emerge represent presumably beneficent applications of knowledge for the prevention and control of diseases and other health problems.[8] Thus, causal inference as practiced in epidemiology involves answering the epistemological question, Is an exposure causal? as well as the related moral question, Should something be done about the exposure?[9] In practice, a firm answer to the first question is not necessary for answering the second. In other words, epidemiologists may recommend reductions in exposure to a factor for which the evidence is insufficient for them to firmly declare causation. Recent examples include recommendations to reduce alcoholic beverage consumption in women at risk of breast cancer.[10,11]

How public health recommendations are made in the face of scientific uncertainty is a methodologic problem that has received little attention in epidemiology. Traditionally, its solution has involved the notion of judgment,[12,13] with little emphasis on what judgment entails, or, for that matter, what constitutes good judgment and bad judgment. One solution, and likely the best, is to use methods of moral reasoning with methods of scientific reasoning when making public health recommendations.

Causal inference is only one example within epidemiology in which epistemological issues are connected to ethical issues, and thus in which methods of scientific and ethical reasoning function well together. The problem of interaction or joint effects is another example.[14,15] Still another involves generalizability—an epistemological concern—and the need to ensure adequate representation of women and minorities in epidemiologic studies—an ethical concern.

The Scope of Scientific and Moral Reasoning in Epidemiology

As Langmuir wryly noted,[16] epidemiologists have struggled with defining their discipline:

Epidemiologists are a unique breed because they are obsessed with trying to define their field. Each of us has spent inordinate amounts of time and emotion on this process. There are so many definitions one wonders if any can be good.

In the first half of the twentieth century, definitions of epidemiology underwent a dramatic change. In 1927, Frost defined epidemiology as the science of the mass phenomena of infectious disease,[17] a meaning subsequently broadened to include noninfectious diseases and injury.[18] In the latter half of the twentieth century, one of the more enduring definitions was proposed by MacMahon and Pugh, who wrote that epidemiology is "the study of the distribution and determinants of disease frequency in man."[19] This definition can be found essentially intact in many textbooks, including those published in the 1970s and 1980s.[20–24] In a recent dictionary, however, it has again been broadened to include the application of the results of scientific study to the control of health problems.[25] This interpretation emphasizes both science and public health practice for epidemiologists and appears to be gaining acceptance.[26] In sum, definitions of epidemiology continue to evolve in response to the dramatic growth and evolution that has characterized the discipline, in methods[27] and in professional obligations.[28] Within this evolution lie clues to the broad scope of epidemiologic reasoning, part science and part ethics.

Scientific reasoning in epidemiology involves a wide range of conditions and exposures, as well as the concepts and methods of other scientific disciplines. Some conditions are physical (such as hepatitis, cancer, cerebral palsy, and hip fractures), some are mental (Alzheimer's disease and depression), and some involve health services (vaccination and screening programs). Many scientific disciplines collect and analyze epidemiologic data, including physics (for example, studies of electromagnetic fields and ultraviolet radiation); chemistry (studies of lead, asbestos, silicates, and air pollution); pharmacology (studies of drug toxicities and hormone replacement therapies); and human biology, at a variety of levels—subcellular (such as oncogenes and biological markers), cellular (white blood cell counts), systemic (height, weight, blood pressure), and behavioral (alcohol-drinking histories and attitudes about screening).

As in medicine, epidemiologists do not only reason *horizontally* within the narrow confines of a single scientific discipline, but also *vertically* from one discipline to another. These disciplines, and the scientific knowledge they represent, can be placed within a hierarchical structure extending from the lowest level of the atom to the highest level of living organisms.[29] Unlike in medicine, however, epidemiologic reasoning goes beyond the level of the individual to that of populations. The entire structure could be reversed, with the "highest" level—meaning to some the most concrete, or the "hardest"—being the molecular level.

For the purposes here, no level will be considered harder or more important than another. Pragmatically speaking, epidemiologists incorporate knowledge at different levels of the hierarchy depending on the circumstances. Thus, in making public health recommendations about a cancer risk factor—say, excessive sun exposure—we consider the extent to which a biological mechanism linking ultraviolet radiation to genetic damage has been demonstrated, along with consideration of the magnitude of relative risks, dose-response curves, and other features of epidemiologic studies in which the relationship between sun exposure and cancer has been examined. Studies may also incorporate knowledge at the biological level. For example, after a new proto-oncogene mutation is identified, it may be combined into the design of studies examining its role in cancer etiology and early detection.[30]

Add to these scientific considerations the concepts and methods of bioethics, and the broad scope of reasoning that could and should be present in epidemiology becomes apparent. Ethics, whether conceived as an appreciation of values or more specifically as guidelines for the conduct of professionals, is a relatively recent addition to the epidemiologic literature, with historical roots traceable to the writings of nineteenth century epidemiologists.[31] Ideally, ethics in epidemiology should be broadly conceived, yet much of the effort to date has been spent on the development and interpretation of brief and underanalyzed ethics guidelines.[28,32–35] Central to many of these guidelines are the bioethical principles developed by Beauchamp and Childress of justice, autonomy, beneficence, and non-maleficence.[36] Other principles, such as fidelity and conscientiousness, and rules and virtues are also relevant.[33,36]

Principles are central concepts in contemporary moral reasoning—less general in some respects than theories, but more general than rules, judgments, or the case studies to which they are applied. Cases are descriptions of specific real-life or lifelike situations. At present, relatively few cases specific to epidemiological practice have been published.[37,38] Others will undoubtedly surface as epidemiologists seek to apply guidelines in professional situations, and as they teach ethics to students of epidemiology. Eventually, many cases relevant to epidemiologic practice will become part of the rich oral tradition of decisionmaking and personal reflection common to those professions defining their obligations and honing their moral decision making skills. Ethical reasoning, moreover, involves ethical theory, including but not limited to theories of justice. Ethical theory is diverse and provides not only the analysis of specific principles but also paradigms and methods for moral reasoning.[39]

Both scientific and ethical reasoning can be represented by methodologic models and many models are relevant to epidemiologic practice. Discussed below are examples describing ways in which we reason from one fact, principle, or conclusion to the next. In practice, epidemiologists may use more than one of these models and may blend them together without formally recognizing the mix. At other times, epidemiologists reason primarily within the narrower confines of one model.

Models of Scientific Reasoning in Epidemiology

A model of scientific reasoning simple and robust enough to permit navigation of the diverse structure of scientific knowledge described above is that represented by hypotheses, observations, and tests of their compatibility. This is the way science functions and there is wide agreement on its general form in epidemiology.[20,23,40] However, its precise role in the acquisition of epidemiologic knowledge, especially causality, has been a source of controversy.

A major aspect of this debate in epistemology began in 1975, with the publication of a paper by Buck on the hypothetico-deductive model of scientific reasoning.[41] In this model, knowledge is tentatively gained as a result of exposing predictions from theory-based hypotheses to rigorous testing. Hypotheses that are rejected (and therefore refuted) reveal errors in the theories from which they were deduced. New theories not subject to those errors but retaining ideas not yet refuted represent progress. These new theories are then subject to testing and potential refutation.[42–44]

Buck's paper is noteworthy because it was one of the first efforts to examine epidemiologic practice in epistemological terms after Susser's book published in 1973.[20] It is also the first paper in a series of articles on causal inference in which the approach sometimes called critical rationalism, or Popper's philosophy, was discussed.[45] As philosophy, the approach not only emphasizes conjecture and refutation, but also regards induction as a dispensable concept and therefore not a major method for acquiring scientific knowledge. Buck's paper emphasized what could be gained from selected Popperian ideas, the need for creativity in science and finding ways to increase the opportunity for refuting a hypothesis when the creator of that hypothesis is personally attached to it. Soon after Buck's paper appeared, critics within epidemiology voiced their concerns, more about Popper's philosophy per se than Buck's limited application of it. Some[46,47] noted the impossibility of dispensing with induction, since statistical inference (and causal inference, for that matter) is a cornerstone of epidemiologic method. Others argued that epidemiology lacks a coherent body of theory, important to the successful application of the hypothetico-deductive method.[48] Francis[49] and Creese[50] emphasized the relevance of other philosophic viewpoints, such as the historical approach of Thomas Kuhn and ideas from earlier philosophers.

The debate on epistemological foundations of epidemiology continued during the 1980s. A handful of investigators, unfortunately labeled "Popperian epidemiologists," examined theoretical and practical facets of two themes: using conjecture and refutation as methodologic guides; and developing theory from which empirically testable conjectures would be deduced.[9,51–57] The ongoing debate has been a contentious one[58–60] and deserves more attention than can be given here, where its complexities are less important than its impact on current practice. Of its several viewpoints, one regarding the need for and use of theory is of interest, because that is also a theme found in a current debate about methods of ethical reasoning.

Epidemiologists have not fully embraced the idea that theoretical development is important. Although several theories of disease causation have been published,[61] epidemiologists typically test hypotheses in relatively simple forms, as potential associations between factors and diseases. These hypotheses may be consistent with causal and biological theories of diseases, but are infrequently related to (much less deduced directly from) such theories. Epidemiologic analysis proceeds more typically in an inductive manner in which the data are collected, with consideration of the "model-in-hand" proceeding if not from the data then from methodologic tradition. Rarely are attempts made to alter the structure of the model during the analysis. Unfortunately, the links between these analytic models and biologic theories are weak,[62] suggesting that use of such models provides for little progress at the level of biologic explanation.

The application of epidemiologic strategies results in the accumulation of factors believed to be important in disease occurrence. Are these factor-disease associations mere conjectures? A new finding, identified in an early epidemiological study, *is* treated solely as a conjecture, that is, as a hypothesis subject to further testing and at risk of refutation. Associations, on the other hand, are treated as something more permanent than conjectures, having survived the testing provided by epidemiologic methods. One of the important considerations in establishing an association, beyond statistical significance, is consistency. In other words, statistically significant findings reported in different studies using different study designs by different investigators are considered associations. Ultimately, any association may be refuted in subsequent prevention trials or if new evidence shows its apparent effects can be better explained by the effects of other factors or bias. But until that time, an association is considered established—a critical rationalist might call it "corroborated." Among established associations, some are considered causal on the basis of decisions made after applying criteria-based methods of causal inference. Others, although not necessarily causal, are judged to be strong enough to warrant action through public health recommendations.

Epidemiologists are almost always ignorant of a theoretical structure within which factor-disease associations fit, hence the term *black box* epidemiology.[63]

Breast cancer, with its list of twenty-three established risk factors, is a good example.[64] To fit them together would require a theory connecting levels of scientific knowledge described earlier in this chapter. The recent trend toward combining laboratory-based research activities with population-based epidemiologic research—*molecular epidemiology*—provides an opportunity to develop such a theory.[65,66] Some breast cancer risk factors, however, are not biological; socioeconomic status and country of birth are two examples. For these factors to be incorporated into a theory of breast cancer occurrence, the theory must incorporate not only biology and lifestyle risk factors, but also "complex systems in which the health-disease process is embedded,"[67] presumably social structures and the like. Given the current status of theory development in epidemiology, this seems a difficult and distant task.

Nevertheless, theoretical development in epidemiology should be encouraged. Theories provide a way to structure the determinants of disease and thus better explain disease occurrence. Better theories may also provide more biologically relevant predictions to be tested as hypotheses in epidemiologic studies.[68] Further, developing theories will not require rejection of the current structure of epidemiologic knowledge, paradigmatically defined as lists of factor-disease associations. Rather, these associations may be integrated within a more biologically and socially relevant framework. Associations will also remain an important way to build bridges between the science of epidemiology and the application of that science in public health policies. Finally, developing theories will increase the scope and scientific relevance of the hypotheses by including factors from a variety of levels of the structure of scientific knowledge. As a result, epidemiology's explanatory power will be expanded.

Models of Ethical Reasoning

Models of scientific reasoning are used to answer questions such as Why does disease occur? and What interventions reduce disease mortality? Models of ethical reasoning are used to answer questions regarding what *ought* to be done in a wide variety of circumstances involving science, technology, related activities of professionals, and how public policy should be formulated to help govern these circumstances.

What methods of ethical reasoning are available and pertinent for epidemiology? Answers to this important question are necessary if we are to connect methods of ethical reasoning with methods of scientific reasoning and use them in causal inference.

The following are some thoughts about method that have been put forward for epidemiologists. Soskolne has emphasized the need for professional guidelines to assist in decision making[69] and has outlined a decision making approach to dilemmas in specific case studies based on the ethical principles found within those guidelines.[37] Principles also figure prominently in decisions to ethically optimize research designs in epidemiology.[35] Beauchamp has stressed the importance of philosophical ethical theories in justifying and analyzing principles. These theories also provide frameworks that can lend support to professional guidelines.[39] Methodologically, he likens ethical reasoning to legal reasoning. Arguments defending specific decisions should be carefully crafted in their appeal to the principles and precedents found in moral theory, analogous to the principles and precedents of law. Maclure has made a similar point regarding the testing of ethical hypotheses.[57]

Although principles figure prominently in many accounts of the role of ethics in epidemiology, methodological dispute has emerged over their role in ethical reasoning. For example, in a discussion of the ethics of communicating health risk information, Jonsen notes that while many questions regarding the right to know and the duty to tell have been answered on the basis of general principles, the specific decisions that emerge in particular cases often remain unsupported by principles as well as theories.[71] He contends that these decisions are made by focusing on the circumstances of the case at hand, paradigm cases parallel to these circumstances, and the moral context within which the case rests. Although some appreciation of the principles and theories of ethics cannot be avoided, Jonsen maintains that direct reference to these more general ideas will be of little assistance in solving the dilemmas central to any case. In sum, he advocates the use of *casuistry*, a case-based method of reasoning, as an alternative to the use of principles or so-called *principlism*. To date, neither of these methods has received much attention in epidemiology.[72,73]

In bioethics, however, these same methods have been at the center of an ongoing controversy. Some discussion of casuistry and principlism is found in Chapter 1, but attention will be given to this debate here to provide a sense of the direction contemporary bioethics is headed *methodologically*. Interestingly, it is, in part, an epistemological debate. One of its characteristic features has been the critical examination of relationships between various structural levels within the hierarchy of ideas central to ethics, especially theories, principles, rules, and cases.

The publication of Beauchamp and Childress's influential text, *Principles of Biomedical Ethics*,[36] is a good starting point. This book, now in its fourth edition, is the first systematic analysis of principles governing a wide range of decisions in biomedicine. Emphasis is placed on how ethical theories do and do not provide justification for the principles of autonomy, nonmaleficence, beneficence, and justice that Beauchamp and Childress developed as a framework. The authors also argue that cases are important both for developing and illustrating the principles and for pointing to ways of resolving conflicts between principles.

Concerns about principles and specifically the approach of principlism surfaced soon after the appearance of the aforementioned text, and a more case-oriented, casuistic approach emerged as a proposed alternative. Toulmin, in a paper titled, "The Tyranny of Principles," compared two approaches to the resolution of ethical issues.[74] One claimed ties to moral objectivity and insisted on absolute general principles; it arose in response to the other approach, which posited moral relativism and the need for cultural dependence on moral decisions. Toulmin believed both approaches to be too radical and proposed a return to casuistry, the practical technique of moral reasoning used by the Jesuits and attacked by Pascal. McCullough[75] described a similar dichotomy: a theory-based method dependent on general moral principles and rules, and another approach that had sprung up from medicine itself and was roughly analogous to casuistry. He argued that both approaches rely on cases.

Elsewhere, Murray[7] criticized theory-based approaches to applied moral judgments within the context of deductivism on the grounds that:

- moral theories are too abstract for direct application to specific cases;
- there is no single overarching moral theory, thus deductivism must select the most appropriate theory and provide justification for that choice;
- an ordering (i.e., lexical ordering) of moral principles is often required to resolve cases, yet neither principles nor most moral theories provide such an ordering;
- moral theories are often insensitive to cultural, social, and historical contexts;
- theories are usually not realistic in their portrayal of how moral decisions are made in practice.

Murray's alternative to theory is a form of casuistry, just as Toulmin advocated casuistry as an alternative to principlism.

The history of casuistry and its reemergence in twentieth century moral thought has been well presented by Jonsen and Toulmin.[76] Jonsen has also described casuistry as a useful approach to practical reasoning,[77] and this description may prove particularly helpful to epidemiologists in search of methods for making ethically informed decisions in real-life situations. In practical terms, an attractive feature of casuistry is its remoteness from ethical theory. Given a case, and within it a decision to be made, the user of casuistry presumably need not refer directly to any type of ethical theory. Rather, the casuist invokes common sense maxims, which are brief rule-like sayings that give the case its moral character. Typically, a case involves more than one maxim.

Jonsen's example, from clinical medicine, is Debbie's Case, published in the *Journal of the American Medical Association* in 1988, in which a resident physician administers a lethal dose of morphine to a young woman with terminal ovarian cancer.[78] For the purposes here, a case more directly related to epidemiologic practice will serve as an illustration of many of the strengths (and some weaknesses) of casuistic reasoning.

Consider the situation faced by an epidemiologist asked to write an editorial for a journal in which the results of a large randomized chemoprevention trial are to be published.[79] These results show that lung cancer incidence and mortality of smokers given beta-carotene supplementation were significantly higher than that of smokers not supplemented. Should the epidemiologist recommend that the public, especially smokers, stop taking beta-carotene supplements?

Casuistry requires a clear exposition of the circumstances of a case, that is, the facts surrounding it. In this illustration, the facts would be the size and duration of the trial, the age and gender of participants, the magnitude of the observed effect, and the evidence on the effects of beta-carotene published prior to the trial. There can be more or fewer facts, depending on the completeness of the description. Maxims in this case could be that "epidemiologists have an obligation to advocate public health actions on the basis of strong scientific evidence" and that "experiments are the strongest evidence of causal effects." Other maxims could include: "epidemiologists should not participate in public health advocacy in any form"; "results of experiments should be biologically plausible"; "unexpected results may be due to chance."

The casuist then must decide which maxims are the most appropriate to rule the case. Differing circumstances (different facts) might require different maxims, for example, if the magnitude of the observed effect was large. The casuist then makes a claim regarding the case, that public health recommendations should or should not be made. This claim is, in essence, the judgment of the individual using the casuist's method, and it is backed by maxims which in turn are supported by more general notions (Jonsen, citing Toulmin,[80] calls them *warrants*). One such general notion could be, for example, the weighing of risks and benefits found within the principle of beneficence.

This case, and its circumstances, maxims, and warrants, provides a brief example of the use of the method of casuistry. The justification for recommending public health action included the principle of beneficence. This is an important methodologic point. Casuistry can be conceived as, and has been promoted as, a useful alternative to principlism and other more theoretical approaches to ethical reasoning—useful precisely because it is far removed from theory and principles. Yet, as seen in this case, principles may lurk at some (higher) level of justification. Thus there may not be as much of a distinction between principlism and casuistry as might be perceived at first glance. They could be considered nearly the same sort of method applied to cases, differing primarily by where the user begins his or her analysis. When employing casuistry, a user begins with the circumstances, proposes maxims, and finds warrants for those maxims in principles. When using principlism, a user begins with the circumstances, proposes the most appropriate principle(s), and then uses rules subsumed by or derived from those principles in making decisions.

In a recent contribution to this methodologic debate, DeGrazia proposes an approach to moral decisionmaking that combines principlism and casuistry.[81] He calls it *specified principlism*. It begins with an initial set of norms—for example, a principle or two—which are then applied toward a solution to an ethical problem in the tradition of principlism. If, however, the norms conflict, then they are balanced intuitively or, better yet, made more specific until the conflict is resolved. The more specific a norm becomes, the closer it resembles a moral maxim of casuistry.

The debate regarding bioethical reasoning may not be over soon.[36,82–85] Nevertheless, for the purposes here we may conclude that in practice a sharp distinction between principlism and casuistry is not helpful. Put another way, both methods of ethical reasoning are likely useful in epidemiologic decisionmaking, as will be shown in the issue of causal inference.

When Models Meet: Links between Science and Ethics in Causal Inference

In the preceding pages, methodologic approaches to scientific and ethical components of epidemiologic reasoning were described, setting the stage for the consideration of a problem central to the practice of epidemiology in which science and ethics are jointly relevant. This is the problem of making public health recommendations in the process of causal inference. Two themes have dominated throughout this chapter. The first concerns the need for theories in the science of epidemiology; the second concerns the apparent lack of a need for theories in the application of models of ethical reasoning, especially in practical decisionmaking. These themes are not as discordant as they may appear. It is possible to apply the basic model of scientific reasoning in epidemiology without explicitly referring to any theory of disease causation. The same holds true for applying specified principlism or another model of ethical reasoning in practical decisionmaking; explicit reference to theory is not often necessary. On the other hand, theories remain important in both science and ethics, either as explanation or as justification for the ideas and concepts at other levels of their respective knowledge hierarchies.

Scientific Reasoning in Causal Inference

Many of those who read this chapter are familiar with how methods of causal inference are applied. Those less familiar with this qualitative and subjective methodology may want to read a classic paper,[86] and a more recent account.[8] Briefly, causal inferences are conclusions about the occurrence of disease in terms of specific factors. These conclusions provide the scientific basis for public health recommendations and are made with the help of criteria-based methods. The two most widely used sets of criteria are referred to as the "Surgeon General's criteria"[87] and "Hill's criteria."[88] The latter include: strength, consistency, biologic gradient, specificity, experimental evidence, biologic plausibility, coherence, temporality, and analogy. The Surgeon General's criteria are a subset of Hill's.

The dominant model of scientific reasoning described in an earlier section of this chapter, comprising hypotheses, observations, and tests of their compatibility, has several roles to play in causal inference. First, it provides the input for methods of causal inference. Thus causal inference is possible after several published studies reveal a reasonably consistent hypothesis—an association—between a factor and a disease. The results of the studies are summarized and criteria are then "applied" to these summary results. Many causal criteria refer directly to this same model of scientific reasoning. Experimental evidence, for example, considered by many to be an important criterion, reflects the idea that randomized prevention trials provide the most valid test of a scientific hypothesis involving populations. The criterion of temporality, in turn, is directly deducible from simple causal hypotheses.[9] The criteria of strength of association and biologic gradient refer to summary observations.

Another role for scientific reasoning in causal inference could be methodologic. Consider, for example, a hypothesis regarding the best subset of Hill's criteria. This hypothesis reflects the fact that no consensus has emerged regarding which criteria should be used in practice.[88] The interpretation of criteria may also differ by user (see Reference 8 for an example of three interpretations of the criterion of consistency). In the face of such theoretical disagreement, both in the choice of criteria and in their interpretation, it is not surprising to encounter different commitments regarding the causal nature of the exposure in question and, as important, regarding the need for public health recommendations. Some disagreement is to be expected and may even be healthy for the discipline, since it may foster attempts to improve methods of inference. Perhaps methodologic hypotheses could be 'tested' by examining the extent to which subsets have been successful in predicting causal associations. Another approach, picking up on the theme of the previous section of this chapter, is for causal criteria to be analyzed theoretically, for example, as deduced from different types of causal hypotheses[9] or as consistent with essential properties of cause.[60] Causal theories may provide justification for particular sets of causal criteria just as ethical theories provide justification for principles and rules.

Ethical Reasoning in Causal Inference: Judgment

Another approach to improving methods of causal inference in epidemiology may be found beyond the concept of judgment in methods of ethical reasoning.

Judgment is important in making public health recommendations, as Hill recognized in the mid-1960s.[86] In his mind, different levels of evidence were required for public health action, depending on who was affected by those actions. Recommendations to avoid pharmaceutical use by pregnant women, for example, generally required a lower standard of evidence than advising healthy, young adult males to change potentially harmful lifestyle behaviors. He did not, however, go beyond this simple relativistic scale and address the methodologic issue of how to judge when recommendations for action were needed in a particular situation. Epidemiologists make such recommendations when they accept an obligation to advocate interventions for the benefit of society.[28] These recommendations, since they describe what *ought* to be done with respect to the exposure under evaluation, are the result of ethical decisions made by epidemiologists. In practice, recommendations appear to emerge from judgments about varying and complex patterns of empirical evidence. In other words, epidemiologists typically apply causal criteria to summary findings from several studies and then make statements either about cause or public health recommendations (or both) without clearly distinguishing which they intend to make.

In a recent description of the practice of causal inference in cancer epidemiology, for example, Weed and Gorelic showed that in series of review papers written on two factor-cancer associations (alcohol and breast cancer, and vasectomy and prostate cancer), some authors make public health recommendations yet ignore causal conclusions, others make causal conclusions yet ignore public health recommendations, and some discuss both.[88] No author in these series of reviews described how he or she came to public health recommendations. How, then, should they be made? It seems reasonable to consider the role that methods of ethical reasoning do and do not play, not only because their advocates often invoke the concept of judgment, but, more fundamentally, because the problem of making public health recommendations (when applying the empirical criteria of causal inference) may be best solved using methods of reasoning appropriate for the task.

Ethical Reasoning in Causal Inference: Methods

Certainly moral principles are at least presupposed in the practice of causal inference. Public health recommendations involve direct applications of knowledge in order to prevent disease or other conditions. For example, a recommendation to reduce exposure to an environmental carcinogen such as radon gas or asbestos is an attempt to reduce the risk of subsequent cancer in those exposed. The principle of beneficence clearly underlies these recommendations, as well as a principle of utility. The principle of nonmaleficence is also relevant, especially when public health recommendations are made involving direct interventions, such as fluoridation of water, in which populations are exposed to a substance or technology presumably in order for that same intervention to subsequently prevent disease. Recommendations to increase exposure to micronutrients or to increase use of early detection technologies are good examples, and one must judge the extent to which harm might occur before making such recommendations. When public health recommendations are taken to the level of public policy, the principles of respect for autonomy and justice are certain to be involved since personal autonomy may be sacrificed in the name of justice or social good.[89]

Thus, principles of bioethics are relevant in making public health recommendations, with beneficence the most prominent. The extent to which the method of principlism is sufficient, however, is not as straightforward as citation of these principles might suggest. Public health recommendations are not likely to be directly constructible from principles, much less from ethical theory, as any principlist would acknowledge.[36] Rather, public health recommendations are formed in league with specification of principles and with reference to the amount and strength of scientific evidence available to the decision maker in the particular situation at hand. Often the summary results of studies of a specific exposure-disease pair are entailed. If these results are considered the facts of a causal inference case, then it is possible to apply casuistic reasoning to causal inference. This is illustrated in a recent paper, in which the method of casuistry is shown to be similar, in basic methodologic form, to the criteria-based methods of causal inference.[90]

Casuistry can be applied to public health recommendations if the empirical evidence are considered the description of the case (a factor-disease pair), while the causal criteria and their interpretative rules are taken as the maxims. The causal association between smoking cigarettes and lung cancer can be considered the paradigmatic case of causal inference in epidemiology. Users of this method then apply judgment to make a public health recommendation based on the relevant circumstances of the case and their interpretation of the criteria chosen, which function as maxims for the decision.

Conclusion

Epidemiology is a search for scientific knowledge about the determinants of disease and a search for ways to improve the public health based on that knowledge. The acquisition and use of epidemiologic knowledge appear to be guided as much by the methods of ethical reasoning as by the methods of scientific reasoning. As a result, the epidemiologist's armamentarium of methods (and need for methodologic expertise) has expanded. The conceptual direction of this expansion is toward more fundamental philosophical concerns because the roots of these methods—their origins, basic assumptions, and structures—are found in philosophy, especially in epistemology and ethics. It follows that epidemiologists have reached an important stage in the development of their professional discipline, a stage in which understanding and contributing to the philosophical foundation is needed.[31] This is a grand task and may be best accomplished with the help of those who have made philosophy their vocation. Nevertheless, epidemiologists must still answer for themselves basic questions: who are we, what is right, how to think, and when to act. The extent to which the answers to these questions can help in making progress in disease explanation and sound prevention policies remains to be delineated. There is reason for cautious optimism.[91]

References

1. Russell, B. *Marriage and Morals*. New York: Horace Liveright, 1929: 301.
2. Healy, M. J. R. "Truth and Consequences in Medical Research," *Lancet* 2 (1978): 1300–01.
3. Hamlyn, D. W. "History of Epistemology." In *Encyclopedia of Philosophy*, ed. P. Edwards. Vol 3. New York: Macmillan, 1972: 8–38.
4. Abelson, R. and Nielsen, K. "History of Ethics." In *Encyclopedia of Philosophy*, ed. P. Edwards. Vol. 3. New York: Macmillan, 1972: 81–117.
5. Brandt, R. B. "Parallels Between Epistemology and Ethics." In *Encyclopedia of Philosophy*, ed. P. Edwards. Vol. 3. New York: Macmillan, 1972: 6–8.
6. Toulmin, S. "Can Science and Ethics be Reconnected?" *Hastings Center Report* 9 (1979): 27–34.
7. Murray, T. H. "Medical Ethics, Moral Philosophy and Moral Tradition," *Social Science and Medicine* 25 (1987): 637–44.
8. Weed, D. L. "Causal and Preventive Inference." In *Cancer Prevention and Control*, ed. P. G. Greenwald, B. S. Kramer, and D. L. Weed. New York: Marcel Dekker, 1995: 285–302.
9. Weed, D. L. "Causal Criteria and Popperian Refutation." In *Causal Inference*, ed. K. J. Rothman. Chestnut Hill, MA: ERI, 1988: 15–32.
10. Graham, S. "Alcohol and Breast Cancer," *New England Journal of Medicine* 316 (1987): 1211–13.
11. Hiatt, R. A. "Alcohol Consumption and Breast Cancer," *Medical Oncology and Tumor Pharmacotherapy* 7 (1990): 143–151.
12. Susser, M. "Criteria of Judgment." In *Causal Thinking in the Health Sciences: Concepts and Strategies of Epidemiology*. New York: Oxford, 1973: 140–62.
13. Susser, M. "Judgment and Causal Inference: Criteria in Epidemiologic Studies," *American Journal of Epidemiology* 105 (1977): 1–15.
14. Weed, D. L., Selmon, M., and Sinks, T. "Links Between Categories of Interaction," *American Journal of Epidemiology* 127 (1988): 17–27.
15. Weed, D. L. and Trock, B. J. "Interactions and Public Health Decisions," *Journal of Clinical Epidemiology* 41 (1988): 207–209.
16. Langmuir, A. D. "The Territory of Epidemiology: Pentimento," *Journal of Infectious Diseases* 155 (1987): 349–57.
17. Frost, W.H. "Epidemiology" (1927). In *Papers of Wade Hampton Frost, M.D.: A Contribution to Epidemiological Method*, ed. K.F. Maxcy. New York: Arno, 1977: 493–542.

18. Gordon, J. E. "The Twentieth Century—Yesterday, Today, and Tomorrow (1920—)." In *The History of American Epidemiology*, ed. F. II. Top. St. Louis: CV Mosby, 1952: 114–67.
19. MacMahon, B. and Pugh, T. F. *Epidemiology: Principles and Methods*. Boston: Little, Brown, 1970: 1.
20. Susser, M. *Causal Thinking in the Health Sciences: Concepts and Strategies of Epidemiology*. New York: Oxford, 1973.
21. Mausner, J. S. and Bahn, A. K. *Epidemiology: An Introductory Text*. Philadelphia: Saunders, 1974: 3.
22. Lilienfeld, A. M. and Lilienfeld, D. E. *Foundations of Epidemiology*. 2d ed. New York: Oxford, 1980: 3.
23. Kleinbaum, D. G., Kupper, L. L., and Morgenstern, H. *Epidemiologic Research: Principles and Quantitative Methods*. Belmont, CA: Lifetime Learning, 1982: 2.
24. Hennekens, C. H. and Buring, J. E. *Epidemiology and Medicine*. Boston: Little, Brown, 1987: 3.
25. Last, J. M., ed. *A Dictionary of Epidemiology*. New York: Oxford, 1988: 42.
26. Beaglehole, R., Bonita, R., and Kjellstrom, T. *Basic Epidemiology*. Geneva: WHO, 1993: 2.
27. Susser, M. "Epidemiology in the United States After World War II: The Evolution of Technique," *Epidemiologic Reviews* 7 (1985): 147–77.
28. Weed, D. L. "Science, Ethics Guidelines, and Advocacy in Epidemiology," *Annals of Epidemiology* 4 (1994): 166–71.
29. Blois, M. S. "Medicine and The Nature of Vertical Reasoning," *New England Journal of Medicine* 318 (1988): 847–51.
30. Taylor, J. A. "Oncogenes and Their Applications in Epidemiologic Studies," *American Journal of Epidemiology* 130 (1989): 6–13.
31. Weed, D. L. "The Merger of Bioethics and Epidemiology." In *Ethics in Epidemiology*, ed. W. E. Fayerweather, J. Higginson, and T. L. Beauchamp. Oxford: Pergamon, 1991: 15–22.
32. Bankowski, Z., Bryant, J. H., and Last, J. M., eds. *Ethics and Epidemiology: International Guidelines. Proceedings of the XXVth CIOMS Conference, November 7–9, 1990 (Summary of Discussions)*. Geneva: CIOMS, 1991: 137–42.
33. Beauchamp, T. L., Cook, R. R., Fayerweather, W. E., Raabe, G. K., Thar, W. E., Cowles, S. R., and Spivey, G. H. "Ethical Guidelines for Epidemiologists," *Journal of Clinical Epidemiology* 44 (Suppl. I) (1991): 151S–69S.
34. "International Epidemiological Association Guidelines on Ethics for Epidemiologists," American Public Health Association. *Epidemiology Section Newsletter* (winter 1990).
35. Coughlin, S. S. and Beauchamp, T. L. "Ethics, Scientific Validity, and the Design of Epidemiologic Studies," *Epidemiology* 3 (1992) 3: 343–47.
36. Beauchamp, T. L. and Childress, J. C. *Principles of Biomedical Ethics*. 4th ed. New York: Oxford University Press, 1994.
37. Soskolne, C. L. "Ethical Decisionmaking in Epidemiology: The Case Study Approach," *Journal of Clinical Epidemiology* 44 (Suppl I) (1991): 125S–130S.
38. Meirik, O., and Cook, R. "Ethical Issues in Epidemiological Research in Human Reproduction: Two Case Studies." In *Ethics and Epidemiology: International Guidelines*, ed. Z. Bankowski, J.H. Bryant, and J.M. Last. Proceedings of the XXVth CIOMS Conference 7–9 November 1990. Geneva: CIOMS, 1991, pp. 117–25.

39. Beauchamp, T. L. "Ethical Theory and Epidemiology," *Journal of Clinical Epidemiology* 44 (suppl. I) (1991): 5S–8S.
40. Rothman, K. J. "Causal Inference in Epidemiology." In *Modern Epidemiology*, ed. K. J. Rothman. Boston: Little, Brown, 1986: 7–21.
41. Buck, C. "Popper's Philosophy for Epidemiologists," *International Journal of Epidemiology* 4 (1975): 159–68.
42. Popper, K. R. *The Logic of Scientific Discovery*. New York: Harper and Row, 1968.
43. Popper, K. R. *Conjectures and Refutations: The Growth of Scientific Knowledge*. New York: Harper and Row, 1968.
44. Popper, K. R. *Objective Knowledge: An Evolutionary Approach*. Oxford: Oxford University Press, 1979.
45. Rothman, K. J. *Causal Inference*. Chestnut Hill, MA: ERI, 1988.
46. Davies, A. M. "Comment on 'Popper's Philosophy for Epidemiologists,' " *International Journal of Epidemiology* 4 (1975): 169–71.
47. Jacobsen, M. "Against Popperized Epidemiology," *International Journal of Epidemiology* 5 (1976): 9–11.
48. Smith, A. "Comment on 'Popper's Philosophy for Epidemiologists,' " *International Journal of Epidemiology* 4 (1975): 171–72.
49. Francis, H. "Epidemiology and Karl Popper," *International Journal of Epidemiology* 5 (1976): 307.
50. Creese, A. "Popper's Philosophy for Epidemiologists," *International Journal of Epidemiology* 4 (1975): 352–53.
51. Rothman, K. J. "Causation and Causal Inference." In *Cancer Epidemiology and Prevention*, ed. D. Schottenfeld and J. F. Fraumeni. Philadelphia: Saunders, 1982: 15–22.
52. Maclure, M. "Popperian Refutation in Epidemiology," *American Journal of Epidemiology* 121 (1985): 343–50.
53. Weed, D. L. "An Epidemiologic Application of Popper's Method," *Journal of Epidemiology and Community Health* 39 (1985): 277–85.
54. Weed, D. L. "On the Logic of Causal Inference," *American Journal of Epidemiology* 123 (1986): 965–79.
55. Lanes, S. F. "The Logic of Causal Inference in Medicine." In *Causal Inference*, ed. K. J. Rothman. Chestnut Hill, MA: ERI, 1988: 59–75.
56. Susser, M. "Falsification, Verification and Causal Inference in Epidemiology: Reconsiderations in the Light of Sir Karl Popper's Philosophy." In *Causal Inference*, ed. K. J. Rothman. Chestnut Hill, MA: ERI, 1988: 33–57.
57. Maclure, M. "Demonstration of Deductive Meta-Analysis: Ethanol Intake and Risk of Myocardial Infarction," *Epidemiologic Reviews* 15 (1993): 328–51.
58. Greenland, S. "Probability Versus Popper: An Elaboration of the Insufficiency of Current Popperian Approaches for Epidemiologic Analyses." In *Causal Inference*, ed. K. J. Rothman. Chestnut Hill, MA: ERI, 1988: 95–104.
59. Pearce, N. and Crawford–Brown, D. "Critical Discussion in Epidemiology: Problems with the Popperian Approach," *Journal of Clinical Epidemiology* 42 (1989): 177–84.
60. Renton, A. "Epidemiology and Causation: a Realist View," *Journal of Epidemiology and Community Health* 48 (1994): 79–85.
61. Olsen, J. and Overad, K. "The Concept of Multifactorial Etiology of Cancer," *Pharmacology and Toxicology* 72 (suppl. I) (1993): 33–38.

62. Greenland, S. "Limitations of the Logistic Analysis of Epidemiologic Data," *American Journal of Epidemiology* 110 (1979): 693–98.
63. Savitz, D.A. "In Defense of Black Box Epidemiology," *Epidemiology* 5 (1994): 550–52.
64. Kelsey, J. L. "Breast Cancer Epidemiology: Summary and Future Directions," *Epidemiologic Reviews* 15 (1994): 256–63.
65. Vandenbroucke, J. P. "Is 'The Causes of Cancer' a Miasma Theory for the End of the Twentieth Century?" *International Journal of Epidemiology* 17 (1988): 708–09.
66. McMichael, A. J. "Invited Commentary: 'Molecular Epidemiology': New Pathway or New Travelling Companion?" *American Journal of Epidemiology* 140 (1994): 1–11.
67. Loomis, D. and Wing, S. "Is Molecular Epidemiology a Germ Theory for the End of the Twentieth Century?" *International Journal of Epidemiology* 19 (1990): 1–3.
68. Skrabanek, P. "The Emptiness of the Black Box," *Epidemiology* 5 (1994): 553–55.
69. Soskolne, C. L. "Epidemiology: Questions of Science, Ethics, Morality, and Law," *American Journal of Epidemiology* 129 (1989): 1–18.
70. MacMahon, B. "A Code of Ethical Conduct for Epidemiologists?" *Journal of Clinical Epidemiology* 44 (suppl. I) (1991): 147S–49S.
71. Jonsen, A.R. "Ethical Considerations and Responsibilities When Communicating Health Risk Information," *Journal of Clinical Epidemiology* 44 (suppl. I) (1991): 69S–72S.
72. Bryant, J.H. "Trends in Biomedical Ethics—Forerunners of Ethical Questions for Epidemiology." In *Ethics and Epidemiology: International Guidelines*, ed. Z. Bankowski, J. H. Bryant, and J. M. Last. Proceedings of the XXVth CIOMS Conference, November 7–9, 1990. Geneva: CIOMS, 1991: 8–13.
73. Weed, D. L. "Bioethical Methods in Epidemiology," *American Journal of Epidemiology* 138 (1993): 671.
74. Toulmin, S. "The Tyranny of Principles," *Hastings Center Report* 11 (December 1981): 31–39.
75. McCullough, L. B. "Methodological Concerns in Bioethics," *Journal of Medicine and Philosophy* 11 (1986): 17–37.
76. Jonsen, A. R. and Toulmin, S. *The Abuse of Casuistry*. Berkeley: University of California, 1988.
77. Jonsen, A. R. "Casuistry as Methodology in Clinical Ethics," *Theoretical Medicine* 12 (1991): 295–307.
78. Anonymous. "It's Over, Debbie," *Journal of the American Medical Association* 259 (1988): 272.
79. Hennekens, C. H., Buring, J. E., and Peto, R. "Antioxidant Vitamins—Benefits Not Yet Proved," *New England Journal of Medicine* 330 (1994): 1080–81.
80. Toulmin, S. E. *The Uses of Argument*. Cambridge: University Press, 1969.
81. DeGrazia, D. "Moving Forward in Bioethical Theory: Theories, Cases, and Specified Principlism," *Journal of Medicine and Philosophy* 17 (1992): 511–39.
82. Arras, J. D. "Getting Down to Cases: The Revival of Casuistry in Bioethics," *Journal of Medicine and Philosophy* 16 (1991): 29–51.
83. Wildes, K. W. "The Priesthood of Bioethics and the Return of Casuistry," *Journal of Medicine and Philosophy* 18 (1993): 33–49.
84. Clouser, K. D. and Gert, B. "A Critique of Principlism." *Journal of Medicine and Philosophy* 15 (1990): 219–36.

85. Lustig, B. A. "The Method of 'Principlism': A Critique of the Critique," *Journal of Medicine and Philosophy* 17 (1992): 487–510.
86. Hill, A. B. "The Environment and Disease: Association or Causation?" *Proceeding of the Royal Society of Medicine* 58 (1965): 295–300.
87. *Surgeon General's Advisory Committee on Smoking and Health. Smoking and Health 1964.* Rockville, MD: Public Health Service; DHEW Publication (PHS)1103.
88. Weed, D. L. and Gorelic, L. "The Practice of Causal Inference in Cancer Epidemiology," unpublished.
89. Pellegrino, E. D. "Autonomy and Coercion in Disease Prevention and Health Promotion," *Theoretical Medicine* 5 (1984): 83–91.
90. Weed, D. L. "Alcohol, Breast Cancer, and Causal Inference: Where Ethics Meets Epidemiology," *Contemporary Drug Problems* 21 (1994): 185–204.
91. Weed, D. L. "Epidemiology, Humanities, and Public Health," *American Journal of Public Health* 85 (1995): 914–918.

II

**INFORMED CONSENT,
PRIVACY,
AND CONFIDENTIALITY**

5

Legal and Ethical Considerations in Securing Consent to Epidemiologic Research in the United States

MARJORIE M. SHULTZ[1]

In recent decades, the science of epidemiology has grown more prominent in health and environmental policymaking. The increasing importance of the field has generated controversy that extends from epidemiology's methods to its outcomes. Epidemiology's relevance to high-stakes conflicts over responsibility for harm (such as toxic, pharmaceutical injuries) has further accentuated debate over the scope and justification of its role and the legitimacy of its procedures. Like scientists in a variety of disciplines,[2] epidemiologists have discovered that public scrutiny and legal regulation accompany greater involvement in political and judicial processes.

Beyond controversies over particular applications of epidemiology lie more fundamental issues. Researchers are skilled professionals who gather and analyze health information, using their findings both to advance scientific knowledge and to further social goals. Although epidemiology serves worthy purposes, it also implicates fundamental moral questions regarding respect for persons, motives and consequences of research, and the distribution of research benefits and burdens. Scientific investigation can pose risks to privacy, autonomy, and justice. It can cause emotional, economic, or even physical harm. But ignorance, too, has costs. Individuals, as well as the research community and society at large, have high stakes in the knowledge generated by research. Absence of research data weakens efforts to prevent or ameliorate health conditions. Research is essential to meaningful assessment of health treatments and interventions. This chapter describes and evaluates legal protection for research subjects against risks arising from epidemiologic research. It cannot, except in general terms, evaluate

the reciprocal gains. It can provide an additional and sometimes cautionary perspective for scientists already aware of benefits they seek to bestow.

American society and its laws place high value on individual rights, striving
never to treat individuals simply as means to an end.[3] Moreover, American experience, as well as events in other countries, warns that even research undertaken in the name of science and the public good can impose unfairness and danger on those it studies.[4]

Multiple sources provide ethical guidance for research, including not only the
law but also professional codes, institutional rules, and individual conscience.
Like each of these others, the law strives to balance competing values. Broadly
speaking, it exercises two forms of authority: (1) articulating and enforcing social norms; and (2) resolving disputes. The legal system is a natural forum for
socially contested questions. Legal analysis draws heavily on ethical traditions
and values, although ethical standards often extend beyond minimum requirements imposed by law. More stringent ethical standards remain supererogatory,
matters of individual aspiration rather than legal duty. Higher standards also fore-
shadow the direction of future legal development.

When a researcher decides whether and how to gain a subject's consent to epidemiologic research, a number of values are at stake. Potentially implicated are
a research subject's bodily integrity, decisional autonomy, expectations about
promise-keeping, privacy of personal information, freedom from avoidable harm,
personal reputation and dignity, and occasionally even rights to property. These
values may be described as interests that are, to varying degrees, legally protected by statutes, regulations, common law, and constitutional rights. Before
turning to specific bodies of law, a brief discussion of the broader legal context
will help set the scene.

Epidemiologic research stands at the juncture between two ethico-legal themes.
One theme involves protecting individual autonomy. How can individuals exercise control over important life choices when they depend on professional elites?
The other theme involves modern information systems and the threats they pose
to personal privacy. Although norms of beneficence and justice are also implicated, preserving respect for individual dignity and autonomy is the primary goal
of legal consent rules.

Lay Control of Professional Experts

In the past half century, the power exercised by professional and technical experts has significantly increased. Recently, strands of disenchantment and skepticism have mixed with those of trust and dependency in public attitudes toward
experts. In medical treatment and research, many factors have contributed to a
stronger emphasis on lay decision making.

Americans jealously guard the benefits of good professional advice and care.

Preferably, such advice would be unequivocal and omniscient. But increasing awareness of the uncertainty of science, of differences of opinion among professionals, of pluralism of relevant values, and of conflicts of interest has undermined public trust in professionals and defeated their hopes for attaining the ideal. Modern consumers recognize a substantial need for lay control over professional experts. Their concerns have encouraged the adoption of more stringent informed consent requirements for medical research and treatment. Risk avoidance is another interest of prospective subjects. The risks posed by epidemiologic investigation are different and often less than those inherent in many other types of research. Epidemiology does, however, study human subjects and does pose risks. Therefore, legal rules governing experimentation on human beings apply.

Safeguards for Privacy Rights of Individuals

Traditionally, legal disputes about privacy have arisen over media investigation and publication, on the one hand, and over the permissible scope of governmental (especially law enforcement) intrusion into personal space and information, on the other. In these contexts, constitutional and common law jurisprudence are richly developed.

Epidemiologic research raises different problems of privacy of information. In legal analysis, context matters. Epidemiologic researchers have little claim to the democracy-sustaining function that justifies journalists' very broad access to information. Epidemiologic investigations also are usually less threatening than those conducted by law enforcement personnel. While legal disputes about information privacy typically involve discrete intrusions on particular individuals, epidemiologic research gathers and stores extensive data about numbers of people. Large data bases pose risks to individuals that mimic classic intrusions, but advancing computer capacities also enable stockpiling of personal information on an unprecedented scale. Traditional privacy law can help assess whether epidemiologic research impermissibly intrudes on individual rights, but inquiries addressed to the special issues in research are also necessary.

These two legal themes—appropriate lay control over professionals and appropriate protection of personal privacy—furnish a foundation for this discussion. The more specific elements of legal protection for research subjects are difficult to establish with precision. Legislation and administrative regulation provide significant guidance but do not exhaust the relevant legal analyses. Constitutional and common law theories also apply.

Decisional law on the rights of research subjects is sparse. Because cases addressing epidemiologic research are rare, some of the following analysis is necessarily a matter of inference. Within the common law, a legal analyst faced with uncharted territory must extrapolate from analogous problems where principles and rules are more fully developed. In drawing analogies, the analyst must closely attend to relevant differences as well as similarities in the new setting. This chapter surveys existing regulations and identifies how common law and constitutional principles may influence the resolution of future disputes about consent.

Federal Regulation of Research on Human Subjects

The most significant source for legal rules governing consent to epidemiologic research is the federal regulatory structure embodied in the Department of Health and Human Services' (HHS) Policy for the Protection of Human Subjects.[5] Many factors engendered this comprehensive regulatory system. Outrage over Nazi "medical" experimentation, anxiety over the European experience with thalidomide, and American research abuses in the post-war era stimulated international discussion regarding ethical standards for research on human subjects. The United States, using federal funding as the entrée for its jurisdiction, adopted human subjects regulations requiring that before any research on humans can begin, institutions must conduct an interdisciplinary review of research protocols to ensure their compliance with ethical standards set forth in federal policy. Federal oversight and funding of research is very substantial, and major research institutions often voluntarily apply federal requirements to all research whether or not it is federally funded. As a result, federal requirements apply in a very large proportion of all research affecting human subjects.

Nazis experimented to determine how long people immersed in freezing water take to die. Government-sponsored research left syphilis patients in the American South untreated after the advent of penicillin. Faced with such atrocities, it is surprising that regulators paid any attention to "mere" informational intrusion, but they did. The final Policy for the Protection of Human Subjects covers protocols proposing to observe behavior, analyze specimens, or gather personal information, as well as physical or interventionist research.

Epidemiologic research uses biological specimens and sometimes entwines with treatment interventions, but the field has historically been concerned primarily with research that is informational and observational in nature. Ethicists and lawyers have paid less attention to issues peculiar to such information research than to those connected with physically risky experiments. For both these reasons, this chapter focuses primarily on the former type of research.

The Basic Regulatory Structure

The Code of Federal Regulations defines research on human subjects to include studies that obtain "(1) Data through intervention or interaction with the individual, or (2) Identifiable private information." The code explains that "intervention includes both physical procedures (for example, venipuncture) and manipulations of the subject or the subject's environment." Further, it defines *interaction* to include "communication or interpersonal contact between investigator and subject," and *private information* to include "information about behavior . . . and information which has been provided for specific purposes by an individual and which the individual can reasonably expect will not be made public (for example, a medical record)."[6]

By broadly defining covered categories of activity, the code extends its reach to most epidemiologic research. The code adjusts its stringency by exempting or expediting review, or by allowing for waivers, for some data analyses and specimen studies. The regulations provide that institutions receiving federal research funds must ensure review of all research protocols by an interdisciplinary Institutional Review Board (IRB). IRBs must make certain that all covered research activity conforms to regulatory requirements.

Requirements concerning the composition and procedures of the IRB are specified by the human subjects policy. The IRB must determine that the research design imposes only risks that are essential and reasonable in proportion to expected benefits. It must also make certain that vulnerable populations such as children or prisoners are especially protected. The foremost IRB priority is to secure compliance with the policy's detailed specifications regarding valid consent by research subjects.

These federal regulations require documented informed consent by research subject-participants. The regulations mandate that researchers seek subjects' or their legal representatives' consent in a manner that enables adequate understanding, reflection, and choice. They specify that each subject shall be provided information about the purposes, methods, and duration of the research; the risks, discomforts or benefits that may reasonably be anticipated; any alternative interventions that may be possible; the study's procedures for maintaining confidentiality of records; the potential for compensation, and for treatment in case of injury incident to the research; and an assurance that refusal to participate will incur no loss of otherwise available benefits.[7]

In addition, where appropriate, researchers must provide information about potential risks to a fetus, the number of subjects involved in the study, potential additional costs, the consequences of withdrawal, and circumstances under which the subject's involvement may be terminated by the researcher. Researchers must promise, if warranted, that research findings that might affect continuing consent will be disclosed to subjects as the research progresses.[8] Finally, the policy provides that under certain circumstances, some or all of these requirements may be waived or altered.[9]

The Code of Federal Regulations elaborates special rules for populations whose vulnerability to coercion (e.g., prisoners) or whose lack of capacity (e.g., fetuses, children) warrants extra protective attention.[10] Pregnant women may participate in research only if it seeks to address health needs of the mother and if risk to the fetus is either minimal or as minimal as is consistent with that purpose.[11] Any research conducted on fetuses in utero must be for purposes that are therapeutic to the patient or that create minimal risks and promise important gains in knowledge.[12] Research on prisoners must use fair selection criteria, must not impose on subjects risks that nonprisoners would refuse, and must not promise to volunteers advantages so substantial as to be coercive in the prison environment.[13] In conducting research on children, researchers are to seek the assent of the minor as well as the permission of parents or guardians. The IRB has special obligations in reviewing the risks and benefits of such child-directed protocols. Research that would be exempt if done on adults requires full IRB review if children are to be subjects.[14]

Institutions in the United States look to these regulations for legal and ethical guidance regarding all research, not just that which is federally funded. Shortcomings in the rules have wide significance beyond their mandatory application. Close examination of the ethical and legal adequacy of the federal requirements is, therefore, extremely important.

A Critical Analysis of the Federal Regulations

Various specific judgments reflected in the regulatory framework can be questioned. For example, there is a worrisome provision that some or all requirements of informed consent may be waived when risk is "minimal" and the research could not otherwise be carried out.[15] Respectable researchers and IRBs will employ this provision rarely—perhaps, for instance, when subjects are dead and no concerns relevant to survivors appear. But the code's language is sufficiently elastic to allow broader uses that do raise ethical questions. How often is any particular research project sufficiently essential that autonomy interests of subjects or their families can be set aside if third parties judge the risk to be "minimal"?[16] Does "could not be carried out" include instances of high expense, difficulty, and likelihood of refusal, or only literal impossibility? If the principle that persons should not be used as means to someone else's end is persuasive, the discretion afforded by this provision is problematic and should be narrowed.

The human subjects policy's blanket exemption for research carried out by federal agencies or under their approval in regard to public benefits programs is also questionable.[17] State or local studies on such programs are identified as likely candidates for waiver of some or all informed consent requirements.[18] Demonstration projects under the Social Security Act, such as those evaluating cost-sharing in the Medicaid program, are explicitly granted waivers from compliance with the policy's requirements.[19] Such exemptions raise doubts even if they are infrequently used. The message they convey—that government can avoid ethical requirements for research on its own programs—is troubling at both substantive and symbolic levels. For example, pursuant to "welfare reform," proposals have been made in some states either to require or to create economic incentives for Aid to Families with Dependent Children (AFDC) recipients to use the long-term contraceptive Norplant.[20] Another problem arises from allowing federal departments and agencies to "adopt such procedural modifications as may be appropriate from an administrative standpoint."[21] This provision leaves the policy vulnerable to subversion by officials not committed to its goals.

Apart from such particular debatable provisions, the regulations reflect one pervasive judgment that is especially consequential for epidemiologic research. Although the policy includes informational research, it manifests a conviction that informational research is less threatening than interventionist research. That assessment is appropriate as a baseline, but there is danger that the comparative judgment will obscure the risks that informational research can impose.

1. *Data without Identifiers.* The policy describes several types of research, such as studies of education or government benefit programs, as "exempt" from IRB review.[22] The guiding principle is that the rules do not apply to information that is not linkable to identifiable individuals. Many people hold an implicit assumption that "impersonal" information cannot be dangerous. The threats traditionally feared are those that endanger *identifiable* individuals. With identifiers removed, what harm could result from analysis of information or specimens?

Private and public data banks covering matters from financial and credit status to medical and genetic data, insurance history, records of entanglement with law enforcement, and status with military services are a fact of modern society. Yet the sheer extent of information as well as the practices through which it is gathered, shared, and used are deeply disturbing to many who have detailed knowledge about such matters.[23] Medical information is particularly sensitive, but is not currently well protected. Insurers, employers, financial institutions, and others have growing incentives to gather medical data. Reorganization of the private health care industry may continue or universal government-based programs may be enacted by states or Congress. Either way, more centralization of data will be required to determine access, ensure quality, evaluate efficacy, and review utilization. That centralization will also exacerbate already severe problems in the management and protection of personal medical information.

Even when data cannot be linked to individuals, data storage *itself* has consequences. The fact of and procedures for collection of data inevitably impinge on privacy, regardless of the controls, cautions, or guarantees of legitimate use that are provided. At the abstract philosophical level, massive collections of data imply certain characteristics in a society. The very existence of data banks increases the potential for oppressive social control now or in the future.[24] Although data collection has benign and valuable uses, some people will have a *frisson* of concern about the flat exemption from regulatory purview of research on nonidentifiable data.

At a more concrete level, use of anonymous data does not guarantee risk-free participation in research, nor does it necessarily maximize patient autonomy judged by a broader perspective. Culpable or careless slips before or during removal of identifiers can never be entirely eliminated. Documentation of consent can itself threaten privacy by allowing identification of otherwise anonymous subjects.[25] The code allows an IRB to waive written consent under such circumstances, but it fails to recognize another ethical problem that can result from such a waiver. If identifiers are *not* retained, research findings cannot be communicated to those studied, nor can counseling or other appropriate follow-up be provided.[26] Also, researchers will be unable to seek further consent from subjects if they or others wish to do unanticipated analyses of the original data.

Researchers are doubtless aware of ways that use of unidentified data can sometimes hamper their work. For example, the adequacy and validity of statistical findings, and consequently of policies based on such findings, would often benefit from continuing access to records and even to subjects. Lack of identifiers can prevent cleaning of samples or elimination of duplication that may in turn increase costs or produce sampling error. It also rules out follow-up linkage of later data sets and studies to earlier ones.

Researchers may be less aware that use of anonymous data neither guarantees risk-free participation nor automatically maximizes autonomy for subjects. Problems described in the preceding paragraphs suggest that while the risks of retaining identifiers usually outweigh the projected consequences of removing them, anonymity is not universally preferable. The argument is not that retention of identifiers is a preferred default position. Rather, the point is that researchers should consciously make, and reviewers review, trade-offs between having and not having identifiers. In particular, evaluators should not simply take for granted that anonymity of data is always the best course of action, even from the research subject's point of view.

The policy's exemption of research on "publicly available" data or specimens[27] raises a related problem. The provision assumes that things either are or are not public. Constitutional law scholar Laurence Tribe criticizes decisions by the Supreme Court regarding the publicness of information.[28] Tribe objects to the binary analysis. For example, the Court has decided that if banks know to whom a person writes checks, or the telephone company has records of whom a person calls, such information is "public" and, thus, legitimately available to anyone. Tribe discusses law enforcement access to such records, but he demonstrates the inadequacy of a simplistic legal conclusion that information is either "private" or "public."

When the policy exempts research on publicly available data, it embraces this oversimplification. One statement in the regulations recognizes that information may be communicated for *some* purposes to *some* persons and still be viewed as private,[29] but that perspective is not consistently displayed. Casting important exemptions in terms amenable to the flawed binary interpretation is particularly problematic. Ethical researchers may already incorporate nuances regarding degrees of publicness and thus of use, but assumptions differ and the elasticity of the language is troubling.

2. *Data with Identifiers.* The code provides that even if identifiers are retained, research on educational tests, survey or interview procedures, and observations of public behavior are exempt from regulatory review unless disclosure of data could "reasonably place the subjects at risk of criminal or civil liability or be damaging to the subjects' financial standing, employability, or reputation."[30] This is the code's most significant and debatable expression of the judgment that informational research usually poses only minor risks. The essential questions are, What counts? and, Who says? in determining potential risk or damage.

Debate over whether assessments should be reached using standards of "objective reasonableness" or on the basis of subjective individualized standards has long plagued the doctrine of informed consent.[31] Subjective standards align more closely with protection of autonomy. Assuming a decision making capacity for autonomy, individuals' decisions need not be either typical or reasonable in the eyes of others. Otherwise, autonomy loses its person-centered meaning.

On the other hand, in medical *treatment*, subjective standards for informed consent place professionals at risk of liability on the basis of hindsight testimony by patients who know at the time of trial that they have incurred medical losses and are themselves parties with high stakes in outcomes of disputes. In treatment cases, judges and legislators have virtually always opted for objective standards of reasonableness both in assessing the adequacy of disclosure and in determining whether omitted disclosures caused an ensuing injury.[32]

Strong justifications support use of objective standards in disputes over consent to treatment, but differences between doctor-patient and researcher-subject relationships may well warrant divergent approaches to consent. Explicit prospective policies govern human subjects research, but judges and juries retrospectively assess malpractice. Compared with treating doctors, researchers have significantly less exposure to liability and little risk from hindsight bias. Research subjects typically receive no therapeutic benefit, but such benefit is the central goal of patients. Patients initiate provision of health care, but researchers enlist subjects. Researchers usually have good intentions, but they are not entitled to a presumption (as are doctors treating patients) that they act in the subject's interest. Together, these factors strongly suggest more stringent requirements for informing and securing consent in research settings than in treatment relationships. They also, to some degree, counter a claim that because epidemiologic research imposes few risks, it should not be rigorously regulated.

Despite these concerns, the federal regulations allow considerable latitude to investigators. For example, unless "otherwise required by [federal] department or agency heads"[33] or unless local institutions or IRBs decide differently, researchers may reach self-executing conclusions about whether their protocols are exempt from IRB review. The possibility that researchers may misguidedly, albeit in good faith, judge their own projects to be exempt from anyone's review of their research design or consent procedures raises significant concern.[34]

Indeed, Carr and Rothman, leading epidemiologists, urge researchers to make greater use of such exemptions and expedited procedures in order to avoid "unnecessary requirements" and "unjustified demands" by IRBs. While a number of their points are well taken—excessive bureaucratization is in no one's interest—these commentators fail to recognize that significant differences in viewpoint exist among the various constituencies involved in research. Moreover, by assuming that federal policies are the only relevant ones, Rothman and Carr disregard legitimate concerns of particular institutions and of state or local governments. By contrast, the federal regulations themselves emphasize that federal human subjects' requirements set minimal expectations and that other decisionmaking entities should feel free to enact further restrictions that they perceive to be important.[35]

Even when an IRB does review a researcher's claim of exemption, the issue simply shifts to another level. The federal policy contemplates "expedited" review by a single member of the IRB for categories of research protocols that involve only "minimal risk."[36] The Code defines "minimal risk" by the yardstick of risks "encountered in daily life" or in "routine physical or psychological examinations," and provides some illustrative and definitional specifications.[37] Efforts to give content to evaluative criteria are praiseworthy. However, under the regulations judgments about minimal risk, like those about exemption, are made not by the persons about whom the information is gathered and to whom the risk or damage may occur, but by third parties. Those third parties are drawn from groups dominated by professionals affiliated with the institutions where the research will be conducted. Professional expertise is central to assessing research design, but it has little salience in judging risk and sensitivity for subjects.

In making decisions, IRB members employ their mostly scientific and professional standards of "reasonableness." The regulations assign responsibility to IRBs for protecting subjects from unethical research, but no third-party proxy is typically as well situated to make judgments about personal interest as are subjects themselves. The code requires some "public" members on an IRB. That representation is merely a token, and typically public members are themselves professionals such as lawyers or ministers. The vast majority of IRB members identify with and share the perspectives of researchers, the institution, and professionals in general. IRBs are unlikely to capture adequately the views and concerns of particular subjects or of lay persons generally.

Alexander Capron persuasively argues that even if no risk of tangible harm is demonstrable, research subjects may still be wronged if they are treated as means, not ends.[38] Judged in terms of respect for human dignity, it is wrong to deny individuals any opportunity to decide who has access for what purpose to their tissues, specimens, and personal information. When the code concludes that protectable personal interests arise only when harmful disclosure actually occurs, rather than also when the opportunity to consent or refuse is denied, it puts societal and scientific needs above individual ones. The gains may outweigh the costs, but the costs are not nothing. Recognition of such costs could not only curb excessive moral glibness, but may also increase researchers' willingness to seek consent or provide notice, at least when the burdens of doing so are not excessive.

A policy provision, similar to that of the code, states that if other "federal statute(s) require(s) without exception that the confidentiality of the personally identifiable information will be maintained throughout the research and thereafter,"[39] such research is exempt from the regulations. Here, as with the code, flexibility presents problems. Confidentiality and autonomy are different goals. They complement but do not substitute for each other.

Modifications of the federal regulations could help to preserve greater personal autonomy without unduly hampering research. At the very least, a right to advance notice (and perhaps, where reporting of information is not legislatively mandated, an opportunity to refuse) regarding possible research uses of patients' specimens and records should be feasible in instances where consent to specific uses is judged too burdensome.[40] IRBs should also devise multiple channels to seek and understand lay concerns about research. Lay representation on IRBs could be increased in number and in category. In addition to requiring careful consent procedures, IRBs should hold public hearings or discussions on examples of research they review in order to get a broad and deep, rather than a token, response about risk and consent from the types of people who are likely to populate research studies. The federal Policy for Protection of Human Subjects takes giant ethical and legal steps forward, but important things remain to be done.

State Regulation of Human Subjects Research

The federal regulations expressly provide that other jurisdictions (such as individual states) may enact additional protections for research subjects.[41] Few states have attempted independent regulation. Those that have tend to track the federal structure, albeit with certain differences of approach. For example, California adopts civil and criminal penalties for careless and willful failure to obtain informed consent, but its statute covers only physically intrusive research.[42] New York's law includes physical and nonphysical intervention, but applies only to nontherapeutic research.[43] Other states have statutes protecting particular subject populations.[44]

Common Law and Constitutional Considerations

Although the Policy for Protection of Human Subjects dominates both legal and ethical discussion, researchers should consider other legal sources that may apply. The federal regulations expressly preserve the applicability of other sources (state, local, foreign) that add further protections for research subjects.[45] Also, the existence of statutory or administrative systems does not preclude common-law claims, although there may be connections between the two. For instance, in a common-law action, evidence about compliance with government requirements might be *relevant*, but is not likely to be the dispositive factor regarding liability.[46] Knowledge of common-law duties is, therefore, vital to understanding legal requirements for consent to research.

Major common-law sources include tort, contract, fiduciary, and, possibly, property doctrines. When researchers or providers of information are government employees or agents, constitutional considerations also apply, particularly to concerns about privacy. A synopsis of these areas of law provides a framework for the discussion that follows.

Tort law protects against intentional or negligent harm caused by one party to another's body, property, reputation, privacy, or other interests. For example, negligence law imposes a duty to act reasonably in securing informed consent[47] and a duty to conduct research in a manner congruent with reasonable professional competence. "Reasonableness" is a pivotal concept in the law, one far too complex to explicate fully here. For purposes of this chapter, suffice it to say that reasonableness is a normative rather than a descriptive standard. Regarding professional behavior, the law defers to the normative judgments of experts within the same profession. The usual measure of reasonableness assesses whether or not the conduct at issue meets the standard of a reasonably competent professional in the same or similar circumstances. A defendant who fails to meet this standard can be liable for harm that proximately results from the breach.

The *constitutional principles* that are most relevant to securing consent to epidemiologic research are closely related to tort law. Constitutional rules prohibit government actors from invading protected individual rights. The Fourth Amendment ban on unreasonable searches and seizures protects some aspects of privacy. In addition, vaguer and more variously rooted norms also guard against government invasions of privacy. Constitutional privacy jurisprudence has been closely connected with medical matters such as access to birth control information,[48] reproductive choice,[49] and refusal of unwanted medical treatment.[50]

Some state constitutions also protect privacy, sometimes more broadly than does the United States Constitution as currently interpreted.[51] Constitutional litigation regarding collection and analysis of information of the types used in epidemiologic research has been sparse. Some commentators suggest constitutional protection for research as a form of information-gathering or expression under the First Amendment.[52] No such right has yet received constitutional recognition, although inferences might be drawn from somewhat analogous contexts like journalism or practice of a profession.

Contracts are voluntary agreements between two or more parties. Unlike tort, where duties are established by public policy, contractual obligations are created by the parties to the agreement and are enforceable by courts if basic standards are met. Contractual liability flows from unexcused failure to keep agreed-to promises. The law views as compensable harm any failure to reap expected benefits of a bargain, or any losses unjustly incurred when foreseeably and reasonably relying on promises made by another.

Fiduciary liability arises from special relationships. A fiduciary is one on whom another depends, one who has undertaken to act in the interest of the other. Typically, fiduciaries are in confidential relationships with dependent parties: doctors and patients, lawyers and clients, trustees and trust beneficiaries, corporate officers or directors and shareholders, *etc*. Fiduciary responsibility demands loyalty to the interests of the dependent party to the exclusion of the fiduciary's own interests. It imposes stringent obligations to disclose to the dependent all information that might be relevant to the dependent's decisions or interests.

Property ownership involves a diverse bundle of legal rights regarding "things." These rights may be exercised by their respective holders. Possession and control are particularly salient aspects of property rights. Property is sometimes tangible and sometimes not. For instance, information is often valuable property. Epidemiologic research deals with information, so disputes over ownership and control of that resource may arise. In addition, analysts currently debate the legal status of body tissues, products, and specimens in contexts as diverse as profitable cell lines created from excised tissue, to transfer of gametes and embryos.[53] Property concepts are relevant in these discussions as well.

Although these common-law principles can be separated on a theoretical level, they overlap and interact when applied. In particular, tort and contract theories combine when a voluntary relationship, such as researcher-subject, involves some risk of personal harm. When that relationship reflects trust, dependency, and an imbalance of power, as is often the case between health scientists and patients or subjects, fiduciary principles also apply. When a researcher is employed, funded, or associated with the government, as many epidemiologists are, constitutional considerations may also arise.

The following discussion divides on the basis of the sources of epidemiologic data. Generally, epidemiologists gather information either *directly* from individual subjects, as when they interview, supply questionnaires, observe or monitor individuals; or *indirectly* from a separate source (such as doctors, data banks, laboratories, hospital records). Sometimes both methods are employed, as when indirect sources provide initial data or help to identify subjects, and then researchers have direct contact with those subjects. All possible scenarios cannot be addressed, but the following discussion can illuminate the types of issues that could arise.

Data or Specimens Gathered Indirectly

Requirements regarding consent might seem to apply only when subjects will have direct contact with researchers. However, issues of consent, disclosure, and notice should be considered even when data will be retrieved indirectly.

At the outset, a patchwork of local, state, or federal statutes, as well as requirements established by particular institutional data holders or professional societies, governs access to data repositories. Many information repositories allow access to researchers but set procedures for and limits on what and how they use data. Many also require review of a project by an IRB. Where the federal human subjects regulations are not applied, or where institutions are lax in their review processes, researchers should police themselves regarding ethical fundamentals like access, consent, and confidentiality.

Professional ethical norms sometimes restrict disclosure of medical information by data banks and individual health workers, even for purposes of research.[54] State laws on the issue vary. For example, the proposed Uniform Health Care Information Act adopts an approach similar to California's Confidentiality of Medical Information Act,[55] but only a few other states have, as yet, adopted the uniform model. When and if Congress acts on health care reform, it must address information privacy, particularly if comprehensive national medical data are gathered, stored, and used. In lieu of Congressional action, current laws governing medical information privacy are fragmented and incomplete. Existing protections are organized around particular *types* of medical conditions (for example, studies funded by alcohol, drug abuse, and mental health agencies[56]) or particular (government) *holders* of data (for example, the Freedom of Information Act (FOIA)[57] and the Privacy Act of 1974[58]). FOIA, for example, generally prohibits government officials from disclosing individuals' medical information, but allows considerable latitude for disclosure to researchers. In addition to whatever sanctions attach to noncompliance with regulatory or professional restrictions, common law principles of liability such as contract or tort may also apply.

Researchers often gain access to individuals' medical records or specimens through an indirect source, such as a primary care doctor or hospital laboratory. If, in seeking a third party source's cooperation, a researcher makes promises regarding the expected uses of data, follow-up contacts, or other assurances, contractual liability for any breach of those promises might ensue. For instance, a promise to give a publication credit to an institutional source, a promise not to contact patients, or a promise not to share data with other researchers could, if broken, give rise to liability for monetary damages. Such damages could arise if the source's loss of expected compliance had value. For example, if patients changed service providers because they felt aggrieved by researcher behavior that deviated from what was promised in the researcher's agreement with the provider, the provider and data source could recover for the economic losses incurred.

Negligence liability could result if personal or economic injury befalls an information source as a result of a researcher's failure to conform to professional standards of care regarding access to and use of information. Further, if irregularities emerge regarding a researcher's claimed credentials, purposes, assertions, or conduct in obtaining information, or if a researcher proceeded in some unauthorized or highly inappropriate fashion, such facts might provide a basis for a claim of tortious intrusion into individual privacy.

The criteria for privacy intrusion are fairly stringent. They require *intentional* intrusion upon the seclusion of another where that intrusion would be highly offensive to a reasonable person.[59] Although such claims in the context of research are likely to be rare, they are not inconceivable. A recently reported incident makes clear that "unthinkable" things can happen. A doctor whose practice included AIDS and HIV+ patients disclosed the names and phone numbers of some of his patients to a political campaign. The campaign staff contacted those individuals on behalf of an openly gay candidate for the California legislature.[60] No researcher was involved, but the actions of the doctor and of the campaign personnel demonstrate that disturbing forms of access to medical information do occur. Tort standards of "reasonableness" evolve as public attitudes change. Facing a modern onslaught of data collection from telemarketers to credit reports to employer and insurer screening of medical histories, the public is experiencing growing concern about the breadth of access to personal information.

Tort law imposes on medical providers an array of fiduciary obligations to individuals whose personal data they hold. If transfer of information by health care providers (either directly to researchers or indirectly to data banks) is not done pursuant to statutory public health mandates, but as voluntary behavior, the providers might well be liable to patients if those disclosures breached fiduciary, tort, or contractual duties of confidentiality.[61] Researchers might also be liable for inducing a provider's breach of duty.[62] The fact that researchers typically have greater familiarity with IRBs and consent requirements than do individual physicians increases the possibility of such claims, because the knowledge accentuates culpability and justifies others' reliance.

So far, litigation about fiduciary duties to maintain confidentiality has occurred mainly when disclosure was for purposes less defensible than medical research. Unfortunately, history demonstrates that even research is neither immune to negligence nor free from unethical conduct. Ethical and legal considerations oblige researchers to be scrupulous themselves. Such constraints also suggest that researchers should encourage their sources to comply with appropriate consent/disclosure practices. In their relations with information sources, researchers should know or inquire about how the source came to hold the information, what the subject-patient knows about uses of such information, and whether the patient has restricted or consented to such uses. Especially where no law mandates release of data, subjects should be notified of and allowed objection to a doctor's, hospital's, or lab's usual practices regarding transfer of personal data or specimens. Failure to do so violates patients' trust, particularly if identifiers are included. Even if no identifiers attach, transfer without *any* notice devalues subjects' personal dignity and autonomy.

If data were collected pursuant to statute, as is often the case when public health is at issue, neither the provider nor the patient has a choice about disclosure. When the state collects information, constitutional issues are raised. In its most analogous decision—*Whalen v. Roe*—the Supreme Court held that no constitutional violation of privacy occurs where a statute requires reporting of information about identifiable patients' prescriptions, as long as the statute includes adequate safeguards for confidentiality and appropriate use.[63] What constitutes "adequacy" is subject to rigorous debate.

Whalen evaluated patients' privacy rights in the context of law enforcement access. That context is not wholly analogous to research access. Law enforcement is more threatening to the individual than is health research, but law enforcement may also offer a more compelling justification for such access than does scientific knowledge.

Constitutional scholar Laurence Tribe has sharply criticized the Supreme Court's views about informational privacy. Tribe believes that information provided for one purpose should not be automatically releasable for different purposes without the knowledge or consent of the individual involved.[64] The Court has not adopted Tribe's approach, but his arguments have relevance to epidemiologic research. Ethically, and perhaps legally as well, someone should make patients aware, perhaps at the time they enter a hospital or a medical practice, of public health reporting requirements. Especially if identifiers are attached, patients should be told that such data are reported and used for research purposes.

Data Gathered Directly from Subjects

Where researchers plan direct written, oral, or observational contact with subjects, important legal and ethical issues arise in securing consent.

OBSERVATIONAL RESEARCH. Where access is gained by observation or surveillance of public behavior, there is arguably no need for consent under the Policy for Protection of Human Subjects. Before reaching that conclusion, however, several questions arise. As already noted, judgments about "publicness" would be more nuanced if made along a continuum rather than pursuant to a binary categorization. Behavior that will be observed should be classified in terms of *degrees* of publicness, and consent procedures should be adjusted accordingly. People do not ordinarily expect systematic observation and recording even when their behavior is "public." Although courts have sometimes treated publicness as a constitutional on/off switch, they have also sometimes used expectations regarding privacy to determine its protection.[65] Observational research on some public conduct (such as use of a public restroom) could violate such expectations and render exemption from consent requirements inappropriate. Intrusive surveillance might also run afoul of common-law safeguards against offensive intrusion into privacy.

APPROACHING SUBJECTS. When research will involve oral, written, or physical contact, someone must make initial inquiries of prospective subjects. Approach through a patient's doctor can assist ethical procurement of consent. Patients will be less startled if approached by their own doctors. In addition to providing reassurance, doctors may offer useful information regarding participation to prospective subjects. A doctor may be able to vouch for a particular researcher's credentials, respect for confidentiality, and legitimacy.

On the other hand, affiliating the researcher with the doctor in the patient-subject's mind could create an inappropriate "halo" effect. For instance, the patient-subject may incorrectly assume that the care-giving doctor *wants* him to cooperate with the researcher, or that the research is connected to or a condition for his continuing care. Even if formal statements to the contrary are made, they may not be absorbed. Or a patient could incorrectly assume that the research offers some therapeutic benefit. Inquiry through a personal doctor could also inaccurately convey that the doctor vouches for the researcher. Particularly if a doctor is unfamiliar with the research and the researcher, the doctor should convey full, accurate, and understandable information about these matters, or the researcher should approach the subject as the stranger that she is. Approaches through other institutions or providers with whom a prospective subject has a preexisting relationship require similar analysis.

SECURING INFORMED CONSENT. Once researchers are dealing directly with subjects, norms of informed consent apply. Ordinarily, epidemiologic research is nontherapeutic, unlike pure treatment or combinations of research and treatment. Because the patient's illness is not a motivator for participation in research, consent to research is more elective than is consent to medical treatment. Researchers have no direct professional responsibility for the best health interests of particular individuals. They are motivated by a desire to gain knowledge and improve policy, as well as by personal reputation and fulfillment of contractual obligations to research sponsors. Researcher-subject relations, therefore, have more arms-length (contractual) characteristics than do doctor-patient relationships.

At the same time, to understand researchers as purely self-interested, in the sense that contracting parties usually are, would be inaccurate. As professionals, researchers are bound by ethical norms and goals that are, to a significant degree, unselfish. Indeed, researchers' association with medical facts, specimens, and contexts could lead prospective subjects to presume a researcher's trustworthiness and expertise, and perhaps to infer a doctor-like fidelity to patients' interests. Subjects may therefore feel some of the dependencies patients experience, even though researchers lack the identity of interest and caretaking obligations of physicians. Because researcher-subject relationships exhibit this mix of elements, courts could impose standards of accountability that typify relationships of dependency and trust, but could simultaneously refuse to allow researchers the same benefit of the doubt that doctors receive when their professional behavior is called into question. In doctrinal terms, nontherapeutic research could accrue duties from *both* contractual and tort-fiduciary doctrines, at the same time that it is denied access to some of the defenses typically available under those same bodies of law. Although courts usually balance duties and defenses, the distinctive logic of the research context makes this type of development entirely possible.

1. *Tort/fiduciary issues*. The Policy for Protection of Human Subjects enumerates minimum standards for securing subjects' consent to research. Several courts have held that the common law imposes higher standards of disclosure and consent in researcher-subject relationships than in doctor-patient relationships. Accordingly, in addition to making disclosures mandated by the policy, epidemiologists also have a duty to disclose what the reasonable researcher knows or should know to be the material risks of study participation from the perspective of the reasonable subject.

Most of the risks in epidemiologic research stem from inappropriate access to or use of personal information. The researcher and her employees constitute the initial layer of such risk. In general, epidemiologists know and guard against problems arising within their own work projects. However, even reputable researchers sometimes violate fundamental ethical and legal standards for consent.[66] On other occasions, researchers have little or no control over unplanned access by third parties. For instance, third parties can sometimes gain access to research data through Freedom of Information Act (FOIA) requests, compulsory court procedures, and physical or electronic theft. The risk of such access is comparatively small, but researchers should sometimes extend disclosure for consent beyond the facts of their own use.

Researchers can seek a Certificate of Confidentiality from HHS, thereby creating a firmer barrier to third-party access, particularly by courts.[67] Careful planning regarding location and rights to research records can also reduce the chances of third-party access. Only data held by federal agencies are subject to FOIA; information in the hands of state agencies is subject only to analogous state statutes. Laws that, like FOIA, require the government to release information usually exempt confidential medical records,[68] although some epidemiologic data may not fall within that category.

Courts have thus far been sensitive to research subjects' desires for confidentiality. An example is a dispute over liability for toxic shock syndrome. Because plaintiffs planned to use Centers for Disease Control and Prevention (CDC) research, the defense argued that it needed access to names and addresses of research subjects in order to prepare for trial. The judge refused defendants' demand but also refused to recognize a general privilege of confidentiality for CDC research data.[69] The appellate court affirmed but declined to make a final or general ruling, stating only that on these facts, the trial judge had properly exercised his discretion.[70] In an action against tobacco companies, another court affirmed subpoenas that required production of research data but allowed redaction of names and other identifiers first.[71] These decisions have precedential value but represent only a few courts balancing particular claims to particular information during particular pretrial motions. Other courts could arrive at different conclusions in different contexts. If researchers have secured a Certificate of Confidentiality, subjects' reliance on representations made when they were asked to participate will strengthen researchers' right to withhold sensitive information. Research data and researchers themselves, however, remain subject to subpoena.[72]

Data-sharing with other researchers raises different questions about third-party access. Professionals sometimes assume that access to one another's confidential information is permissible. Subjects may not share that assumption. Desire to facilitate research relations with colleagues, and to gain reciprocal access to others' data, may blind some researchers to the problems of confidentiality and consent that this practice raises. Subjects' consent should be sought by each researcher. At the least, practices and intentions regarding confidentiality and data-sharing should be fully disclosed when consent is initially sought.

Some recent decisions governing consent broaden duties of professional disclosure in ways that could eventually be applied in research contexts as well. Requirements that physicians disclose conflicts of interest have particular significance. Several cases suggest required disclosure to patients regarding both a treating doctor's personal health status[73] and her financial interests.[74] Ethical traditions, and some institutional or statutory rules as well, affirm a researcher's duty to disclose the sponsorship and funding of research, as well as any personal stakes (such as employment, consulting arrangements, continuation of grant funds) that the researcher has in the project or outcome. Several courts have required more disclosure in nontherapeutic research than in treatment.[75] If these expanded-disclosure cases are widely followed, that principle will likely be applied to epidemiologic research as well.

Legal duties to warn of harm can add to disclosure requirements both at the time of consent and afterward. Once again, cases decided in other contexts portend more obligations for researchers. For example, even where no treatment relationship exists, courts have imposed on health professionals responsibilities to warn of known risks, particularly where a "medicalized" context could induce an assumption that professionals will act as fiduciaries for the well-being of the individual.[76] In the decided cases, greater reasons for such reliance existed than is typical in epidemiologic research. Nevertheless, if the researcher were a doctor, or were introduced to the subject through the patient's doctor, analogous policies would come into play. For example, if epidemiologic research involved determination of HIV status, or if the subject might not otherwise receive notice of dangerous health data, courts could hold that a researcher is obligated to warn subjects about such matters.[77] Similarly, the federal human subjects regulations suggest that researchers have a responsibility to warn when their research conclusions have significance to their subjects' well-being.[78] General recognition of patients' right to review their medical records further supports the view that research subjects should, if they wish, have access to their personal data and to the study's results.

Duties to warn sometimes extend beyond study subjects to third parties. In *Tarasoff v. Regents of the University of California*,[79] the California Supreme Court held that psychiatrists had a duty to warn a young woman that their patient had threatened to harm her. Although such duties are typically imposed only when the threat is severe and the target is clearly identified, similar rules might well apply to research, for example, regarding AIDS. Disclosure about HIV status is often regulated by statute, but explicit requirements regarding other dangerous diseases are more common. A growing consensus of health workers and policy analysts views doctors as having discretion to disclose risks of transmission to known sexual partners of HIV+ patients if the patients refuse to do so. This consensus implies a similar obligation for researchers.[80] A researcher often reasonably assumes that someone else, notably a treating doctor, is in a better position to provide such warnings. Where no primary care giver is at hand, however, researchers' responsibilities would likely expand, especially if identities are available.

Studies of genetic pedigree raise analogous problems regarding whether to inform or warn subjects and relatives about discovered defects. Because time pressure is less likely to be a factor in genetic disclosure situations, courts would probably require higher standards for disclosure and consent between researcher and subject than they would in circumstances known to pose the extreme and immediate risks of AIDS transmission. Even when a policy of warning third parties has been disclosed and agreed on in advance, discovery of genetic defects will typically allow for discussion with particular subjects regarding who should be told and how. Because many genetic defects have no means of treatment presently available, disclosure is even more problematic. Nevertheless, respect for the autonomy of persons argues for disclosure in most instances. These situations require difficult tradeoffs between a research subject's right to confidentiality and others' right to be warned of impending harm.

Researchers should consider duties to warn subjects and third parties when consent procedures are designed. Duties to warn also have ramifications regarding retention of identifiers.[81] The ability to warn subjects or third parties—whether by researchers or through treating doctors—requires retention of identifiers. Yet identifiers increase risks to confidentiality and heighten requirements in IRB review. There are no perfect solutions, but researchers and reviewers should assess with care how duties to warn should shape disclosure practices.

Finally, the problem of deception in research requires examination. If researchers intentionally deceive subjects about the purposes or risks of their research or about other relevant matters, they may commit common-law fraud. Fraud—defined as the knowing misrepresentation of a fact or, occasionally, as a failure to speak when there exists a duty to do so—is legally actionable. Fiduciaries, on whom others depend, bear greater than ordinary affirmative obligations to speak. Tort law provides compensatory damages for harm incurred through fraud, sometimes allowing punitive damages as well. Any decisions based on misrepresentation or culpable omissions may be invalidated.

Some investigators defend deception as essential to certain types of research and support relaxation of, or exemption from, consent requirements in such instances.[82] The federal regulations explicitly allow some limited waivers of consent requirements where subjects' ignorance is essential to research design and risks are minimal.[83] Yet the common law treats fraud very seriously. Common-law courts could be considerably less flexible regarding deceptive research than federal regulations or scientific norms. Even when truth-telling about purposes or hypotheses threatens scientific validity, researchers have little right to usurp volunteer subjects' autonomy, especially given the speculative nature of many justifications for deception.

2. *Contract issues.* Both research and treatment relationships typically rest on consensual agreement. However, patients' dependence on professionals causes courts to supply the substantive terms of most doctor-patient agreements through public policy rather than through the arms-length private choices that (theoretically) characterize contracts.[84] Even in treatment relationships, courts sometimes employ contract principles to analyze doctors' duties to patients.[85] As already noted, nontherapeutic research shares features of fiduciary dependency but is also a more voluntary and arms-length transaction than is treatment. Accordingly, in ordinary consensual agreements researchers should comply with standards for voluntariness, as well as with those added within fiduciary relationships.

The law presumes that individuals are competent unless shown to be otherwise. Researchers must be alert to problems of competency or voluntariness when subjects are vulnerable people such as minors, the mentally disabled, the seriously ill, or the incarcerated. Beyond basic competency, contract doctrine demands a voluntary bargaining process. Lies or culpable omissions vitiate consensual assent. Courts may void an agreement if bargaining power is extremely disparate, if terms are unreasonably tilted to favor the more powerful side, or if the subject lacks meaningful choice or is unduly pressured to agree. When consent fails to satisfy these criteria, courts may grant restitution of benefits unjustly conferred, compensation for detrimental reliance, or other forms of equitable relief.

Researchers should remember that, if broken, promises to subjects may be enforced by compensating for loss of expected benefits. On occasion, disclosures made during the informed consent process can function as promises about the researcher's future conduct. For example, if a researcher states that data will not be shared with other researchers, or that court processes seeking access to data will be resisted, the subject may recover damages flowing from the researcher's failure to keep the promises of confidentiality. If a researcher promises to provide a full report about significant findings, a breach of that promise creates liability for loss of whatever benefit the subject would have accrued from such a report. A researcher's promise to assist a subject in gaining access to care, or to help him in litigation in exchange for participation, could also result in liability for benefits lost as a consequence of breaking the promise. Ordinarily, promises are explicit, but they may also be inferred from conduct and circumstances. Subject to certain exceptions, promises need not be written to be enforceable.[86] Finally, although courts rarely characterize *treating* doctors' reassurances as enforceable promises, they are more likely to hold researchers to their word because the researcher-subject relationship lacks the therapeutic and care-giving character that defines the doctor-patient connection.

3. *Property theories.* Information has value as property. Trade secrets are business property, as are mailing lists. Lawyers describe property ownership as having a diverse bundle of rights in something. Such rights may be held by a single owner or by several different people. For instance, medical records and information typically belong to individuals or organizations that create, gather, and store them—doctors, hospitals, laboratories, etc. In many states, however, patients have a right of personal access and some control over others' access to personal medical records. Release of confidential medical information without the consent of the patient is, with certain exceptions, proscribed by law as well as by professional ethics. Many of the previously discussed tort and fiduciary duties regarding consent and disclosure could, alternately, be characterized as mechanisms protecting property-like rights over personal information. Use of one label as compared with another can affect the substance of obligations, but is more

prone to influence such technical but significant matters as the availability of remedies or the length of time during which a claim can be brought. Researchers should recognize that concepts of property ownership—at least in the sense of control over access—can be applied to information as well as to things.

Recent disputes have questioned whether live tissue, organs, and biological products should be conceptualized and regulated as property. Contexts as diverse as patentability of nonhuman organisms,[87] control over organs for transplant and donation,[88] testamentary disposition of semen,[89] and control over *in vitro* embryos[90] implicate property issues. This newly emerging body of law has relevance for gaining research subjects' consent. In *Moore v. University of California Regents*, plaintiff alleged that researchers had converted (that is, intentionally interfered with possession of) his property when they used tissue from his excised cancerous spleen to create a cell line valuable in cancer research. The physician-researchers, together with their university employer, patented the cell line and sold a license for its exclusive use, allegedly without having informed the patient or sought his consent to their proprietary activities.[91] The California Supreme Court rejected the appellate court's view that spleen cells could be characterized as property. Instead, California's high court described plaintiff's grievance as a possible breach of a fiduciary duty to disclose the physician-researchers' proprietary activities.

Despite the final *Moore* decision, the issues are new and choices about what legal categories should be applied in regulating such research remain contentious. Researchers who utilize human biological specimens may soon have ethical and/or legal duties to ensure that research subject-sources are informed of, and their consent sought for, research using tissue or body products.[92] If duties like the one articulated in *Moore* were widely adopted and were combined with increased recognition that information itself has proprietary value, epidemiologic researchers might eventually be required to inform regarding such matters as their research purposes and any conflicts of interest (such as the employer as source of research funding, and further grants contingent on research success) in order to obtain valid consent from research subjects. This might be true even when data collection and analysis involve no physical specimens, but only information. However, society's perceived need for research knowledge will likely outpace societal fears about intrusive data collection. If so, legislative, administrative, or judicial decision makers could prevent such restrictions from being imposed.

Reflections on Legal and Ethical Meanings of Consent

Throughout this chapter, the stated imperative has been to obtain ethically and legally valid consent. Yet the material primarily addresses duties to disclose information. The emphasis on disclosure stems partly from the law's focus on the obligations of the more active and more powerful party to a transaction—here, the researcher. But the emphasis also reflects a recognition that specifying check lists of information "inputs" is easier than describing qualitative outcomes of a complex human process. Were the law to evaluate the quality of *consent*, rather than simply of *disclosure*, it would enter a murky terrain of weighing competency, assessing relationships, and determining what is understood rather than simply what is said.

Determining how people understand and use information is difficult.[93] Often, individuals themselves do not know what they mean or want. Wishes and meanings waver and shift. The law avoids more difficult and nuanced judgments, settling instead for indices that are more readily assessed. The law presumes competence unless incapacity is proved. The law holds people accountable for measurable efforts rather than for less determinate outcomes. Less constrained by systemic limitations, ethical deliberation cannot so easily escape. Ethical norms extend beyond the law and strive to consider not just what is and is not said, but by whom, in what context, and with what result. Ethics must ask deep questions regarding what is understood and what is meant.

Finally, ethical researchers should feel responsibility for those who surround and assist their work. Where data are accessed through intermediate sources, the likelihood of a researcher being held liable for wrongs of other professionals is low. Nevertheless, a scrupulous investigator will be attentive to subjects' knowledge about the research and the scope of their permission for using personal medical data. Especially troublesome are uses by third parties for purposes beyond those originally intended by the giver. Researchers' greater knowledge of ethical requirements for research allows attentive investigators to contribute substantially to the ethical management of data by sources, data-entry personnel, and publishers.

Conclusion

Ethical discussion about consent to epidemiologic research has increased, but judicial precedents are sparse. Currently, the principal legal constraints on epidemiologic research are established by the federal Policy for the Protection of Human Subjects. That policy uses the carrot of federal funding to require peer review of research value and to ensure the adequacy of disclosure and consent. The policy applies to epidemiologic research that uses information or specimens gathered from human beings. Some may believe that the policy ought not extend to epidemiologic research because surveys and analysis of specimens or records pose less risk than interventionist research. The regulations note that concern by allowing greater flexibility of review and requirements for consent to such research. In addition to the policy's regulatory rules, common-law principles governing deceit, broken promises, misplaced trust, and carelessly engendered harm also apply, as, in some instances, do constitutional protections for individual privacy.

Much within the legal framework parallels the ethical norms of professional conduct. To that extent, compliance with legal requirements should be unobjectionable to researchers. However, to a greater degree than professional codes, the law requires professionals to be aware of and responsive to the concerns of research subjects and the public at large. A lawyer's job includes thorough analysis of potential problems and scrupulous attention to alternate arguments and points of views. Those whose gaze is focused on gaining knowledge and solving problems can easily forget the autonomy, privacy, and harm-avoidance concerns noted here.

Investigators sometimes fail to consider or even to see potentially differing viewpoints. They need to step back from the urgency of their own agendas—however altruistic and vital those may be—to recognize the enormous degree to which the modern world uses information to intrude. An individual may object on religious grounds to use of bodily tissue or specimens for study, but the research community may see only harmless or "minimal" risk in such analysis. Others may suffer inward wounds or debilitating fears about researchers' use of information that epidemiologists deem "not damaging" to reputation, financial status, or liability. Individuals may perceive calls or letters from epidemiologists as violations of trust by doctors who provided their names and health data. Scientists may view the same transactions as simply allowing greater efficiency and accuracy in their work.

Although epidemiologists possess essential knowledge and professional judgment regarding the conduct of their research, other viewpoints also matter. For instance, as Carr and Rothman note, high rates of nonparticipation may reduce or taint scientific validity. However, a lawyer-ethicist would likely disagree with their suggestion that when large numbers of potential subjects choose not to participate, different and potentially less stringent consent procedures should be used.[94] Substantial nonparticipation strikes one who is legally trained as a reason to give greater rather than lesser protection to subjects' rights to refuse involvement in a study. Carr and Rothman use survey information to suggest that resistance or refusal to volunteer may not be "real." They suggest that methods of gaining consent that yield higher rates of participation should be substituted. Without doubt, individuals' "true" preferences are exceedingly difficult to assess. Reactions are ambivalent and changeable, varying with context and circumstance. Although Carr and Rothman are forceful in arguing for their vision of the public good, their perspective reflects the limits of their professional acculturation, as does anyone's. Multiple and varied perspectives in formulating review procedures offer the best route to research that will optimize both knowledge and fairness.

Epidemiologic investigators may assert a right to research under concepts like academic freedom or a First Amendment right to know.[95] These are certainly relevant concerns, but courts have not, as yet, recognized such a right. In addition, individuals including research subjects, scientists, policy analysts, and other decision makers have interests in the knowledge that epidemiologists generate. Research also gives subject-volunteers meaningful opportunities to contribute to others. Despite the importance of these various interests, they must be balanced against subjects' rights to autonomy, privacy, and avoidance of harm. Because individualist values are so central to our society, subjects' legal rights to privacy and autonomy will likely take precedence over researchers' and public claims, except in instances where the need to know is extreme and exigent, once a dispute has become public.

Legal and ethical requirements can render regulation more obstructive without making it better. In the realm of bureaucracy, lose-lose outcomes are all too common. Many researchers already chafe at IRB review or the involvement of courts and lawyers, seeing them as generating unnecessary delay, obstruction, and expense.[96] Sometimes they are right. The goal is to ensure rigorous, appropriate standards for consent while streamlining unnecessary bureaucratic impediments—something more easily said than done.

Lawyers perceive a need for checks and balances on any person or group. They value vigorous assertion of alternative viewpoints, particularly where multiple interests are at stake. Law plays a vital role of ensuring varied input and dispersion of power. But externally imposed procedures, however essential, are insufficient. Only when researchers fully understand and genuinely internalize the principles expressed in legal and ethical requirements will those principles be wholly realized. When that is achieved, detailed oversight will be less necessary and compliance with rules less onerous.

Epidemiology can do enormous good. It informs public choice and individual decisions. It enlarges understanding of health conditions and causes. It shapes problem solving and evaluates the efficacy of interventions. It increases the accuracy of assessments about responsibility for causing harm. But along with expanding opportunity and mandate go increased legal and ethical accountability. Profound attention to legal and ethical norms regarding informed consent to research is essential to the legitimacy of the epidemiologic profession.

Notes and References

1. I greatly appreciate the capable research assistance of Tom Oscherwitz and Duane Valz. I am also grateful to Dr. Elizabeth Holly, Dr. Art Reingold and Dr. Guy Micco for the helpful comments they made on earlier drafts of this chapter.

2. One recent example involves forensic use of DNA. See generally *DNA On Trial: Genetic Identification and Criminal Justice*, ed. Paul R. Billings. Cold Spring Harbor, NY: Cold Spring Harbor Laboratory Press, 1992.

3. Kant, Immanuel. *Foundations of the Metaphysics of Morals* (1785). Reprinted in *Philosophical Writings*, ed. Ernest Behler (New York: Continuum, 1986) p. 94. For commentary on the ethical centrality of this principle generally, see Alasdair MacIntyre, *After Virtue: A Study in Moral Theory* (Notre Dame: University of Notre Dame Press, 1981). For discussion of the means-ends principle in consent to medical research, see Ruth R. Faden and Tom L. Beauchamp, *A History and Theory of Informed Consent* (New York: Oxford University Press, 1986), pp. 354–55.

4. Influential commentary on research abuses includes Henry K. Beecher, "Ethics and Clinical Research," *New England Journal of Medicine* 274 (1966): 1354; Jay Katz, with the assistance of Alexander M. Capron and Eleanor Swift Glass, *Experimentation with Human Beings* (1972); James Jones, *Bad Blood* (New York: The Free Press, 1981).

5. 45 C.F.R. §§46.101–46.409 (1992).

6. 45 C.F.R. § 46.102 (f).

7. *Id.* at § 46.116.

8. *Id.* at § 46.116 (b).

9. *Id.* at 46.116 (c)(d).

10. *Id.* at §§ 46.201–211 (fetuses, pregnant women), at §§ 46.301–306 (prisoners), at §§ 46.401–409 (children).

11. *Id.* at § 46.207.

12. *Id.* at § 46.208.

13. *Id.* at § 46.305. The IRB must also include a prisoner-member, and a majority of members must have no association with the prison.

14. *Id.* at §§ 46.404, 46.405 (c), and at § 46.406 (d).

15. *Id.* at § 46.116 (d).

16. The regulations define "minimal risk" as "the probability and magnitude of harm or discomfort anticipated in the research are not greater in and of themselves than those ordinarily encountered in daily life or during the performance of routine physical or psychological examinations or tests." 45 C.F.R. § 46.102 (h)(i). Tom L. Beauchamp et al. "Ethical Guidelines for Epidemiologists," *Journal of Clinical Epidemiology* 44 (suppl. 1991): 151S, 157S (no absolute right to conduct research).

17. 45 C.F.R. §46.101 (b)(5)(i).

18. *Id.* at § 46.116 (c)(1).

19. 45 C.F.R. Part 46 at p. 118 (Editorial Note) and DHHS Notice of Waiver, 47 Fed. Reg. 9208 (March 4, 1982).

20. See, e.g. H.B. 3207, Statewide Session (1993 South Carolina). New Jersey adopted a different method (the Child Exclusion barring some children from eligibility for benefits) to encourage reduction in the size of welfare families, and HHS granted a waiver of federal policy to allow New Jersey's "experiment." A current challenge to that New Jersey provision attacks the Child Exclusion as, among other things, a violation of federal rules requiring informed consent to research on human subjects. However, because the human subjects regulations exempt research on public benefits programs from IRB scrutiny, plaintiffs have had to rest that challenge on a different and much narrower statutory base. See Brief in Support of Plaintiff's Motion for Summary Judgment, *C.K. et al. v. Shalala*, No.

93–5354 (D.N.J. 1993). These developments demonstrate how significant and problematic the exemption of public benefits research from the human subjects regulatory framework can be.

21. 45 C.F.R. § 46.101(e) and § 46.101(a).

22. *Id.* at § 46.101(b).

23. Alpert, S. "Smart Cards, Smarter Policy: Medical Records, Privacy and Health Care Reform," *Hastings Center Report* 23 (1993): 13–23.

24. See generally, James Rule et al. *The Politics of Privacy: Planning for Personal Data Systems as Powerful Technologies* (New York: Elsevier, 1980); and James Rule, *Private Lives and Public Surveillance* (New York: Schocken Books, 1974).

25. 45 C.F.R. § 46.117 (c)(1).

26. See Ronald Bayer, et al., "The American, British and Dutch Responses to Unlinked Anonymous HIV Seroprevalence Studies: An International Comparison," *Law, Medicine, and Health Care* 19 (1991): 222–23. Of course, lack of appropriate follow-up can occur even where identifiers are retained, as in the infamous Tuskegee Syphilis Study, where researchers acted to prevent treatment of subjects so their research design would not be disrupted. See Jones, *Bad Blood, supra* note 4.

27. 45 C.F.R. § 46.101 (b)(4).

28. Tribe, Laurence H. *American Constitutional Law*, at §§ 1390–93. 2d ed. 1988.

29. 45 C.F.R. § 46.102(f)(5).

30. *Id.* at § 46.101 (b)(2)(i).

31. Jay Katz, "Informed Consent—A Fairytale? Law's Vision," *University of Pittsburgh Law Review* 39 (1977): 137; Marjorie M. Shultz, "From Informed Consent to Patient Choice: A New Protected Interest," *Yale Law Journal* 95 (1985): 219, 248–50.

32. President's Commission for The Study of Ethical Problems in Medicine and Biomedical and Behavioral Research. *Making Health Care Decisions*, Washington, D.C.: U.S. Government Printing Office 1984: 206–45.

33. 45 C.F.R. § 46.101(b).

34. For a cogent critique on this point, see Judith P. Swazey, "Professional Protectionism Rides Again: A Commentary on Exempted Research and Responses to DHEW's Proposed Regulations," *IRB* 2 (1980): 4.

35. Carr, C. I. and Rothman, K. J. "IRBs and Epidemiologic Research: How Inappropriate Restrictions Hamper Studies," *IRB* 6 (1984): 5–7.

36. 45 C.F.R. § 46.110.

37. *Id.* at § 46.110 and 46 *Federal Register* 8392 (1991).

38. Capron, A. M. "Protection of Research Subjects: Do Special Rules Apply in Epidemiology?" *Journal of Clinical Epidemiology* 44 (suppl. 1991): 81S–89S.

39. 45 C.F.R. § 46.101 (b)(3)(1).

40. Holder, A. R. and Levine, R. J. "Informed Consent for Research on Specimens Obtained at Autopsy or Surgery: A Case Study in the Overprotection of Human Subjects," *Clinical Research* 24 (1976): 68. See also National Commission for the Protection of Human Subjects of Biomedical and Behavioral Research, *Institutional Review Boards: Report and Recommendations*, DHEW Pub. No. (OS) 78-0008 (Recommendation 4II and commentary) (1978).

41. 45 C.F.R. § 46.101(f).

42. See *California Health & Safety Code*, §§ 24170–24179.5 (West 1992).

43. *N.Y. Public Health Law*, §§ 2440–2446 (McKinney 1985).

44. See, e.g., *D.C. Code Ann.* §§ 6–1969 (1989).
45. 45 C.F.R. § 46.101(f) and (g).
46. Compare *Whitlock v. Duke University*, 637 F. Supp. 1463 (M.D.N.C. 1986) (adopting federal regulations as minimum standard of disclosure in nontherapeutic research).
47. Significant analyses of informed consent include Faden and Beauchamp, *supra* note 3 (philosophy); Jay Katz, *The Silent World of Doctor and Patient* (1984) (medicine); Katz, *Fairytale*, *supra* note 31 (medicine and law); Shultz, *Patient Choice*, *supra* note 31, (law); and Peter Schuck, "Rethinking Informed Consent," *Yale Law Journal* 103 (1994): 899 (law).
48. *Griswold v. Connecticut*, 381 U.S. 479, 85 S.Ct. 1678, 14 L.Ed.2d 510 (1965).
49. *Roe v. Wade*, 410 U.S. 113, 93 S.Ct. 705, 35 L.Ed.2d 147 (1973).
50. *Cruzan v. Director, Missouri Dept. of Health, et al.*, 497 U.S. 261, 110 S.Ct. 2841, 111 L.Ed.2d 224 (1990).
51. See, e.g., *California Constitution.* art. I. § 1.
52. See John A. Robertson, "The Scientist's Right to Research: A Constitutional Analysis," *Southern California Law Review* 51 (1977): 1203 (analogizing research to freedoms of speech and press).
53. *Moore v. Regents of the University of California*, 51 Cal.3d 120, 271 Cal. Rptr., 146, 793 P.2d 479 (1990) (cell line from spleen tissue) and *Davis v. Davis*, 842 S.W.2d 588 (Tenn. 1992) (contested disposition of frozen embryos at divorce).
54. One commentator notes that "the two most recent AMA statements not only fail to address disclosure (by doctors) to medical researchers but also seem to preclude such disclosures. . . . [T]hey do not appear to permit disclosures of identifiable medical information for uses that are generally accepted by the medical establishment. . . ." Robert M. Gellman, "Prescribing Privacy: The Uncertain Role of the Physician in the Protection of Patient Privacy," *North Carolina Law Review* 62 (1984): 255, 270–71.
55. See, e.g., *California Confidentiality of Medical Information Act*, Cal. Civ. Code §§ 56–56.35 (West 1982) (makes research an exception allowing disclosure of medical information without patient's authorization).
56. 42 U.S.C. § 242m (1988).
57. 5 U.S.C. § 552 (1982).
58. 5 U.S.C. § 552a (1982).
59. *Restatement (Second) of Torts* § 652 B (1977).
60. Spiegel, C. "Patient Privacy Is Breached in Political Race," *Los Angeles Times*, (July 28, 1991): A3. Although the doctor admitted releasing the names, he denied any wrongdoing.
61. See, e.g., *Humphers v. First Interstate Bank*, 298 Or. 706, 696 P.2d 527 (1985) (en banc) (doctor's provision of false medical information to adopted child seeking biological mother held actionable breach of confidentiality).
62. Compare *Alberts v. Devine, et al.*, 479 N.E.2d 113 (Mass. 1985) (doctor's unauthorized disclosure of medical information to patient's employer allows action for doctor's breach of confidentiality and for employer's inducement of such breach).
63. *Whalen v. Roe*, 429 U.S. 589, 97 S.Ct. 869, 51 L.Ed.2d 64 (1977).
64. Tribe, *supra* note 27, at §§ 1389–1400.
65. See *Katz v. United States*, 389 U.S. 347, 88 S.Ct. 507, 19 L.Ed.2d 576 (1967) (privacy interest should reflect individual's reasonable expectations).
66. For instance, in the largest-ever study of lumpectomy conducted by the National

Surgical Adjuvant Breast and Bowel Project, medical data on at least three dozen women was collected and analyzed against their express wishes. John Crewdson, "Breast Cancer Study Ignored Privacy Rights," *Chicago Tribune* (December 17, 1995): 1.

67. 42 U.S.C. § 241 (d) (1988).

68. See, e.g., *Freedom of Information Act*, 5 U.S.C. § 552 (a)(6)(C)(b)(6) (1988).

69. *Lampshire v. Procter & Gamble Co.*, 94 F.R.D. 58 (N.D.Ga 1982) (issuing protective order preventing release of research subjects' names).

70. *Id.* at 60–61. Rule 26(c) of the Federal Rules of Civil Procedure gives the court discretion to issue protective orders to prevent "annoyance, embarrassment, oppression, or undue burden or expense. . . ."

71. Application of the American Tobacco Company et al., in *Mount Sinai School of Medicine and the American Cancer Society v. American Tobacco Co., R.J. Reynolds Tobacco Co., and Philip Morris, Inc.*, 880 F.2d 1520 (2d Cir. 1989).

72. See *American Tobacco*, 880 F.2d 1520 (2d Cir. 1989); Angela R. Holder, "Research Records and Subpoenas: A Continuing Issue," *IRB* 15 (Jan.-Feb. 1993): 6.

73. *Hidding v. Williams*, 578 So.2d 1192 (La.Ct.App. 1991) (doctor's failure to disclose own alcohol abuse actionable under doctrine of informed consent). Compare *Estate of Behringer v. The Medical Center at Princeton*, 249 N.J.Super. 597, 592 A.2d 1251 (1991) (hospital's requirement that surgeon disclose own HIV+ status justified under informed consent doctrine).

74. *Moore v. Regents of University of California*, 51 Cal.3d 120, 271 Cal.Rptr. 146, 793 P.2d 479 (1990).

75. See, e.g., *Whitlock v. Duke University*, 637 F. Supp. 1463 (M.D.N.C. 1986) (greater disclosure required in nontherapeutic research than in treatment); *Weiss v. Solomon*, R.J.Q. 731 (1989) (patient died from allergic reaction to injection during nontherapeutic research); *Halushka v. Univ. of Saskatchewan*, 53 D.L.R.2d 436 (1965) (paid subject suffered cardiac arrest from catheterization during experimental anesthesia). Compare *Estrada v. Jaques*, 70 N.C.App. 627, 321 S.E.2d 240 (Ct. App. 1984) (higher duty of disclosure for research than for treatment where the two combine).

76. See, e.g., *Betesh v. United States*, 400 F. Supp. 238 (D.D.C. 1974) (selective service induction exam raised duty to disclose irregularity in X-Ray); *Tresemer v. Barke*, 86 Cal.App.3d 656, 150 Cal.Rptr. 384 (1978) (although he had not seen her in 3 years, doctor had duty to notify patient of later-discovered danger of IUD).

77. See C. Levine, "Has AIDS Changed the Ethics of Human Subjects Research?" *Law, Medicine, and Health Care* 16 (1988): 167, 170 (notice of intent to do HIV screening required in consent process); Leon Gordis, "Ethical and Professional Issues in the Changing Practice of Epidemiology," *Journal of Clinical Epidemiology* 44 (suppl. 1991): S9–S11 (should disclosure be made if interviews with HIV+ subjects who were promised confidentiality reveal that subjects had recently donated blood).

78. 45 C.F.R. § 46.116 (b)(5). The Tuskegee Syphilis Study involved abuse of a similar duty. See A.M. Brandt, "Racism and Research: The Case of The Tuskegee Syphilis Study," *Hastings Center Report* 8 (1978): 21.

79. 17 Cal.3d 425, 131 Cal.Rptr. 14, 551 P.2d 334 (1976).

80. See Levine, *supra* note 76, at 170.

81. Responsibilities to inform subjects or third parties could be contingent on whether identifiers are kept, as one Public Health Service communication implies. See

Levine, *supra* note 76, at 170, n.13. Such an approach seems less ethically appropriate than full initial consideration of both issues.

82. See Stanley Milgram, *Obedience to Authority: An Experimental View*, (New York: Harper & Row, 1974), pp. 193–202; S.C. Patten, "The Case that Milgram Makes," *Philosophical Review* 86 (1977): 350–64; L. Humphreys, *Tearoom Trade: Impersonal Sex in Public Places* (Chicago: Aldine Publishing Co., 1970); D.P. Warwick, "Tearoom Trade: Means and Ends in Social Research," *Hastings Center Studies* 1 (1973): 27.

83. 45 C.F.R. § 46.116(d).

84. Typically, these characteristics yield tort rather than contractual analysis. *See* Shultz, *supra* note 31, at 223–24. Public policy may also be invoked in analyzing a health care contract. *See Tunkl v. Regents of University of California*, 60 Cal.2d 92, 82 Cal.Rptr. 33, 383 P.2d 441 (1963).

85. See Shultz, *supra* note 31, at 264–65.

86. See Melvin A. Eisenberg, *Basic Contract Law*, 5th ed. 1990, pp. B13–B15.

87. *Diamond v. Chakrabarty*, 447 U.S. 303, 100 S.Ct. 2204, 65 L.Ed.2d 144 (1980) (living organism patentable).

88. *Brotherton v. Cleveland*, 923 F.2d 477 (6th Cir. 1991) (widow's quasi-property right in husband's corneas protectable under due process). *Cf.* Uniform Anatomical Gift Act, 8 U.L.A. 15 (1968) (procedures allowing organ donation after death).

89. *Hecht v. Superior Court*, 16 Cal.App. 4th 836, 20 Cal.Rptr.2d 275 (1993).

90. See, e.g., *Davis v. Davis*, 842 S.W.2d 588 (Tenn. 1992) (divorce dispute over frozen embryos); *Del Zio v. The Presbyterian Hospital*, 74 Civ. 3588 (memorandum decision S.D.N.Y. 1978) (parents claim conversion of property based on destruction of embryo); A.C. Roark, "Couple Back Home with Their Embryo," *Los Angeles Times*, Sept. 26, 1989, at p. 2, p. 3 (infertility center must release frozen embryo to couple that moved out of state).

91. *Moore v. Regents of the University of California*, 51 Cal.3d 120, 271 Cal.Rptr. 146, 793 P.2d 479 (1990).

92. Contra Holder and Levine, *supra* note 39 (arguing NIH wrong to demand specific consent for research specimens). This discussion antedates litigation of most disputes over property rights in human tissue.

93. See, e.g., William C. Thompson, "Psychological Issues in Informed Consent," in President's Commission for the Study of Ethical Problems in Medicine and Biomedical and Behavioral Research. *Making Health Care Decisions: The Ethical and Legal Implications of Informed Consent in The Patient-Practitioner Relationship: Appendices* (1982); *Judgment Under Uncertainty: Heuristics and Biases* (Daniel Kahneman et al., eds., 1982).

94. Carr and Rothman, *supra*. note 35.

95. See Robertson, J.A., *supra* note 50; Tribe, *supra* note 27, at 812 n.32, 944–65 (discussing constitutional status of right to know information); Beauchamp et al., *Ethical Guidelines supra* note 16 (". . .[T]hese guidelines presume that there is no absolute right to scientific investigation . . .").

96. See, e.g., I. de Sola Pool, "The New Censorship of Social Research," *The Public Interest* 59 (spring 1980): 57–65.

6

Confidentiality and Privacy Protection in Epidemiologic Research

ELLEN B. GOLD

Experience should teach us to be most on guard to protect liberty when the government's purposes are beneficent. Men born to freedom are naturally alert to repel invasion of their liberty by evil-minded rulers. The greatest dangers to liberty lurk in insidious encroachment by men of zeal, well-meaning but without understanding.
—Louis D. Brandeis, Associate Justice of the Supreme Court
Olmstead v. United States, *1928*

Webster defines the word *confidential* as "entrusted with private or secret matters" and *privacy* as "withdrawn from public view or company, seclusion."[1] The concept of privacy of information, specifically, protecting the privacy of health information, has been developed largely from the common-law right of privacy (the right to be left alone and to keep personal information inaccessible to others)[2] and the principles of respect for autonomy (allowing individuals to make their own choices) and nonmaleficence (not doing harm).[3]

Much of epidemiologic research, especially the collection of personal information about individuals, involves invasions of privacy. However, particularly since the passage of the Privacy Protection Act in 1974 and the report of its Privacy Protection Study Commission,[4] assurances that confidentiality will be maintained are generally provided in informed consent statements for epidemiologic study participants. Investigators assure subjects that their private information will not be disclosed in individually identifiable form. If informed consent cannot be obtained, researchers must document the reasons for institutional review boards (IRBs) as to why it will not be obtained, and substantive methods for maintaining confidentiality and protecting privacy must be instituted.

In the two decades since the passage of the Privacy Protection Act, however, some controversies have not entirely abated, such as the implications of situations in which informed consent cannot be obtained.[5] A number of new issues have also arisen as epidemiology, along with the rest of society, has entered the information and technology age. In 1974, many epidemiologists were still using card sorters for analyzing data; gigabyte hard drives, personal computer networks, the Internet, and facsimile machines were but twinkles in their eyes. These and other advanced technologies have raised new challenges regarding confidentiality and privacy protection in epidemiologic studies. Such challenges have also been presented by a host of recent issues such as the growing prevalence of AIDS and of teenage pregnancy; scientific interest in mental disorders and aging; adverse health effects of occupational exposures; proliferation of chemical and physical agents without prior testing for long-term human health effects; ethnic and cultural diversity in the population; health care reform; and the unlocking of secrets of the human genome.

Many of the issues surrounding special circumstances and vulnerable populations, such as AIDS victims, children, the elderly, and the mentally ill or disabled, will be covered in detail elsewhere in this volume. This chapter will focus on the more general issues, as well as their underlying principles and backgrounds, that epidemiologists confront in attempting to safeguard confidentiality and privacy protection as we embark on the twenty-first century.

Balancing Benefit and Harm

As Canadian cancer epidemiologists have recently noted,[6] investigators are often faced with obtaining the proper balance between a number of sets of considerations: individual privacy rights and rights of researchers to access records and information,[7,8] individual rights and social benefits, potential risks and benefits, and the various ethical guidelines that affect the validity of research and influence our ability to answer important questions regarding the public's health. Balancing individual and societal or group rights is not unique to epidemiologic research. It is well-grounded in health policy and in public health practice, such as requiring vaccinations of children for entrance into public school, collection of vital statistics that remain in the public domain, banning the sale of commercial products that are potentially contaminated, and identifying and treating sexual contacts in sexually transmitted disease control programs. Often in these circumstances, the individuals who are giving up some rights, or innocent individuals such as unborn children, also obtain some benefit and the risks are usually minimal.[9]

In the past, the courts have frequently permitted the collective good of society to outweigh infringement of individual rights, although any such infringement must be solicited voluntarily or, if mandated, must be either temporary or demonstrated to achieve a public benefit. Individual rights in general and privacy rights in particular are thus conditional. When societal benefits outweigh these rights, incursions on autonomy and privacy by health professionals may be permissible. For example, the right of an individual to refuse vaccination for a highly infectious disease may be superseded by the right of the state to ensure protection of the public health. However, while public good is often given priority over that of the individual, public good alone is not sufficient reason for privacy rights to be overridden. Thus, in some recent instances, individual rights of mental patients or of genetic screenees have been permitted to supersede societal rights or benefits if the risks to society are minimal. The right of public health intervention to take precedence over privacy rights depends on the balance of the nature and magnitude of the public benefit, the degree of restriction of individual rights, and the distribution of both benefits and risks.[9]

Basic Principles

Behind the notion of seeking proper balance are the four principles developed for biomedical ethics by Beauchamp and Childress: nonmaleficence, beneficence, respect for autonomy, and justice.[10] It is largely held by society and most scientists that the obligation of research and researchers extends beyond nonmaleficence (not doing harm) to beneficence (trying to remove harm and provide benefits).[3] In addition, respect for individuals participating in research dictates that such individuals not be a means to an end, but that each should be an end in himself or herself and a partner with the investigators in research.[11] Finally, justice requires that all human beings be treated equitably and share benefits and burdens equally, unless there is a strong ethical justification for differences. Thus the distribution of benefits and burdens of research must be equitable and shared.

Informed Consent

The 1977 report of the Privacy Protection Study Commission made good progress in balancing the need for access to records by legitimate researchers with the individual's right to privacy, thereby attempting to balance research requirements with the need for informed consent.[2,12] The consensus is that consent is not required for legitimate epidemiologic research involving the use of records of patients who are not currently receiving care and are not placed at risk by the research, and that such a requirement would not only make the costs of some research prohibitive[13] but also impossible.[14] For example, in some case-control studies the only way to know whom to include and contact is to review medical records. Nonetheless, not obtaining informed consent can violate the principle of respect for autonomy. Obtaining consent from patients who are currently receiving care also raises important issues. Although current patients generally do not have to be traced, medical records may still need to be reviewed to determine appropriate contacts. Knowledge of this procedure can be disconcerting to the patient who believes that access to records is limited to treatment staff, but such review is often essential for conducting research.

In addition, attempts to partially address issues of privacy protection and confidentiality in informed consent are not only of ethical concern, they may also affect the validity of epidemiologic research, as is reflected in decreasing response rates with reduced levels of assurances of confidentiality.[15] If patients are routinely *informed* at their first visit or at admission that their records will be reviewed by research personnel, but are not required to provide consent, the obligation to inform can sometimes be met[13] without compromising the validity of the sample and study design. Alternatively, general or blanket *consent* for research access to records could be obtained, which recognizes the privacy interests of the patient. However, this approach could compromise study validity if consent is withheld; moreover, blanket consent does not constitute adequately informed consent, because the details of any specific project would not necessarily be known.[16,17] Still another option, which has been used in the past, is to obtain the physician's consent. Although consistent with the notion of one person coordinating (and controlling) access to records, this paternalistic approach does not recognize or address the patient's right to autonomy.

Individual Identifiers

The validity and quality of research can be compromised if removal of identifiers is required. Certainly confidentiality is better maintained and privacy better protected without identifiers, and courts have upheld this practice on a number of occasions when private companies have sought raw research data.[11,18] However, such removal precludes follow-up of the study population or linkage with additional data sources (such as registries or the National Death Index), the need for which may be recognized after publication or analysis of the original study data. Removal of identifiers may also preclude replication of study analyses or results by other investigators.[11] Thus, again the need for balance arises: to develop means of maintaining confidentiality and protecting against unwarranted or illegitimate disclosure, while providing for methods to maintain scientific validity and rigor.

Individual Harm and Group Harm

In general, participation in epidemiologic research does not involve risk of physical harm (although recent trials, such as that involving the Women's Health Initiative, and the Tamoxifen chemoprevention trial, raise this possibility).

Nonetheless, harm can occur to individuals or groups who participate in epidemiologic research if private or identifiable information is disclosed, not only in the form of invasion of privacy but also in the forms of social ostracism, embarrassment, discrimination, or loss of employment or housing. Protection against harm in epidemiologic studies has largely been addressed by requiring review by IRBs, which assess the risks and benefits and restrict those studies in which the risk outweighs the benefit, and by obtaining the informed consent of study participants. With regard to assessing risks and benefits, it is imperative that researchers and IRBs explore all potential risks both to individuals and to groups. In the context of informed consent, it is important that researchers avoid overstating claims that the research is for the good of society and that no harm will come to participants. In recent decades, many courts have set standards of informed consent on the basis of what a reasonable person would want to know, rather than on the basis of what a physician or researcher believes is necessary,[19] which moves in the direction of circumventing the paternalistic or altruistic approach.

On the other hand, researchers often take concerns about confidentiality very seriously but are impeded in their efforts to protect privacy by legal actions (usually taken by parties with financial interests at stake).[7,11,18,20,21] In the public arena, the individual's right to privacy and the public's right to know about government-supported research are often simultaneously vigorously supported and in apparent conflict.[22] This tension becomes evident in investigations of epidemics involving vulnerable populations, as in the AIDS epidemic,[23] and specific measures have been taken in AIDS surveillance offices to maintain confidentiality and protect privacy.[24,25] Alternatives to using individually identifiable information in research, such as anonymous or alias or randomized responses,[26] may be considered.[27] (In randomized response techniques, by the roll of a die the respondent answers either a sensitive or an unrelated, innocuous question, without giving the interviewer any indication of which is being answered. When this process is used with large groups, the proportion of individuals in the sample who answered the sensitive question and the proportion who answered in the affirmative or negative can be known without individually identifiable responses.) However, these alternative methods are cumbersome and generally make validation of information very difficult, if not impossible.

Proper handling of sensitive information also must be considered, and what constitutes sensitive information differs among individuals and populations. Sensitive information linked to an individual, or injurious information about groups, can lead to discrimination by employers, educators, landlords, or insurers, or can result in stigmatization, embarrassment, shame, or a sense of being wronged.[28,29] Respect for privacy reflects respect for the individual and the information that he or she provides, as well as respect for the dignity of groups. When disclosure of sensitive information may put a group at risk of adverse treatment or criticism, communication of study results must be carefully planned and executed to avoid such harms. The duty of researchers to communicate results must be balanced against the potential harm of disclosure, which in turn must be mitigated by interpretations that protect the dignity of those at risk, while at the same time maintaining scientific integrity.

Modern Confidentiality and Privacy Concerns

Many of the privacy and confidentiality issues described in the foregoing pages have been addressed in epidemiologic research for decades. However, with the rapidly paced introduction in the past two decades of new technologies to transmit and store large amounts of information, it is appropriate to examine some of the new issues these innovations raise. The special circumstances created by molecular epidemiology and occupational research, by the increasing diversity in our population, and by health care reform also need to be considered.

The Information Technology Age

In the past, much of the information used in epidemiologic studies originated in paper form and was coded and entered for computerized manipulation. Thus, provisions for maintaining confidentiality and protecting privacy included storing identifiers separately from the paper or electronic versions of the information generated,[15] keeping written records in locked cabinets, password-protecting computerized data files, stressing to research staff the importance of maintaining confidentiality and requiring pledges from them to do so, and furnishing only aggregated data in published analyses.[5] All of these provisions still apply, but emerging technologies present new challenges to maintaining privacy and confidentiality in epidemiologic studies, such as: security of paperless record stores, unauthorized decoding of passwords and the threat of computer "viruses," sharing and transmitting data through networks and modems, printer and facsimile machine outputs lying unattended in common and unsecured areas, and the implications of privatization of the Internet.

Many technological advances have been made in the interests of reducing paper files, transmitting data faster, making information available to more users, and storing larger amounts of information. Medical offices and hospital record rooms, for example, are moving to paperless records,[30] stored on personal computer or network hard drives with tape or diskette back-up. To provide privacy protection for such records, some have suggested removing identifiers,[30] or restricting access to use only for clinical purposes and obtaining prior patient consent for any other uses.[31] Technological advances raise many of the same concerns for epidemiologic research that were discussed in the context of written records two decades ago.[32] Data files are readily available to multiple users over networks, sometimes requiring password entry (perhaps at multiple levels) or data encryption,[15] and can be transmitted quickly in electronic forms through networks or in hard-copy version through facsimilies, which are often located in unsupervised public areas.[33] Thus, the opportunities for breaches of confidentiality are numerous. In addition, with probable privatization of the Internet, invasion of privacy and breach of confidentiality by unauthorized parties become possible, as do threats to validity of data by means of interception or censorship by the private parties with ownership shares of the Internet.

In the face of multiple opportunities to breach confidentiality, additional precautions must be taken to protect the privacy of study participants and the confidentiality of the information they have entrusted to investigators. These measures include: transmission over networks only of study data without individual identifiers, and with appropriate password and encryption protection; transmission of data over networks only when the sending and receiving ends are monitored by authorized study personnel; storage of data on nonnetworked devices with appropriate password and encryption protection; transmission by facsimilie and to printers in unsecured areas only when authorized study personnel are monitoring receipt of the output; prominent marking of printed material as confidential; and regular emphasis on and retraining of study personnel in confidentiality procedures.

In addition, new legislation may be required to regulate use of the Internet for research purposes in order to prevent interception, intrusion, and censorship by private owners or unauthorized parties. It is also important to note that the motivation for the passage of the 1974 Privacy Protection Act was to curb invasion of privacy by the government. In this context, the government's development of the encryption systems for future use in monitoring and decoding information on telephones, computers and digital set up boxes for interactive television, and all data that will be transmitted on the Internet[34] and on the National Information Infrastructure (the "information superhighway") may indicate the need for further regulation to guard against government intrusion. Such measures may be necessary not only to maintain confidentiality and protect privacy, but also to preserve the integrity of scientific data. It is interesting to note the potential for abuse of these new, unregulated government-sponsored technologies have in light of the concern over lack of uniform privacy protection standards for health data (see below). As William J. Brennan, associate justice of the Supreme Court, stated seventeen years ago, "The central storage and easy accessibility of computerized data vastly increase the potential for abuse of that information, and I am not prepared to say that future developments will not demonstrate the necessity of some curb on such technology."[4]

Health Care Reform

Interest in health care reform is such that some type of modifications seems inevitable in the near future. This reform is likely to raise a number of privacy and confidentiality issues relevant to epidemiologic research. Comprehensive, uniform privacy standards, rules, and guidelines for health care information may well need to be established.[35] Some proposals, such as the now-failed American Health Security Act of 1993, suggest that every citizen have a health security card and a unique identifier to register for and receive health services.[36] The identifier could be used to establish links among health records in order to monitor quality, allow for the analysis of patterns of care and patient outcomes, and conduct scientific research. In Canada and the Scandinavian countries, much valuable epidemiologic research has been made feasible by the ability to link health data sets through unique identifier systems.

The Social Security Number (SSN) has been proposed for use as this identifier in the United States, although the SSN is not always a unique identifier, and verification of identities would be costly. Privacy risks also exist with the use of the SSN for this purpose, since the SSN is also used by debt collectors, commercial interests, the Internal Revenue Service, other federal and state agencies, law enforcement, employers, and schools. Furthermore, with the enhanced computer linkages discussed earlier, the opportunities are almost limitless for intrusion into and interception of private health data linked to the SSN by any number of unauthorized persons. Such intrusions and interceptions would be possible with any identifier, but use of the SSN raises the specter of health information being linked to other private information, such as employment history, income, assets, and debtors.

The Supreme Court has ruled that when the government collects health information, it must have standards and procedures for protecting privacy. However, this does not necessarily pertain to nongovernment researchers, and the rule has been inconsistently applied. Even the Privacy Protection Act of 1974 does not regulate nongovernmental institutions. Some states have amended their constitutions or passed laws to protect medical information against breaches of privacy by government agencies, but not necessarily by nongovernmental parties and not necessarily for electronic records.[36] Some states also have specific provisions for protecting privacy regarding specific illnesses such as AIDS or sexually transmitted diseases, but not for most other conditions. In addition, some states codify the physicians' obligation to protect patient privacy, but do not extend these legal obligations to other health care providers, insurers, or researchers. Thus, given the likelihood of adoption of an individual identifier for a reformed health care system and the widespread national (and international) accessibility of computerized information, the need exists for institution of uniform national (rather than state-by-state) privacy protection regulations. Such measures should also provide for access to individually identifiable health information by legitimate health researchers. General informed consent standards should be adopted as well for future disclosure under an individual-identifier system.

Research to Decode DNA

The mysteries encoded in DNA are rapidly being unlocked and revealed, both by the Human Genome Project and by government-sponsored research designed to identify the genetic codes that place individuals at high risk for conditions such as breast cancer, colon cancer, and hypercholesterolemia. The major goals of such efforts are largely beneficent, that is, to identify individuals at high risk to enable early detection through screening and, with the development of newly emerging gene therapies, to intervene and prevent serious disease or its sequelae. However, accompanying these potential benefits are many of the potential social and legal risks already discussed—such as discrimination, stigmatization, embarrassment, and ostracization—as more is learned about individuals from DNA samples. Thus, suggestions have been made for the regulation of DNA data banks,[2] including: public disclosure of intent to establish the data bank; justification for establishing the data bank; prior written authorization and approval that set forth the uses and purpose of the data bank; guaranteed individual access to the sample and the records, and the right to request return or destruction of the sample; protection of individuals' rights to correct inaccurate information; strict security measures and protection against unauthorized or third-party access; and notification of new information with potential impacts on health. These proposals warrant discussion, before regulations are put in place, by all interested parties—researchers, potential subjects (and their spouses, heirs, or family members), government representatives, medical care providers, criminal justice officers, employers, employees, and ethicists—in order to advance research, provide appropriate access by authorized investigators, and protect against unauthorized intrusion.

Occupational Epidemiologic Studies

Although the study of occupationally related disease dates back centuries, this area of epidemiologic investigation has grown in recent decades with the introduction into the workplace of thousands of untested chemicals and physical agents (such as microwaves, electromagnetic fields, hazardous equipment, and ergonomic stressors). Perhaps in no other area of epidemiologic investigation is the tension between paternalism, autonomy, and privacy protection more salient.

Administrative occupational standards in which priority is given to limiting worker exposure are examples of beneficent though paternalistic approaches.

Indeed, some industry representatives have criticized selected occupational health policies on this basis, maintaining that workers ought to take some responsibility for their own protection.[9] However, it is not uncommon for industry management to assume they know what is best for their workers. Such actions abrogate workers' autonomy by not permitting them to decide about participation for themselves.

Similar areas of concern arise in occupational epidemiologic studies. First, individual rights to autonomy should not be sacrificed with regard to informed consent. The decision to participate in a study should be the worker's, not the employer's. As in all epidemiologic studies, workers should be informed of potential risks and benefits of participation, and assured that individually identifiable information will not be provided to employers and that participation (or nonparticipation) in a study will not affect their jobs. Obtaining informed consent to participate in studies in the occupational setting may be difficult owing to workplace pressures to produce and because of cultural diversity in the workplace[37] (see below). Nonetheless, it is unethical to conduct occupational or other epidemiologic studies that involve individual contact with worker participants without obtaining their informed consent.[38]

The potential for job discrimination, job loss, and wage loss if individual information is not adequately protected poses severe hazards. These risks are particularly pronounced in occupational studies of hazards to reproductive health. Title VII of the Civil Rights Act as amended in 1978 and recent Supreme Court rulings, such as the *Johnson Controls* decision in 1991, have codified as discriminatory and illegal the practice of transferring women of childbearing age to lower paying jobs, or of firing pregnant workers or workers who might become pregnant.[39] Further, employers have an obligation under the Occupational Safety and Health Act to take affirmative steps to remove or mitigate workplace risks, rather than to transfer such responsibility to employees.

Nonetheless, epidemiologists and other researchers have to maintain extraordinary vigilance in protecting the privacy and confidentiality of sensitive information, such as fertility and other medical data, about workers in occupational studies. Providing this protection may well create tension between the investigator's ethical responsibility and the industry's or company's paternalistic approach. It may also conflict with desires on the part of industry, government, insurers, or individuals to know specific health hazards associated with specific workplace activities or exposures.[40] Often an observed excess risk of an adverse health outcome, even if statistically significant, may involve only a few workers. In this instance, subgroup analyses of specific work sites or activities may be desired to enhance the specificity of knowledge regarding the exposure-outcome relationship. The public's right to know about specific plants or occupational activities that put workers at risk must then be balanced against both the individual's right to privacy and confidentiality of study information, and the scientific validity of disaggregating data into subgroups of such small sample size as to be uninterpretable. Further, if reanalysis of data is desired by industry, government, or individual (for example, worker or advocacy) interests, it may be possible for individual privacy or confidentiality to be breached, as when data on confounding variables such as age, gender, and race/ethnicity are provided. Careful consideration of these potential breaches must be undertaken before data are furnished and reanalysis permitted.

Federal courts have generally ruled that researchers are entitled to protect the privacy of study participants against third-party intrusions, but this principle is not uniformly applied.[21,36] When privacy issues arise in occupational epidemiologic studies, they often place the principles of justice, respect for autonomy, beneficence, and nonmaleficence in conflict. Disclosing information on plant-specific or job-activity-specific risks, particularly for rare outcomes, may jeopardize privacy and confidentiality of workers who provided the information, particularly if further separation of these outcomes by age and/or gender and/or race/ethnicity are considered. As is true in all epidemiologic research, individual privacy protection and maintenance of confidentiality in occupational studies must be weighed against potential societal benefits.

Population Diversity

As the population of the United States has increased and as technology has improved, the population has grown more diverse in the racial and ethnic groups represented. Contact with and investigation of populations outside the United States have also increased. In addition, federal research policy now mandates the inclusion of minority populations in health-related research. As a result, investigations here and abroad must address the acceptability and appropriateness of the language for informed consent statements and data collection instruments for various population subgroups. Moreover, the special sensitivities of such populations must be considered with regard to privacy, confidentiality, and specific information obtained in epidemiologic studies.[40] Because respect for personal autonomy is the ethical foundation for privacy, the principle of respect for autonomy applies. Appropriate phrasing is required to ensure that local or cultural customs and traditions relevant to consent and privacy protection are respected.[38] Illiteracy or cultural differences do not equate with inability to make informed decisions.[28]

Respect for autonomy and nonmaleficence for all populations also means that researchers must be sensitive to information or activities that must be kept confidential and that stigmatize, harm, or demean in these different cultural settings.[28] Each study should develop protections for the dignity of all study participants, and pay particular attention to vulnerable groups such as those who are poor, compromised, restricted, persecuted, or in other ways disenfranchised. The payment of money or other inducements to participate in research must be carefully examined and balanced—appropriate remuneration for the time and inconvenience required must be considered, as well as the need to avoid reimbursement that would be coercive.[28] At the same time, while investigators must respect the customs, practices, and sensitivities of different cultural and ethnic groups, these too must be balanced so as not to override concerns related to justice and autonomy.

Conclusion

Epidemiologic research by its nature involves invasion of privacy when investigators examine personal aspects of the lives of study participants. Such invasion is normally disclosed and justified in informed consent statements and in review of study protocols by institutional review boards. The conduct of epidemiologic and biomedical research should be guided by the principles delineated by Beauchamp and Childress of beneficence, nonmaleficence, respect for autonomy, and justice.[10] Often these principles highlight the need to balance conflicting interests or rights: privacy rights and rights of health researchers to health information, individual rights and societal benefits, paternalism and autonomy, potential risks and benefits, and the conduct of valid research versus unaddressed public health questions. In addition, information of public health importance can be so sensitive to an individual or a group that the potential can be substantial for discrimination, stigmatization, embarrassment, shame, or harm. Thus, researchers must protect the integrity of scientific research but also the autonomy of the individuals and groups they study. Further, modern advances in technology, in unlocking the secrets of the genetic code, in increasing cultural and ethnic diversity in study populations, in studying workplace hazards, and in health care reform present new challenges to maintaining confidentiality, protecting privacy, and balancing risks and benefits. Some of these challenges have not yet been addressed in the form of privacy regulations. Uniform standards to protect privacy and confidentiality in the face of modern challenges need to be considered as epidemiologic and other biomedical research progresses into the twenty-first century.

References

1. McKechnie, J. L., ed. *Webster's New Universal Unabridged Dictionary*. New York: Simon and Schuster, 1983: 382.
2. Annas, G. J. "Privacy Rules for DNA Databanks: Protecting Coded 'Future Diaries,' " *Journal of the American Medical Association* 270 (1993): 2346–350.

3. Capron, A. M. "Protection of Research Subjects: Do Special Rules Apply in Epidemiology?" *Law, Medicine and Health Care* 19 (1991): 184–90.

4. Privacy Protection Study Commission. *Personal Privacy in an Information Society.* Washington, D.C.: U.S. Government Printing Office, 1977.

5. Gordis, L., Gold, E., and Seltser, R. "Privacy Protection in Epidemiologic and Medical Research: A Challenge and a Responsibility," *American Journal of Epidemiology* 105 (1977): 163–68.

6. Clarke, E. A., Darlington, G., Holowaty, E. J., Kreiger, N., Marrett, L. D., McLaughlin, J., Parkes, R., Sloan, M., and Theis, E. "Confidentiality and Research," *Canadian Medical Association Journal* 149 (1993): 792–93.

7. Holder, A. R. "The Biomedical Researcher and Subpoenas: Judicial Protection of Confidential Medical Data," *American Journal of Law and Medicine* 12 (1986): 405–21.

8. Berger, P. M., and Stallones, R. A. "Legal Liability and Epidemiologic Research," *American Journal of Epidemiology* 106 (1977): 177–83.

9. Lappé, M. "Ethics and Public Health." In *Public Health and Preventive Medicine*, ed. J. M. Last. 12th ed. Norwalk: Appleton-Century Crofts, 1986: 1867–77.

10. Beauchamp, T. L. and Childress, J. T. *Principles of Biomedical Ethics.* 4th ed. New York: Oxford University Press, 1994.

11. Brennan, T. A. "Ethics of Confidentiality: The Special Case of Quality Assurance Research," *Clinical Research* 38 (1990): 551–57.

12. Curran, W. J. "The Privacy Protection Report and Epidemiological Research," *American Journal of Public Health* 68 (1978): 173.

13. Applebaum, P. S., Roth, L. H., and Detre, T. "Researchers' Access to Patient Records: An Analysis of the Ethical Problems," *Clinical Research* 32 (1984): 399–403.

14. Waters, W. E. "Ethics and Epidemiological Research," *International Journal of Epidemiology* 14 (1985): 48–51.

15. Nehls, G. J., Hayes, C. G., and Nelson, W. C. "Confidentiality and Freedom of Information for Epidemiological Data in Governmental Research," *Environmental Research* 25 (1981): 160–66.

16. Wallace Jr., R. J. "Privacy and the Use of Data in Epidemiology." In *Ethical Issues in Social Science Research*, ed. T. L. Beauchamp, R. R. Faden, R. J. Wallace Jr., and L. R. Walters. Baltimore: The Johns Hopkins University Press, 1982: 274–91.

17. Baldwin, J. A., Leff, J., and Wing, J. K. "Confidentiality of Psychiatric Data in Medical Information Systems," *British Journal of Psychiatry* 128 (1976): 417–27.

18. Curran, W. J. "Protecting Confidentiality in Epidemiologic Investigations by the Centers for Disease Control," *New England Journal of Medicine* 314 (1986): 1027–28.

19. Meisel, A. and Kabrick, A. "Informed Consent to Medical Treatment: An Analysis of Recent Legislation," *University of Pittsburgh Law Review* 41 (1980): 407–40.

20. Marwick, C. "Epidemiologists Strive to Maintain Confidentiality of Some Health Data," *Journal of the American Medical Association* 252 (1984): 2377–383.

21. Marshall, E. "Court Orders 'Sharing' of Data," *Science* 261 (1993): 284–86.

22. McMichael, A. J. "Ethics in Epidemiological Research," *Medical Journal of Australia* 142 (1985):537–38.

23. Levine, C. "Has AIDS Changed the Ethics of Human Subjects Research?" *Law, Medicine and Health Care* 16 (1988): 167–73.

24. Bayer, R., Lumey, L. H., and Wan, L. "The American, British and Dutch Responses

to Unlinked Anonymous HIV Seroprevalence Studies: An International Comparison," *Law, Medicine and Health Care* 19 (1991): 222–30.

25. Torres, C. G., Turner, M. E., Harkess, J. R., and Istre, G. R. "Security Measures for AIDS and HIV," *American Journal of Public Health* 81 (1991): 210–11.

26. Warner, L. "Randomized Response," *Journal of the American Statistical Association* 60 (1965): 63–69.

27. Boruch, R. F. "Methods for Resolving Privacy Problems in Social Research." In *Ethical Issues in Social Science Research*, ed. T. L. Beauchamp, R. R. Faden, R. J. Wallace Jr., and L. R. Walters. Baltimore: The Johns Hopkins University Press, 1982: 292–314.

28. Gostin, L. "Ethical Principles for the Conduct of Human Subject Research: Population-based Research and Ethics," *Law, Medicine and Health Care* 19 (1991): 191–201.

29. McCarthy, C. R. and Porter, J. P. "Confidentiality: The Protection of Personal Data in Epidemiological and Clinical Research Trials," *Law, Medicine and Health Care* 19 (1991): 238–41.

30. Andrews, G. and Wilkins, G. E. J. "Privacy and the Computerised Medical Record," *Medical Journal of Australia* 157 (1992): 223–25.

31. Anonymous. "Confidentiality, Records, and Computers," *British Medical Journal* 1 (1979): 698–99.

32. Gordis, L. and Gold, E. "Privacy, Confidentiality, and the Use of Medical Records in Research," *Science* 207 (1980): 153–56.

33. Lawler, P. G. "Faxes Breach Confidentiality," *British Medical Journal* 307 (1993): 1426.

34. Krol, E. *The Whole Internet: Users Guide and Catalogue.* Sebastopol, CA: Nutshell Handbook O'Reilly Associates, 1992.

35. White House Domestic Policy Council. *The President's Security Plan: The Clinton Blueprint.* New York: Times Books, 1993: 136–38.

36. Gostin, L., Turek-Brezina, J., Powers, M., Kosloff, R., Faden, R., and Steinauer, D. D. "Privacy and Security of Personal Information in a New Health Care System," *Journal of the American Medical Association* 270 (1993): 2487–493.

37. Saiki, C. L., Green, R., Gold, E. B., and Schenker, M. B. "Communication Issues in a Multi-Component Study of Semiconductor Employees," *American Journal of Industrial Medicine* (1995).

38. Hessel, P. A. and Fourie, P. B. "Ethical Issues in Epidemiological Research," *South African Medical Journal* 72 (1987): 863–65.

39. Saiki, C. L., Gold, E. B., and Schenker, M. B. "Workplace Policy on Hazards to Reproductive Health," *Occupational Medicine: State of the Art Reviews* 9 (1994): 541–50.

40. Council for International Organizations of Medical Sciences. "International Guidelines for Ethical Review of Epidemiological Studies," *Law, Medicine and Health Care* 19 (1991): 247–58.

III

BALANCING RISKS AND BENEFITS

7

Ethically Optimized Study Designs in Epidemiology

STEVEN S. COUGHLIN

It is generally accepted that epidemiologists have a moral and professional obligation to maximize the potential benefits of research studies to subjects and to society, and to minimize potential risks, as enjoined by the ethical principle of beneficence (which requires providing benefits and balancing benefits against risks).[1,2] An example is found in the rule that the confidentiality of medical information used in epidemiologic research should be conscientiously protected.[3–5] Other moral obligations of epidemiologists are grounded in the principle of nonmaleficence (which requires that we avoid causing harm), a principle that has often been associated with the Hippocratic injunction to do no harm.[1,2] For example, in carrying out studies in developing countries, there is a need to avoid harming members of impoverished communities by diverting scarce health personnel from their routine activities in order to meet the needs of research studies.[6]

Epidemiologists also have an obligation to respect the autonomy of individuals who participate in research studies, a principle that underlies rules of privacy and confidentiality. These rules should not be violated without first obtaining the informed consent of research subjects, except under exceptional circumstances when that is impractical and the potential risks and benefits of the research have been carefully considered by an independent review committee.[1,5] A further obligation is the need to ensure that the burdens and benefits of epidemiologic research are distributed in an equitable fashion, which is grounded in ethical principles of justice (principles of fairness in the distribution of benefits and risks).[2] Recent efforts to ensure that women and minorities are adequately represented in research projects funded by the National Institutes of Health (NIH) are well-known examples.[7]

As these illustrations suggest, the ethical principles of beneficence, non-maleficence, justice, and respect for autonomy provide a useful framework through which many moral problems surrounding epidemiology may be understood and evaluated. Careful specification of these principles helps ensure that the welfare and rights of individuals and communities are protected in the design and conduct of epidemiologic studies.[2,8] Further, these principles are reflected in ethics guidelines for epidemiologists such as those developed by the Council of International Organizations of Medical Sciences, the International Epidemiological Association, and the Industrial Epidemiology Forum.[9-11] Specific understandings of these principles have contributed to the presentation below, although this chapter does not overtly reflect or engage in the kind of philosophical argument that analyzes or specifies these principles.

With the possible exceptions of safeguards for protecting privacy and the confidentiality of information obtained from research subjects (topics considered by Ellen Gold in Chapter 6 and Tom Beauchamp in Chapter 2), there has been inadequate discussion of specific recommendations that can be made to ensure that epidemiologic studies are ethically optimized. In the discussion that follows, specific improvements in design are considered that may minimize potential risks to subjects and groups of individuals, maximize the potential benefits of nonexperimental epidemiologic studies to individuals and to communities, and increase the likelihood that the benefits and burdens of the research are distributed in an equitable fashion. The adequacy of provisions for obtaining the informed consent of subjects is also considered below in relation to epidemiologic study design.

Minimizing Risks to Subjects and Groups

The risks posed by nonexperimental epidemiologic studies are often minor compared with those that must be considered in designing and conducting clinical trials and other experimental studies, and surveys of respondents' attitudes toward participation in epidemiologic studies have suggested that many subjects find the experience personally satisfying or rewarding.[12,13] Nevertheless, individuals participating in epidemiologic research may be burdened by a loss of privacy (the condition of limited access to a person), by time spent completing interviews and undergoing examinations, and, in some instances, by adverse psychological effects such as anxiety and grief.[2] Other potential risks in some studies include stigmatization and loss of employment or insurance resulting from breaches of confidentiality, although these are admittedly remote possibilities in most epidemiologic studies because of regulatory controls and organizational safeguards.[14] On the other hand, there may be risks to privacy from disclosure of confidential information to third parties in the institution at which the research is conducted.

Measures that may be taken to protect individual privacy and ensure the confidentiality of health information are well known to most epidemiologists and are considered elsewhere in this volume. Examples of such protective measures include keeping records with personal identifiers under lock and key, limiting access to confidential records to selected members of the research team on a need-to-know basis, discarding personal identifiers from data collection forms and computer files whenever feasible, reinforcing the importance of maintaining the confidentiality of health records at the time of orientation and training sessions for study personnel, and various safeguards to prevent data from publication or release in a form that would allow previously undisclosed identifications to occur.[3,4,15]

In addition to measures for ensuring confidentiality, a number of other specific steps may be taken to minimize risks to individuals participating in epidemiologic studies. For example, potential risks and inconveniences may be reduced by restricting the length of questionnaires and examinations, by allowing maximum flexibility in scheduling interviews, and by not scheduling interviews on holidays or anniversary dates that are likely to enhance grief.[2] It may also be important to postpone surrogate interviews until after a reasonable amount of time has elapsed since the death of the respective family member.

Although such protective measures may currently be widely practiced in epidemiology, exceptions do occur. For example, in a recent case-control study of sudden infant death syndrome in two counties in Great Britain, the parents of deceased infants were interviewed within seventy-two hours of their child's death, most within twenty-four hours.[16] The parents were questioned about social factors, family history, maternal medical history, details of the pregnancy and perinatal period, and the infant's medical history, including recent signs of illness, feeding habits, precise details of the infant's last sleep, the position in which he or she had been found, the precise quantity and nature of the clothing and bedding, whether the baby had been swaddled, whether the bedclothes had been over the baby's head when found, how the baby's room was heated, and the time the heat had been on.[16]

It might be argued that any psychological distress resulting from participation in studies of this nature is likely to be relatively minor and transitory, and that the potential social benefits of the study must also be taken into account. Further, the reliability and validity of some information obtained from next-of-kin are likely to decline over time. However, principles such as beneficence and respect for autonomy suggest that recently bereaved individuals and other vulnerable populations are deserving of protective measures such as obtaining epidemiologic data in a less intrusive fashion. The principle of nonmaleficence, which demands the noninfliction of harmful acts that may impair health or lead to mental distress,[1,2] also bears on this discussion, although nonmaleficence—when conjoined with the principle of beneficence—does not preclude balancing potential harms against potential benefits. Other case-control studies of sudden infant death syndrome have examined similar associations while delaying interviews of bereaved parents until six weeks after their baby's death.[17] Prospective studies of high-risk infants have also been undertaken,[18] and such studies may avoid the need to interview recently bereaved parents.

Further, epidemiologic research can inadvertently pose potential risks to groups of individuals and communities. For example, populations defined by race, ethnicity, or lifestyle may suffer stigmatization or lowered self-image following the publication and dissemination of research findings that create or reinforce negative cultural stereotypes.[19,20] A related problem is the way in which epidemiologic research findings are presented to the public by the media. For example, shortly after the initial reports of an epidemic of respiratory distress syndrome among adults residing in the American Southwest, the *Washington Post* reported concern among Navajos that inaccurate talk of a "Navajo flu" or more broadly "Navajo illness" might lead to unfounded efforts to segregate or otherwise avoid contact with that community.[21] Disparaging information about a group can result in harms such as discrimination in employment, housing, or insurance, or lowered self-esteem and racial or cultural pride.[19] The problems encountered by Haitians following their identification as a risk group for HIV infection and AIDS further illustrates such harms.[20,22]

As an example of how risks to groups can be minimized through improvements in study design, epidemiologic studies of racial or ethnic differences in disease associations or risk factors can sometimes adopt more scientifically valid measures of income, educational attainment, and other indices of socioeconomic status. This enables investigators to better examine whether socioeconomic factors or other exposures account for any observed associations with race or ethnicity.[23] In some instances it may also be desirable to apply statistical methods that correct risk estimates for imprecision in the assessment of exposure variables,[24,25] or to present findings using alternative classifications such as socioeconomic status or geographic locality, particularly when this is both scientifically and ethically defensible.[20,26]

The identification of disparities in health or the maldistribution of health services across groups defined by race, ethnicity, or lifestyle can serve as a basis for health planning and policy making, and thereby contribute to improving the health of those who are less well-off in society.[27] For example, recent surveys have suggested that lesbians may be more likely to develop cancer of the breast as a result of reproductive decisions, increased alcohol consumption and body mass, underutilization of screening mammography, and attitudinal, economic, and provider-related barriers to receiving quality preventive health care.[28–30]

However, few surveys of lesbian health practices have been undertaken and scientifically valid data with which to plan cancer-control interventions in this possible high-risk population are currently limited. Indeed, data from the SEER cancer registries[31] and most large scale epidemiologic studies of women do not include information about sexual orientation. In view of the overwhelming evidence that sexual orientation and sexual activity are related to health behaviors and risk factors for disease, the absence of questions about sexual orientation in many large-scale epidemiologic studies seems unscientific. Of course, decisions to include questions about sexual orientation must take into account concerns about privacy and the *possible* impact of such questions on response rates.

It is also conceivable that studies of the health practices of lesbians could inadvertently contribute to discrimination against them in employment or insurance. For example, some early surveys of lesbians were limited to small samples of women encountered at bars—an approach likely to introduce study bias and to convey negative impressions of this diverse community of women. Such risks can be minimized by ensuring that scientifically valid sampling procedures are used, similar to those applied in more recent surveys of lesbians and gay men.[28,32] In some studies it may also be helpful to include questions about sexual activity rather than orientation, to avoid the need for labeling respondents according to their sexual orientation. For example, in interviews that are planned as part of the Womens' Health Initiative, the respondents will be asked if they are sexually active, and, if so, whether they prefer having sex with men, women, or both.

As this example illustrates, epidemiologic research does not take place in a social vacuum, and areas of ethical conflict may exist between the need to obtain scientifically accurate information about the health of population subgroups and the moral imperative to avoid harming populations that already suffer stigmatization and discrimination from the mainstream societies in which they live.[22] Many competing values may have moral weight equal to or greater than the freedom of scientific inquiry. Which values should be put in the balance and how much weight they should be given will often be controversial, and a consensus may not emerge. Nonetheless, recent developments, such as the decision by the NIH Office of Research on Womens' Health to designate lesbians as a population subgroup worthy of further study, suggest that these challenges can be met and that positive professional and social change is possible.

Maximizing Benefits to Subjects and to Society

The potential benefits of epidemiologic research are largely societal in nature and include obtaining new information about the etiology and preventive aspects of important causes of morbidity and mortality, and about the utilization of health care resources.[27,33] The promotion of the common good is an important aspect of beneficence and provides strong justification for many public health measures.[1,34] The individuals who participate in epidemiologic studies often derive no direct benefit from the research.[33] Nevertheless, opportunities sometimes exist for subjects to receive some personal gain from participation, such as when previously unrecognized disease is detected during health examinations and individuals are then referred to private physicians for treatment.[27]

Many other opportunities exist to maximize the usefulness of epidemiologic studies. One example concerns a multicenter epidemiologic study of HIV infection in women in the Washington, DC, area as part of the Womens' Interagency Health Study. The investigators agreed to provide previously unavailable data on the health care utilization of these women to the DC Commission of Public Health (with personal identifiers removed) in order to assist the DC Office of AIDS Activities in planning and allocating future AIDS services to area residents. In view of the cost of many epidemiologic studies and the increasing scarcity of health care resources, such opportunities to extend the potential benefits of epidemiologic research to local communities should not be overlooked.

A further area in which improvements in study design may maximize the potential benefits of epidemiologic research is the combination of large observational studies with randomized clinical trials. For example, in a recent multicenter study by the Vaginal Infections and Prematurity Study Group, an observational study of *Ureaplasm urealyticum* among 8287 pregnant women was followed by a randomized controlled trial of erythromycin for the prevention of premature delivery.[35] Women who had *Ureaplasm urealyticum* discovered at the screening visit and who were eligible for enrollment in the trial were asked to sign a second informed consent form.[35] By combining observational and randomized study designs, the investigators increased the likelihood that some subjects would benefit from the research, and decreased the likelihood that clinical practice would be inappropriately changed due to the dissemination of observational research findings alone. Although the results of the trial were negative, this study still illustrates how the efficiency of epidemiologic research can be enhanced—and potential benefits to subjects and to society maximized—through the use of innovative study designs.

As part of some population-based studies, it may be feasible to plan some health care advantage to the community following completion of the study, such as epidemiologic research that leads to the establishment of a local disease registry or the training of members of a community in basic methods of population research.[20] The indirect benefits of epidemiologic studies may be particularly important to consider in planning and carrying out studies in socioeconomically disadvantaged populations, such as research conducted in some developing countries and in some urban and rural areas of the United States.

A Just Distribution of the Burdens and Benefits of Research

The historical practice of relying on patients treated at inner-city teaching hospitals for experimental studies has been criticized since low-income minority patients tend to be overrepresented and therefore bear a greater share of the potential risks of the research.[2] Such arguments call upon an egalitarian theory of justice, which implies that each person or class of persons in society should receive an equal share of the potential burdens (and benefits) of health research.[1,2]

Different considerations may apply to epidemiologic research because the risks associated with nonexperimental studies are relatively minor, and the evidence suggests that, if anything, minority populations were often underrepresented in epidemiologic studies until recently.[2] Nonetheless, the potential risks and benefits of epidemiologic studies to different social subgroups are partly determined by the nature of the study population and the generalizability of the findings. To cite one example, most studies of factors associated with survival in idiopathic dilated cardiomyopathy have been carried out in predominately Caucasian patient populations, and little is known about racial differences in mortality in idiopathic dilated cardiomyopathy.[36] Results from the Washington, DC, Dilated Cardiomyopathy Study suggest that black patients with this poorly understood cause of heart failure may be substantially more likely to die in the first two years following diagnosis than are whites, even after other prognostic factors are taken into account.[36]

Studies that draw their subjects from an entire community or geographic locality, such as the Bogalusa Heart Study[37] and the Atherosclerosis Risk in Communities (ARIC) Study,[38] are more likely to distribute the benefits and burdens of research equitably than are studies of relatively selected patient populations. Studies that select subjects from several hospitals in an attempt to reduce referral bias and increase the representativeness of the sample may also treat subjects more equitably.[2]

Obtaining Informed Consent

A further consideration in designing epidemiologic studies is the adequacy of provisions for obtaining the informed consent of subjects. (A topic considered by Tom Beauchamp in Chapter 2 and Marjorie Shultz in Chapter 5.) The ability of individuals to reach an autonomous decision regarding their participation in a research study may be diminished during hospitalization as a result of illness, medication, or dependence on physicians and other health care providers.[1] For example, patients may feel obligated to participate in the study or feel that their relationship with their physician will be harmed by failure to participate, even when their right to withhold consent is carefully explained to them. Individuals are therefore motivated to do something they wish not to do, even though the agent seeking a consent does not intend to so manipulate them.

In light of this observation, when feasible it is both prudent and respectful to request consent from potential subjects only after they have recovered or have been discharged from the hospital. The informed consent of individuals who have already been released from the hospital may be obtained verbally over the telephone, or by mailing a consent form to their home address. The informed consent of nonhospitalized individuals may also be obtained in person if the interviews are conducted in the subjects' homes. A further issue is whether the quality of informed consent obtained by telephone or in person is likely to be increased or diminished. Written informed consent statements are easier for some individuals to understand, but not for others.

A case-control study of breast cancer and exposure to hair dye carried out at the Sloan-Kettering Cancer Center illustrates several issues about informed consent.[39] The subjects were interviewed in the hospital during the course of their admission. Interviews were obtained from 89.5 percent of 448 eligible cases, and 92.6 percent of 675 eligible hospital controls who were primarily women with other types of cancer.[39] The most common reasons for refusal given by nonconsenting subjects were "too many interviews," "too ill," and "don't like to be interviewed." The scientific validity of this study was enhanced by showing the subjects photographs of hair dye brands as a memory aid. If the subjects had been interviewed at home following discharge, by telephone or in person, their ability to reach an autonomous decision regarding participation in the study might have been improved, but alternative interviewing procedures of this nature might have been overly costly or logistically difficult, and telephone interviews would not have allowed for the use of visual aids. Nevertheless, in other case-control studies of this association, the subjects have been interviewed at home by telephone. For example, in a study by Nasca et al.,[40] telephone interviews were obtained for 96 percent (118 of 123) of the breast cancer patients. The response rate among the potential neighborhood controls identified by random digit dialing was only 77 percent, however.

Some patients have such limited knowledge bases that communication about alien or novel situations is difficult, especially if new concepts are involved.[41] But even under difficult circumstances, enhanced understanding and adequate decisions are often possible. Successful communication of unfamiliar and specialized information to laypersons can often be accomplished by drawing analogies between new information and more ordinary events familiar to them.[41] Similarly, professionals can express risks in both numeric and nonnumeric probabilities, while helping the patient or subject to assign meanings to the probabilities through comparison with more familiar risks and prior experiences.

At the same time, obligations to obtain informed consent have limits. Consent requirements imposed by institutions should be formulated and evaluated against a range of social and institutional considerations. The preservation of autonomous choice is the first, but certainly not the only, consideration. For example, a patient's need for education and counseling in order to achieve a substantial understanding of a medical situation must be balanced against the interests of other patients and of society in maintaining a productive and efficient health care system.[41] Accordingly, institutional policies must consider what is fair and reasonable to require of health care professionals and researchers, what the effect would be of alternative consent requirements on efficiency and effectiveness in the advancement of science, and—particularly in medical care—what the effect of the requirements would be on the welfare of patients. Nowhere is this problem better illustrated than in epidemiology.

Summary and Conclusions

This chapter has considered a number of steps that may be taken in the design and conduct of nonexperimental epidemiologic studies to ensure that such studies are ethically optimized. Although some of the suggested improvements in design exceed the minimum regulatory requirements of many institutional review boards and funding agencies, they are still morally defensible and, at the very least, consistent with morally justified procedures in the conduct of epidemiologic science. Of course, some of the recommended study design elements may already be commonly practiced in epidemiology, or may not be practical in all research settings.

This overview has drawn from a rich and growing literature on the ethics of epidemiologic research, including recently formulated ethics guidelines for epidemiologists.[9–11] Nevertheless, existing guidelines do not provide an exhaustive set of specific recommendations for how epidemiologists can best meet their obligations to identify solutions to important public health problems, while protecting their subjects from morally inappropriate requests and methods.

References

1. Beauchamp, T. L. and Childress, J. F. *Principles of Biomedical Ethics.* 4th ed. New York: Oxford University Press, 1994.
2. Coughlin, S. S. and Beauchamp, T. L. "Ethics, Scientific Validity, and the Design of Epidemiologic Studies," *Epidemiology* 3 (1992): 343–47.
3. Gordis, L., Gold, E., and Seltser, R. "Privacy Protection in Epidemiologic and Medical Research: A Challenge and a Responsibility," *American Journal of Epidemiology* 105 (1977): 163–68.

4. Kelsey, J. L. "Privacy and Confidentiality in Epidemiological Research Involving Patients," *IRB* 3 (1981): 1–4.

5. McCarthy, C. R. and Porter, J. P. "Confidentiality: The Protection of Personal Data in Epidemiological and Clinical Research Trials," *Law, Medicine and Health Care* 19 (1991): 238–41.

6. Council for International Organizations of Medical Sciences. "International Guidelines for Ethical Review of Epidemiological Studies," *Law, Medicine and Health Care* 19 (1991): 247–58; and *International Ethical Guidelines for Biomedical Research*. Geneva: CIOMS, 1993.

7. U.S. House of Representatives, Committee on Energy and Commerce. *National Institutes of Health Revitalization Amendments of 1990* (report 101-869). Washington, DC: U.S. Government Printing Office, 1990.

8. Weed, D. L. and Coughlin, S. S. "Ethics in Cancer Prevention and Control." In *Cancer Prevention and Control*, ed. P. Greenwald, B. F. Kramer, and D. L. Weed. New York: Marcel-Dekker, 1995.

9. Bankowski, Z., Bryant, J. H., and Last, J. M., eds. *Ethics and Epidemiology: International Guidelines. Proceedings of the XXVth Council for International Organizations of Medical Sciences Conference*, November 7–9, 1990 (Summary of Discussions). Geneva: CIOMS, 1991: 137–42.

10. American Public Health Association. *Epidemiology Section Newsletter* (winter 1990).

11. Beauchamp, T. L., Cook, R. R., Fayerweather, W. E., et al. "Ethical Guidelines for Epidemiologists," *Journal of Clinical Epidemiology* 44 (1991): 151S–69S.

12. Savitz, D. A., Hamman, R. F., Grace, C., et al. "Respondents' Attitudes Regarding Participation in an Epidemiologic Study," *American Journal of Epidemiology* 123 (1986): 362–66.

13. Taylor, C., Trowbridge, P., and Chilvers, C. "Stress and Cancer Surveys: Attitudes of Participants in a Case-Control Study," *Journal of Epidemiology and Community Health* 45 (1991): 317–20.

14. Greenwald, R. A., Ryan, M. K., and Mulvihill, J. E., eds. *Human Subjects Research: A Handbook for Institutional Review Boards*. New York: Plenum Press, 1982.

15. NCHS Staff Manual on Confidentiality. Hyattsville, MD: National Center for Health Statistics, 1984: DHHS Publ. No. (PHS) 84–1244.

16. Fleming, P. J., Gilbert, R., Azaz, Y., et al. "Interaction Between Bedding and Sleeping Position in the Sudden Infant Death Syndrome: A Population Based Case-Control Study," *British Medical Journal* 301 (1990): 85–89.

17. Ponsonby, A. L., Dwyer, T., Gibbons, L. E., et al. "Thermal Environment and Sudden Infant Death Syndrome: Case-Control Study," *British Medical Journal* 304 (1992): 277–82.

18. Gibbons, L. E., Ponsonby, A. L., and Dwyer, T. "A Comparison of Prospective and Retrospective Responses on Sudden Infant Death Syndrome by Case and Control Mothers," *American Journal of Epidemiology* 137 (1993): 654–59.

19. Gostin, L. "Ethical Principles for the Conduct of Human Subject Research: Population-based Research and Ethics," *Law, Medicine and Health Care* 19 (1991): 191–201.

20. Dickens, B. M. "Issues in Preparing Ethical Guidelines for Epidemiological Studies," *Law, Medicine and Health Care* 19 (1991): 175–83.

21. "Navajos Fight Fear With Faith. Tribe Shadowed by Strange Illness," *The Washington Post* (June 3, 1993): 1.

22. Dickens, B. M., Gostin, L., and Levine, R. J. "Research on Human Populations: National and International Ethical Guidelines," *Law, Medicine and Health Care* 19 (1991): 157–61.

23. Stern, M. P. "Invited Commentary: Do Risk Factors Explain Ethnic Differences in Type II Diabetes?" *American Journal of Epidemiology* 137 (1993): 733–34.

24. Kleinbaum, D. G., Kupper, L. L., and Morgenstern, H. *Epidemiologic Research Principles and Quantitative Methods.* Belmont, CA: Lifetime Learning Publications, 1982: 220–41.

25. Rosner, B., Spiegelman, D., and Willett, W. C. "Correction of Logistic Regression Relative Risk Estimates and Confidence Intervals for Measurement Error: The Case of Multiple Covariates Measured With Error," *American Journal of Epidemiology* 132 (1990): 734–45.

26. Freeman, H. "Race, Poverty, and Cancer" (Editorial), *Journal of the National Cancer Institute* 83 (1991): 551–57.

27. Last, J. M. "Epidemiology and Ethics," *Law, Medicine and Health Care* 19 (1991): 166–74.

28. Bradford, J. and Ryan, C. "The National Lesbian Health Care Survey," National Gay and Lesbian Health Foundation, 1987.

29. Bybee, D. "Michigan Lesbian Health Survey," Michigan Organization for Human Rights, 1990.

30. Warchafsky, L. "Lesbian Health Needs Assessment," Los Angeles Gay and Lesbian Community Services Center, 1992.

31. Miller, B. A., Ries, L. A. G., Hankey, B. F., et al. Cancer Statistics Review, 1973–1989. Bethesda: National Cancer Institute, 1992: NIH Publ. No. 92–2789.

32. Munoz, A., Schrager, L. K., Bacellar, H., et al. "Trends in the Incidence of Outcomes Defining Acquired Immunodeficiency Syndrome (AIDS) in the Multicenter AIDS Cohort Study: 1985–1991," *American Journal of Epidemiology* 137 (1993): 423–438.

33. Gordis, L. "Ethical and Professional Issues in the Changing Practice of Epidemiology," *Journal of Clinical Epidemiology* 44 (1991): 9S–13S.

34. Lappé, M. "Ethics and Public Health." In *Public Health and Preventive Medicine*, ed. J. M. Last. 12th ed. Norwalk: Appleton-Century-Crofts, 1986: 1867–877.

35. Eschenbach, D. A., Nugent, R. P., Rao, A. V., et al. "A Randomized Placebo-Controlled Trial of Erythromycin for the Treatment of *Ureaplasma urealyticum* to Prevent Premature Delivery," *American Journal of Obstetrics and Gynecology* 164 (1991): 734–42.

36. Coughlin, S. S., Gottdiener, J. S., Baughman, K. L., et al. "Black-White Differences in Mortality in Idiopathic Dilated Cardiomyopathy: The Washington, DC Dilated Cardiomyopathy Study," *Journal of the National Medical Association* 86 (1994): 583–91.

37. Berenson, G. S., Srinivasan, S. R., Webber, L. S., et al. "Cardiovascular Risk in Early Life: The Bogalusa Heart Study." In *Current Concepts*. Kalamazoo: The Upjohn Co., 1991.

38. The ARIC Investigators. "The Atherosclerosis Risk in Communities (ARIC) Study: Design and Objectives," *American Journal of Epidemiology* 129 (1989): 687–702.

39. Wynder, E. L. and Goodman, M. "Epidemiology of Breast Cancer and Hair Dyes," *Journal of the National Cancer Institute* 71 (1983): 481–88.

40. Nasca, P. C., Lawrence, C. E., Greenwald, P., et al. "Relationship of Hair Dye Use, Benign Breast Disease, and Breast Cancer," *Journal of the National Cancer Institute* 64 (1980): 23–28.

41. Faden, R. R., and Beauchamp, T. L. *A History and Theory of Informed Consent.* New York: Oxford University Press, 1986.

8

Ethical Issues in the Design and Conduct of Community-Based Intervention Studies

KAREN GLANZ
BARBARA K. RIMER
CARYN LERMAN

Community-based health intervention research includes studies with several different labels: community health research, public health intervention research, behavioral research, health education research, and health promotion research, to name a few. Our definition of community-based intervention research and our use of this term and of the others just mentioned are intentionally broad. For the purposes of this chapter, *community-based intervention research* is research that investigates strategies designed to improve the health of individuals and populations through: promoting wider adoption of efficacious prevention, early detection, and therapeutic practices; increasing availability of and reducing barriers to services and conditions that influence healthful behaviors and optimal health status; and reducing distress or improving psychological status through information, counseling, or services. The term includes research on defined populations in a wide variety of settings (work sites, health care environments, communities, schools, the consumer marketplace) and covers the continuum from disease prevention and health promotion to treatment, rehabilitation, and long term care. Excluded from this broad category of intervention research are: (1) clinical trials that test the efficacy of medical, such as pharmaceutical and surgical, techniques for treating disease or improving health status (even though these studies may be conducted partly in community settings); and (2) laboratory studies of human cognitions and behaviors.

156

Much community health research has been stimulated by the relatively high prevalence of chronic diseases such as heart disease, cancer, and stroke. Two areas of chronic disease control have dominated. The first concerns individuals' lifestyle behaviors such as smoking, diet, and physical activity in order to prevent disease onset. The second is aimed at screening, early detection, and management of risk factors for chronic illness. The latter include, as major areas of research interest, hypertension and cholesterol screening and management, and early detection of breast cancer through mammography screening.[1] Additional areas of interest in community health research are injury prevention, AIDS prevention, and prevention or cessation of drug and alcohol abuse.[2] An emerging area of community-based research involves genetic testing for disease susceptibility and targeted prevention and surveillance strategies for persons identified as at increased risk.[3] All of these facets have broad social, ethical, and economic implications for communities beyond their impact on individuals.

Health research in community settings has increased and diversified dramatically over the past twenty-five years.[4,5] Much of the heightened interest in community-based health interventions has been stimulated by the epidemiologic transition from infectious diseases to chronic diseases as the leading causes of death, rapidly escalating health care costs, and data linking individual behaviors to increased risks of morbidity and mortality.[2,6] Advances in medicine have also drawn attention to the need for compliance with proven therapeutic regimens, participation in screening programs for early detection of disease, and appropriate use of health services. With these advances have come new dilemmas involving ethics, law, and the study of human behavior.[3,7,8]

During this period, public and professional concern about ethical issues in research have grown. New ethical considerations have arisen out of new health-related problems addressed by research and the expanded repertoire of methods used by community health researchers.[9,10] In addition, fresh information about past research (such as government-sponsored radiation experiments) has created a need for reevaluation of the ethical safeguards for some earlier studies. The challenge of balancing scientific rigor and dynamic community research environments with ethical concerns has become increasingly complex. Until recently, most attention on research ethics focused on clinical research involving individuals; the emergence of ethical examinations of preventive, educational, and health promotion research in communities are new developments.

In this chapter, we will examine the scientific and methodological foundations of community-based intervention research that bear on ethical concerns. We will also discuss key ethical issues related to research participants, researcher-community partnerships, professional relationships, and relationships of science to society.

Methodological Foundations and Ethical Concerns in Community-Based Intervention Research

To introduce this analysis of ethical issues in community-based health intervention research, we briefly describe the range of methodologies currently being used in these studies. The field is marked by tremendous diversity of intervention strategies, data collection techniques, and study designs.

Intervention Strategies

Contemporary community interventions may address health problems at one or more levels. They may focus on intrapersonal factors (such as knowledge, attitudes, affect, behavior), interpersonal processes (family relationships, social support, social networks), institutional factors (organizations and their norms or rules), community factors, and public policy.[11] Interventions generally labeled as health promotion include not only educational and motivational strategies but also organizational change, policy directives, laws, economic supports, and community activation.[6,12] For example, community smoking cessation programs have used a variety of strategies, such as behavior modification, mass media, citizen participation, delivery of self-help materials in clinic settings and by mail, involvement of health professionals to identify smokers at high risk, and regulations.[6,13] Programs aimed at increasing utilization of mammography screening and Pap tests among women have also used diverse approaches: printed and audiovisual materials, risk assessment and counseling, cost reduction in order to increase access, outreach and advocacy, telephone counseling, education of community physicians, and modification of delivery system factors.[3,14,15]

Methods of Data Collection

The unit of observation in community-based intervention research may be individuals, groups, organizations, or communities defined by geographic or political boundaries. In addition, data may be collected both directly (by asking questions or conducting observations) and indirectly (by reviewing records and archival sources). The most common methods for collecting data from individuals is survey research using self-administered written questionnaires, and telephone or face-to-face interviews. However, the use of medical, educational, occupationally related, or public record sources may allow for unobtrusive measurement[16] and verification of self-reported data.[17] Linkages are increasingly being made to large data bases such as Medicare files. Biologic information such as blood pressure, serum cholesterol levels, body weight, saliva thiocyanate levels, and urinary cotinine may serve as proxy measures of behavior, indicators of risk level, or biomarkers of behavior change.

At the organizational or community level, information about social structure and the physical environment may be obtained by interviews with key informants or by direct observation. Indirect indicators of enforcement of tobacco control policies or of consumers' eating patterns might include measures such as environmental tobacco smoke or cafeteria plate waste. These data collection approaches raise ethical concerns about informed consent and privacy.

Community intervention researchers are increasingly using qualitative methods to obtain greater in-depth information and to learn about unique cultural groups or high-risk populations.[4] These methods, including focus group testing and open-ended questions, can also be combined with more quantitative measurement techniques to provide a more valid and complete assessment of the process and impact of programs.[6,18]

Study Designs

Randomized, controlled experiments remain the most rigorous type of design in community-based intervention research. However, numerous variations on randomized controlled trials also are employed because of practical and political considerations. In some studies, randomization to different conditions is performed on a unit larger than the individual, for example, by family, organization, or community. This technique is both practical and necessary if the intervention involves organizational change, and where social networks would create excessive contamination between groups (such as cross-talk within the organization), which happens in many worksite health intervention studies. However, when an "organization" is the unit of randomization, individuals may be prevented from having a personal choice about whether to participate, even though community-level interventions may be directed at these individuals. It can be difficult or ethically unacceptable to recruit groups or individuals to participate in research without their receiving the benefit of some type of intervention or service. Hence, additional design variations may include using modified control groups (such as usual care or "wait-list" control), before-after comparisons, and combinations of cohort and cross-sectional samples for evaluation.

Multidisciplinary Health Research Traditions and Ethical Concerns

Community-based intervention research is, by its nature, eclectic and multidisciplinary. It is at the intersection of biological and social sciences, and draws on theoretical perspectives and tools from such diverse disciplines as psychology, sociology, anthropology, communications, statistics, biology, epidemiology, and marketing.[6] An important consequence of this multidisciplinary approach is that the codes and standards of conduct, as well as the identification and resolution of ethical dilemmas, may differ among the professional groups involved. The field of psychology, with its emphasis on individual behavior, has been the basis for many of the research studies and methodologies used; sociological approaches are particularly important to the study of organizations and social structures within communities. Many of the classic experimental studies that are central to the body of knowledge about human behavior come from social psychology.[19–22]

There is substantial overlap between public health and medicine in health interventions carried out in clinical settings. However, the ethical issues most salient for community-based intervention research are derived *primarily* from the traditions of the social sciences and public health sciences, and only secondarily from biomedical ethics. A fundamental distinction has been made between public health ethics and traditional medical ethics.[23] Medical ethics has its roots in the rights and respect due to *individuals* in their relationships with physicians and other health care professionals,[24] whereas many view the central concern of public health ethics to be maximizing the welfare of the community or society as a whole.[23,25–28]

Ethical conflicts arise in public health interventions when decisions must be made about distribution of health resources and priorities for programs, and when standards for health protection are at stake. They also occur in public health research due to concerns about privacy, autonomy, and the equitable treatment of individuals.[23,26] In both medicine and public health, conflicting obligations sometimes result from the dual roles of practitioner and scientist.[29] From a public health viewpoint, the decisions about community research design depend primarily on three factors: (1) the anticipated kind and extent of benefit to the public (and to scientific knowledge); (2) the degree of restriction of individual rights needed to achieve the benefit; and (3) the ultimate distribution of both benefits and harms attendant to participation.[23,26] An emphasis on community or public health has been used to justify many health and safety measures that are considered by some to be paternalistic (such as smoking and seat belt regulations).[30] While it seldom warrants entirely sacrificing individual rights and liberty for the public good, this perspective of public health as an independent value does influence decisions regarding the design and conduct of community health intervention research.

Ethical Issues Related to Research Participants

Ethical considerations impose both restrictions and responsibilities on researchers. Ethical guidelines are vital to community intervention research for ensuring that studies have worthwhile goals, and for protecting the welfare of research participants.[21] Several ethical principles in community-based intervention research relate to research participants. They are respect for autonomy, benefi-cence, justice, privacy, and deception.[10,20,21,31,32]

Respect for Autonomy

Autonomy involves respect for the rights of individuals and groups to make de-cisions for themselves.[23,31] In public health, it is accepted that there are some situations in which autonomy must be limited to protect the public's health, such as the requirement of immunization against communicable diseases. But in most cases, autonomy is a central ethical principle and infringements of autonomy are not permitted.

In community-based intervention research, autonomy is relevant to informed consent, voluntary data provision and participation in interventions, and the avoidance of excessive incentives to research subjects. Elements of disclosure in informed consent include a statement of purpose, explanation of procedures, and a description of discomforts and risks that participants might experience. Standards of disclosure may be community standards or "reasonable person" stan-dards.[33] One ethical question regarding informed consent concerns how specific a researcher needs to be about the study aims when the provision of complete information may lead to refusal to participate, behavior change in anticipation of the study, or biased responses to measures used for evaluation.[33,34] For example, it is common for consent forms in randomized trials to state that participants will be assigned to one of two different educational programs, without reference to specific differences or the fact that one program is enhanced in some manner. Decisions regarding disclosure should be carefully weighed so that information is as complete as possible without severely compromising research methodology.

In some cases, consent for participation is obtained for the group, organiza-tion, or community, and individuals become research subjects without their ex-plicit consent by virtue of belonging to a group or community. However, they do have free choice about participating in terms of whether they answer question-naires or interviews. But when information contained in medical records or em-ployment records on factors such as absenteeism are used as measures, individ-ual subjects may not be approached directly for their permission. While these assessment methods may seem ethically questionable, they are justified in some circumstances—for example, when research questions are significant and the risk of harm to subjects is very low. However, minorities and other underserved pop-ulations may be especially sensitive to being unwitting participants in studies conducted by outsiders.

Program or study attrition compromises the internal and external validity of community-based intervention studies. Attrition is the result of inherent attitudi-nal and behavioral differences between individuals who remain and those who drop out (for example, those who are achieving less benefit may be more likely to stop participating). In one community cardiovascular disease prevention program for ninety-six black families in a Southwestern city, program attendance fell to less than half after only four weeks of the fourteen-week program because of time conflicts and dislike for assigned dietary self-monitoring forms.[35] This posed insurmountable problems to the analysis and interpretation of the program's impact.

One strategy to ameliorate the problem of attrition is the use of incentives such as small gifts, payment to participants, or reimbursement for inconvenience or travel expenses. Although this practice may be perceived as manipulative or restrictive of freedom to participate, such compensation usually does not compromise ethics if incentives are not so strong that they involve unreasonable enticements or so threatening that they constitute coercion. It is even possible that, for some groups, small incentives covering extra expenses of time or effort involved in the research enable a broader base of subjects to take part. While this example should probably be regarded more as a reimbursement than an incentive, different institutional review boards (IRBs) may take different stands on the issue of incentives. Some view any compensation as potentially coercive or manipulative. It is true that a small incentive for a poor person could have a very different impact than the same incentive offered to a middle-class person.

Beneficence

The principle of beneficence requires that researchers minimize risk to participants and maximize the potential benefits both to subjects and to society.[23,31] Potential risks to participants include psychological distress resulting from participation in research, physical danger, respondent burden, and loss of self-esteem and anxiety.[21] In chemoprevention studies, there may be a risk of toxicity associated with the drugs. The potential *benefits* of the research should be judged in terms of the direct benefits to participants, as well as the prospects that the findings will improve the health of subjects and other populations. One group of people should not be expected to bear risks unduly; this is especially true for socioeconomically disadvantaged and underserved populations.

The concept of beneficence has unique implications for community-based intervention research in which screening or health examinations might result in the identification of cases of at-risk individuals. In such situations, provisions should be made for referral and follow-up to protect the welfare of the participants, even if it means violating the study plan. It is unethical to recruit people into screening programs without providing for treatment should abnormalities be detected. Investigators are responsible for minimizing risks to participants by examining the potential risks, and ensuring that they are unlikely, minor, and reversible if they occur. Measures for the early detection of any physical or psychological harm should also be taken.[10,21]

Another aspect of beneficence in the conduct of health-related research is the obligation to act on important interim findings. For example, in interim analysis a fear-arousing communication designed to motivate smoking cessation could be found to generate significant anxiety but minimal behavior change. Under such circumstances, it would be unethical to continue the trial without substantive modification to the intervention. Alternatively, interim analysis could show a clear improvement in psychosocial or medical outcomes associated with an intervention. It would then be reasonable to offer the more effective strategy to all communities or participants. Accordingly, the research questions could focus on identifying subgroups that are most or least likely to benefit, based on individual or organizational factors.

Justice

Ethical principles of justice concern the fair distribution of benefits and burdens of research among potential subjects.[31] According to utilitarian theories of justice, the public benefit should be maximized, potentially justifying a relaxing of the requirement that *each subject* receive an equal share of the benefits from the research.[23,32] Justice-based considerations are relevant to selection of research subjects and communities, and to the randomization of subjects or organizations to receive different interventions. For example, investigators may need to make a choice between studying those most in need of an intervention and selecting a more accessible or practical population. Further, such decisions may be imposed by funding sources, such as government research set-asides that are available only for studying selected minority groups or women.

Meeting requirements of distributive justice is particularly challenging when individuals or communities are assigned to control or comparison groups that do not receive the intervention hypothesized to be most effective. The control subjects may be burdened disproportionately by data collection requirements without receiving the benefit of services or resources. The use of a minimal intervention such as an educational brochure may provide an acceptable level of benefit. Another common solution to this problem is the use of a delayed control group design, wherein the intervention is delivered during a later phase of the study, or the intervention materials or services found most effective are provided to all groups at the conclusion of the investigation. However, this solution may require special resources that are not always available as part of research funding. Investigators should take particular care not to make promises they cannot keep. It is easy to offer delayed treatment and much harder to follow through.

Privacy

Conflicts can arise in research when individuals' rights to privacy are at odds with the goal of obtaining important knowledge to improve public health.[15] Dimensions of privacy include the sensitivity of the information, the setting being observed, and plans for dissemination of information and its linkage to the subjects' names.[13,36] Anonymity may not always be possible in cohort studies or record linkages; however, privacy should be protected to the extent feasible, names should be destroyed as soon as they are no longer needed, and the anonymity of individuals should always be protected in reporting results. Early community health research often involved fictitious names for communities being studied, though the location of community research is not usually concealed today. Currently, the use of pseudonyms for research communities may not accomplish its intended purpose because of the difficulty of maintaining secrecy. An alternative is to use a general description of the study's locale (such as region or state).

Community-based intervention studies that use indirect data collection methods and unobtrusive measures preserve privacy if they collect data at the level of the environment, community, or other aggregate unit of observation, and if individuals cannot be identified. These may be appropriate techniques for testing environmental interventions. For example, Ellison et al.[37,38] worked with food service personnel to reduce fat and sodium in two New England boarding schools. Their analysis of meal consumption patterns (without surveying students) showed that the foods eaten by students contained significantly less sodium and saturated fat, even without including a direct education component for the students.

Guarantees of confidentiality are essential when research is being conducted in settings where individuals work, receive services, and are educated. For example, employees may be reluctant to respond to surveys or obtain screening in worksite health promotion research if they have reason to believe that management will have access to personal information that they provide.[39] Employer access to risk-factor information could lead to job discrimination and loss of insurance. Although the provision of aggregate data to cooperating organizations is usually justified, it is critical that participants be protected from any possible repercussions of disclosure of information they provide in the course of research. In community studies, investigators should avoid situations in which workers are collecting personal data on people they know. This is a very real issue since researchers are increasingly hiring indigenous community workers.

It is also ethically unjustified to study very private areas of life without subjects' prior permission. Research on AIDS risk reduction, as well as studies of other sexually transmitted diseases and unwanted pregnancy, which are potentially of great public health importance, often entail highly personal questions about sexual practices and drug use.[40,41] Participants must be assured of strict confidentiality, and any exceptions should be disclosed. One way to address this problem is to study repeated cross-sectional samples of anonymous subjects rather than identifiable cohorts.[42] However, sampling error could lead to erroneous interpretations of behavior change.

Deception

Several types of deception are of particular concern in community-based intervention research, for example, deliberately lying about the research purpose[10] and manipulation of information within an intervention involving persuasive communication.[27] Deception is common in laboratory-based psychological experiments, and in fact was used in some classic social psychological investigations such as Milgram's[43] studies of obedience to authority and Asch's experiments on the effects of social pressure.[10,21,22] In community-based studies of human behavior, deception has been used in studies of response to simulated emergencies, discrimination, and prejudice.[21]

Deceptive research methods have revealed important problems in health care that would probably not have been acknowledged if deception was totally avoided. Rosenhan[44] used eight "pseudopatients" to study the treatment of patients confined to mental health facilities and to evaluate how normal behavior would be interpreted by hospital staff following a psychiatric diagnosis. He found that the treatment environment and diagnostic labels were more powerful determinants of staff treatment of patients than their actual behavior. In another classic health care experiment that seems questionable by today's standards, Hofling et al.[45] examined how nurses' unquestioning compliance with physicians' orders to administer medication improperly (excessive dose, ordered by telephone in violation of hospital policy) might endanger patients' well-being. To avoid actual harm, the experiment was halted as soon as it was clear that the nurse (subject) was about to comply with the order.

Reasons for deception in community research include methodological control, external validity, and pragmatic factors (time, money, access).[21] Alternatives such as forewarning participants, role-playing, or use of hypothetical scenarios are methodologically weaker. A review of studies using deception found that, while it is considered "morally wrong," research participants often say that they enjoy it, do not mind being deceived, and do not mind the invasion of their privacy.[22] As long as potential risks and harms are minimal and the protocol has been approved by an independent review committee, short-term deception is sometimes a justifiable technique for answering important research questions than cannot otherwise be resolved.[10,21,22]

Ethical Issues Related to Researcher-Community Partnerships

Effective community health interventions and intervention research call for scientists to collaborate with organizations that provide access to information about research subjects, and that serve as gatekeepers for both interventions and data collection. Partnerships between scientists and these organizations present challenging and often neglected problems regarding researchers' responsibilities to the subjects and to the intermediary organizations or communities. These concerns include the extent of collaboration, the risk of raising false hopes when preparing grant proposals, the timing of feedback, and the responsibility to leave the community with increased capacity or services. The primary emphasis in community-based intervention research should not be on the advancement of researchers' careers or advances in scientific knowledge alone, but on the individuals and communities whose health is at stake.

Partnership Models: A Continuum

At every stage of planning and conducting community-based research, investigators should engage in partnership activities. There is a broad continuum of possible degrees of involvement and interaction with communities. In the extreme case of minimal involvement, researchers may recruit participants through mass media advertising, and seek cooperation from existing organizations only to increase the appearance of legitimacy in their outreach efforts to research subjects and to avoid conflicts with established service providers. Another model of minimal involvement is merely to obtain the cooperation of a government or health agency, hospitals, schools, employers, or insurers to provide demographic data and information about how to contact potential participants, and to deliver intervention materials and messages through telephone or mail channels.

Organizational or community participation will be greater when interventions are aimed at engaging social networks or influencing organizational factors to promote desirable health practices or conditions. Such "citizen participation" often occurs through structures such as task forces or advisory boards.[46] It has been suggested that the most effective vehicle for community health intervention is through some type of group or defined community, so that the advantages of social support and organizational power can be invoked.[47,48] Members of the community possess the greatest expertise in the social meanings of health and disease, and can help researchers identify relevant issues, implement acceptable interventions, and gather meaningful data.[48] Investigators who collaborate actively with community or organization members may use a participatory research, or action research, approach. Key characteristics of action research are that it is collaborative, an interactive learning process, an empowering process, and that it develops competencies in the community.[5,48-52] Research models that involve greater community participation and collaboration have the greatest potential to provide long-term benefit to research participants and the community, and demand special efforts by researchers to fulfill their ethical responsibilities to community partners.

Responsibility to Community Partners

Before actively beginning a research project, investigators should initiate working relationships with community partners, obtain their input on proposed methods and operational issues, and sometimes conduct preliminary studies to assure funding agencies that the proposed study is feasible. This work must often be completed with few financial resources, and requires time, effort, and emotional investment from both scientists and community members. In promoting enthusiasm and cooperation, scientists risk raising false hopes in the community about funding or other future resources. While there is no easy solution to this dilemma, it is incumbent on investigators to be open about the possibility of not receiving funding, and to make contingency plans for pursuing alternative resources to carry out some or all of the proposed project.

The research process involves substantially delayed gratification. As was noted in a recent journal article, "The community is more likely to be attracted to the potential of using research to solve immediate social problems, whereas the researcher and the funding agency seek information for scientific or policy purposes."[48] It is essential that researchers recognize these value differences, and seek methods to increase the mutual benefits of cooperation and decrease the possibility of exploitation of community members. This give and take may assume many forms: informal provision of valuable expertise to the community, contributions of technological resources or advocacy that yield immediate results, and offers to collect data of special interest to community leaders (but marginal to the research focus) as part of a project. What is of value to the community will vary based on the unique situation of the research institution and community needs; creative and energetic efforts may be necessary to develop a mutually satisfying relationship.

In experimental research, communities assigned to "control" conditions may experience the burden of participation without receiving tangible benefits. Two solutions are possible: use of comparison groups that receive a different type of treatment, unlikely to influence the main research outcome variable; and provision of delayed treatment. The former method can sometimes enhance the rigor of the research design by controlling for attention and support. For example, in a study of interventions to increase use of cancer screening services among older adults through programs in senior centers, the control groups received a physical activity program of equal length that participants viewed as valuable.[53] The latter approach can be incorporated into a study design that evaluates short-term versus long-term impact of the main intervention.

The responsibility to build the community's capacity for self-help and to leave something after conclusion of the formal study has made program institutionalization a central issue in intervention research. Three large community cardiovascular disease prevention projects in Minnesota, Rhode Island, and California funded by the National Heart, Lung, and Blood Institute all struggled to design interventions that would outlive their funding periods.[54] Successful institutionalization needs to begin early in the program and must involve the community partners in defining objectives, identifying resources, and implementing worthwhile activities that build on the experience of the research project. It also requires foresight of the researchers to ensure that some resources can be devoted to this purpose.[55] In one cancer prevention and early detection trial now in progress, the investigators obtained a commitment from their institution to leave the data systems and computer equipment behind at the end of the study period.

A final ethical responsibility of scientists to their community partners is providing them with feedback about research results.[56] The community should not be the last to learn the findings through subsequent publications or media attention. Interim feedback about results may be important to help participants feel that data are not being collected and "thrown into a black hole," and to see some concrete product of their participation. It may be necessary to take precautions about who receives this information when feedback could threaten the integrity of the research design. Scientists also need to make special efforts to provide feedback about research findings in terms that the community can understand and use for their own future development.

High-Risk and Vulnerable Communities

Due to the disproportionate burden of disease, disability, and premature death, we will continue to see increased intervention research directed to minority and low-income communities.[2,48] Despite the structures and policies of organized science that are designed to protect study populations, many members of minority and disadvantaged communities have a fundamental distrust of scientific research directed at them.[48] This is particularly evident in African-American communities, where the abuses of the Tuskegee Syphilis Study (which documented the natural history of syphilis among poor black men in Alabama) have led to distrust of health researchers.[57] Formal safeguards and reforms in research may be insufficient to change fears of exploitation and harm in vulnerable communities. The needs of communities to protect the welfare of their members and ensure long-term social benefit make community partnerships and sensitivity in design, conduct, and interpretation of findings especially important. Studies using deception are often particularly ill-advised in such communities because of the potential for loss of trust. In order to produce high-quality, ethical research in minority and disadvantaged communities, both researchers and funding institutions need to overcome objections that community partnerships introduce unacceptable biases and compromise methodological rigor.[58]

Reconciling Multiple Scientific and Community Agendas

Even when the value of collaboration between researchers and the communities they study is recognized, many complicated pragmatic issues remain. As Dressler[58] notes, "Negotiating such a collaborative relationship can demand skills, time, and patience perhaps notably lacking in some academic researchers. Similarly, the willingness of the community to enter into the long-term pact required for high-quality research can oftentimes necessitate a difficult shift in values." With their different agendas, researchers have legitimate reasons for conflicts with community leaders and residents. However, the multiple needs of scientists and the participating communities can be reconciled with attention to three areas: (1) increased sensitivity to ethnic and cultural habits and norms; (2) instilling trust through better communication, particularly with minorities; and (3) understanding and addressing important problems of communities such as crowding, crime, poverty, racism, and violence.[59]

Ethical Issues Related to Professional Relations and Interactions

Researchers who conduct community-based intervention research interact not only with research participants and their communities, but also with other professionals both within and outside their primary disciplines, and with the public at large. Relationships with funding sources, professional colleagues, practitioners, and legislators and policy makers may present ethical dilemmas related to conflict of interest, as well as biased conduct and interpretation of research and the use of research findings in practice and policy arenas. Professional codes of ethics include attention to principles of research integrity in areas of funding, relationships, data use, and communication.[10,20,21,60]

Funding and Sponsorship

When financial support for research comes from sources with economic interests or image investments in the research outcomes, this may produce a conflict of interest for the scientist. Private sector sources may place explicit restrictions on design, measurement, or disclosure of findings that are ethically untenable for researchers.[60,61] Implicit restrictions may also exist because researchers do not want to alienate their funding sources. Employers that contribute resources to research could demand a degree of control over the study design or data that interferes with protection of the welfare of individual research participants.[36] An additional constraint might relate to restrictive funding from agencies or organizations with disease-specific missions. Such a constraint may prevent researchers from engaging in community partnerships that help define the problem and intervention methods. For example, a corporate conglomerate that manages tobacco interests might disallow programs that include tobacco-control efforts. In another scenario, a health maintenance organization could threaten to discontinue a collaboration if researchers publish data that reveal inadequate diagnostic follow-up of abnormal screening results.

In each of these situations, investigators must carefully review both the legal and implied contract involved in accepting funding or sponsorship for community-based intervention research. If such matters are discussed before the research begins, it may be possible to identify ways to satisfy the sponsor while adhering to professional ethical standards.

Publications and Reporting

While scientific fraud in publications of community health intervention research is relatively rare, several instances have occurred in which ethics in reporting research findings warranted attention. Researchers have an obligation to disclose their findings honestly, which also carries the responsibility to acknowledge weaknesses or shortcomings of study design or implementation.[10,21,60] When a study yields important yet serendipitous findings, they should be presented as such, not as a priori hypotheses.[10] In addition, negative findings as well as positive findings should be published to advance scientific knowledge and avoid bias in the professional literature.[10] Community intervention studies that have negative results often provide secondary gains in scientific understanding and other indirect benefits.

Researchers may be reluctant to report that an intervention in which they have invested large amounts of time and money was ineffective or minimally effective, and some journals have a bias against accepting articles about such studies. A related issue has to do with overstating conclusions based on statistical significance versus "clinical" or practical significance, and the need to address both types of significance.[62] To cite an example, the Stanford Five City Project was a multimillion-dollar study that compared treatment and control cities for changes in risk-factor knowledge, blood pressure, cholesterol, smoking, weight, and resting pulse using representative cohort and cross-sectional surveys at baseline and three later occasions.[63] The intervention was a five-year comprehensive program based on social learning theory, community organization principles, a communication-behavior change model, and social marketing. Community residents participating in the experiment were exposed to about twenty-six hours of education.[64] After thirty to sixty-four months of intervention, statistically significant net reductions in community averages were observed that favored treatment, for plasma cholesterol (2%) and blood pressure (4%). Weight gain occurred in all communities, but there was a trend toward greater weight gain in the control communities.[64]

These results might be interpreted as either impressive, given that they were distributed across large, diverse populations, or as disappointing, given the major financial investment in research and intervention activities. Findings from such large, long-term community demonstration evaluation projects have the potential to lead to conclusions regarding the possible impact of preventive and health-promoting interventions, and pose complex reporting problems for the investigators. Analysis of the cost-effectiveness of intervention programs can yield information about the overall value of a particular approach.

Use of Research Findings to Influence Practice and Policy

The results of community-based health intervention studies are often complex, making it difficult to draw succinct conclusions with clear implications for public health, health care, and public policy.[6,27] Nevertheless, the topics and problems studied are frequently of considerable significance, and the conduct of this type of applied research carries a responsibility to provide guidance to practitioners and policy makers regarding the implications of investigations. The researcher's challenge in communicating with practitioners relates to deciding when to speak out (if all the data are not available to provide definitive answers); whether to provide unsupported opinions on research-related issues about which the investigator has strong personal feelings; and the degree of certainty of expression that is justified.[21,65]

Additional ethical concerns involve managing interactions with "allies" (other scientists, journalists, policy makers, legislators) who present science-based opinions in inaccurate or exaggerated ways. The press may try to push the researcher to make more of her findings than warranted in order to craft an exciting story. Further, the scientist must decide when the evidence justifies communicating directly with the general public, in a manner that makes a dramatic and compelling case, and how to convey information about the scientific limitations of the work.[10,21]

Increasingly, researchers are being forced into policy battlegrounds. Some commentators have argued that prevention policy should be based only on the results of prevention trials, preferably randomized controlled trials.[62] The recent debate about the value of mammography for women in their forties was argued loudly in a variety of fora, including the print and broadcast media. Some contended that it is unethical to recommend mammography to all women in their forties in the absence of definitive data. Others argued that it is unethical to "withdraw" a test that might be of value. The level of evidence that is acceptable becomes, in itself, a matter of controversy. When large populations are involved, especially when interventions are being applied to healthy people, the maxim to "do no harm" takes on greater importance. Chemoprevention trials are a further example of community-based studies in which these issues are present.

Emerging Ethical Issues: Technology and Protection of Subjects

New technologies have the potential for remarkable advances in health and social welfare, but they also raise new ethical questions for community intervention researchers. Emerging information and communication technologies make it increasingly possible to collect data about individuals' personal behaviors without their consent. Highly sensitive screening tests have made feasible the detection of behaviors such as past substance abuse, and of biologic factors such as early HIV infection and genetic predisposition to disease. As screening tests for genetic markers are developed and become more widely available for cancer and other diseases, a variety of challenging ethical issues will emerge.

Issues of informed consent and the voluntary nature of participation in research are particularly pertinent to community-based genetic testing programs. A major challenge to these programs is ensuring sufficient participant education about the benefits, limitations, and risks of genetic testing. To make an informed decision, individuals must understand that genetic information is probabilistic, and they also should be aware of the potential for adverse psychological, social, and economic consequences of participation in these programs.[66] Family members of individuals who receive genetic test results may unwittingly discover information about themselves that could be damaging, despite the fact that they have not provided prior consent. Special efforts must be made when obtaining consent from minors and persons who are more psychologically vulnerable or have different cultural backgrounds.[3]

Confidentiality and protection of privacy are critically important in programs that involve collection of genetic information. However, in exceptional circumstances, information may sometimes be disclosed in order to prevent grave harm to other family members.[67] Ethical problems arise when screening employees for genetic susceptibility to occupational exposures. Under these circumstances, safeguards must be in place to protect against unfair employment discrimination. Concerns have also been expressed about the risk of loss of health and life insurance among persons identified as carriers of major disease genes.[68]

Summary and Conclusions

Ethical principles are vital to community-based intervention research, to ensure that the research addresses worthwhile goals, to protect the welfare of individuals and communities participating in the research, and to help establish and maintain effective community partnerships and professional relations. Technical proficiency must be accompanied by a sensitivity for values and ethics and a sense of social responsibility. There are few ready-made formulas for making difficult decisions. In this chapter we have tried to present some familiar issues and to analyze new problems of growing concern to community researchers.

As health investigators strive to conduct innovative and high-quality research, they should take precautions to safeguard participants' privacy, autonomy, and receipt of benefits from the research. Special care should be exercised to protect the rights and interests of vulnerable populations, including children, older adults, minorities, and high-risk populations. Deception should never be used without a thorough ethical analysis of the situation and consideration of alternative research strategies. The targets of interventions—communities and individuals—should be consulted and their wishes respected in the conduct of research. At the conclusion of a study, efforts should be made to offer the most effective treatment to all participants. Bias in reporting results should be avoided, and the scientists should fulfill their obligations for responsible use of research knowledge for public health, medical practice, and social policy. Moreover, public health investigators should form partnerships with ethicists or members of IRBs to identify proactively the ethical implications of research and to ensure that basic ethical principles are not violated. Finally, there should be a continuing search to improve the nature of information provided to participants in studies and to preserve informed consent as one of the ethical foundations of community-based research.

ACKNOWLEDGMENTS

The preparation of this chapter was supported in part by the University of Hawaii Development Fund. The authors acknowledge the assistance of Gwen Ramelb with word processing.

References

1. Rimer, B. K., Glanz, K. and Lerman, C. "Contributions of Public Health to Patient Compliance," *Journal of Community Health* 16 (1991): 225–40.
2. U.S. Department of Health and Human Services, U.S. Public Health Service: "Healthy People 2000," National Health Promotion and Disease Prevention Objectives (DHHS Publ. No. 91–50212). Washington, DC: U.S. Government Printing Office.
3. Lerman, C., Rimer, B. K. and Engstrom, P. F. "Cancer Risk Notification: Psychosocial and Ethical Implications," *Journal of Clinical Oncology* 9 (1991): 1275–82.
4. Green, L. W. and Lewis, F. M. *Measurement and Evaluation in Health Education and Health Promotion.* Palo Alto: Mayfield Publishing Co., 1986.
5. Argyris, C., Putnam, R. and Smith, D. *Action Science: Concepts, Methods, and Skills for Intervention.* San Francisco: Jossey-Bass, 1985.

6. Glanz, K., Lewis, F. M. and Rimer, B. K. *Health Behavior and Health Education: Theory, Research and Practice.* San Francisco: Jossey-Bass, 1990.

7. Smith, H. L. *Ethics and the New Medicine.* Nashville: Abingdon Press, 1970.

8. Daniel, E. L., ed. *Taking Sides: Clashing Views on Controversial Issues in Health and Society.* Guilford, CT: Dushkin Publishing Group, 1993.

9. McLeroy, K. R., Gottlieb, N. H., and Burdine, J.N. "The Business of Health Promotion: Ethical Issues and Professional Responsibilities," *Health Education Quarterly* 14 (1987): 91–109.

10. Babbie, E. "The Ethics and Politics of Social Research." In *The Practice of Social Research*, ed. E. Babbie. 6th ed. Belmont, CA: Wadsworth Publishing Co., 1992: 462–82.

11. McLeroy, K., Bibeau, D., Steckler, A., and Glanz, K. "An Ecological Perspective on Health Promotion Programs," *Health Education Quarterly* 15 (1988): 351–77.

12. Green, L. W. and Kreuter, M. *Health Promotion Planning.* Mountain View: Mayfield Publishing Co., 1991.

13. Mittlemark, M. B., Luepker, R. V., Jacobs, D. R., et al. "Community-wide Prevention of Cardiovascular Disease: Education Strategies of the Minnesota Heart Health Program," *Preventive Medicine* 15 (1986): 1–17.

14. Lerman, C., Rimer, B. K., Trock, B., Balshem, A., and Engstrom, P.F. "Factors Associated With Repeat Adherence to Breast Cancer Screening," *Preventive Medicine* 19 (1990): 279–90.

15. Rimer, B. K. "Understanding the Acceptance of Mammography by Women," *Annals of Behavioral Medicine* 14 (1992): 197–203.

16. Webb, E. and Campbell, D. *Nonreactive Measures in the Social Sciences.* 2d ed. Boston: Houghton Mifflin, 1981.

17. King, E. S., Rimer, B. K., Trock, B., Balshem, A., and Engstrom, P.F. "How Valid are Mammography Self-Reports?" *American Journal of Public Health* 80 (1990): 1386–88.

18. Glanz, K., Brekke, M., Harper, D., Bache-Wiig, M., and Hunninghake, D.B. "Evaluation of Implementation of a Cholesterol Management Program in Physicians' Offices," *Health Education Research* 7 (1992): 151–163.

19. Aronson, E. and Carlsmith, J. M. "Experimentation in Social Psychology." In *The Handbook of Social Psychology*, ed. G. Lindzey and E. Aronson. 2d ed. Reading, MA: Addison-Wesley, 1968.

20. Sobal, J. "Research Ethics in Nutrition Education," *Journal of Nutrition Education* 24 (1992): 234–38.

21. Diener, E. and Crandall, R. *Ethics in Social and Behavioral Research.* Chicago: University of Chicago Press, 1978.

22. Christensen, L. "Deception in Psychological Research: When is its Use Justified?" *Personality and Social Psychology Bulletin* 14 (1988): 664–75.

23. Lappé, M. "Ethics and Public Health." In *Maxcy-Rosenau Public Health and Preventive Medicine*, ed. J.M. Last. 12th ed. Norwalk, CT: Appleton-Century-Crofts, 1986: 1867–77.

24. Veatch, R. M. A Theory of Medical Ethics. New York: Basic Books, 1981.

25. Pellegrino, E. D. "Autonomy and Coercion in Disease Prevention and Health Promotion," *Theoretical Medicine* 5 (1984): 83–91.

26. Brett, A. S. "Ethical Issues in Risk Factor Intervention," *American Journal of Medicine* 76 (1984): 557–61.

27. Faden, R. R. "Ethical Issues in Government Sponsored Public Health Campaigns," *Health Education Quarterly* 14 (1987): 27–37.

28. Riis, P. "Mass Screening Procedures and Programmes." In *Ethical Dilemmas in Health Promotion*, ed. S. Doxiadis. Chichester: John Wiley and Sons, 1987: 171–82.
29. Schafer, A. "The Ethics of the Randomized Clinical Trial," *New England Journal of Medicine* 307 (1982): 719–724.
30. Beauchamp, D.E. "Community: The Neglected Tradition of Public Health," *Hastings Center Report* 15 (December 1985): 28–36.
31. Beauchamp, T. L. and Childress, J. F. *Principles of Biomedical Ethics*. 4th ed. New York: Oxford University Press, 1994.
32. Coughlin, S. S. and Beauchamp, T. L. "Ethics, Scientific Validity, and the Design of Epidemiologic Studies," *Epidemiology* 3 (1992): 343–47.
33. Levine, R. J. *Ethics and Regulation of Clinical Research*. 2d ed. Baltimore: Urban & Schwarzenberg, 1986.
34. Faden, R. R. and Beauchamp, T. L. *A History and Theory of Informed Consent*. New York: Oxford University Press, 1986.
35. Baranowski, T., Henske, J., Simons-Morton, B., et al. "Dietary Change for Cardiovascular Disease Prevention Among Black-American Families," *Health Education Research* 5 (1990): 433–43.
36. Powers, M. "Privacy, Justice, and the Uses of Genetic Information." In *Proceedings of the Committee on Assessing Genetic Risks*. Washington, D.C.: Institute of Medicine, National Academy of Sciences, 1994.
37. Ellison, R. C., Capper, A.L., Goldberg, R.J., Witschi, J.C., and Stare, F.J. "The Environmental Component: Changing School Food Service to Promote Cardiovascular Health," *Health Education Quarterly* 16 (1989): 285–97.
38. Ellison, R. C., Goldberg, R.J., Witschi, J.C., Capper, A.L., Puleo, E.M., and Stare, F.J. "Use of Fat-modified Food Products to Change Dietary Fat Intake of Young People," *American Journal of Public Health* 80 (1990): 1374–1376.
39. Roman, P. M. and Blum, T. C. "Ethics in Worksite Health Programming: Who is Served?" *Health Education Quarterly* 14 (1987): 57–70.
40. Osborn, J. E., "AIDS, Social Sciences, and Health Education: A Personal Perspective," *Health Education Quarterly* 13 (1986): 287–99.
41. Solomon, M. Z. and DeJong, W. "Recent Sexually Transmitted Disease Prevention Efforts and Their Implications for AIDS Health Education," *Health Education Quarterly* 13 (1986): 301–16.
42. Martin, J. L. "AIDS Risk Reduction Recommendations and Sexual Behavior Patterns Among Gay Men: A Multifactorial Categorical Approach to Assessing Change," *Health Education Quarterly* 13 (1986): 347–58.
43. Milgram, S. "Behavioral Study of Obedience," *Journal of Abnormal and Social Psychology* 67 (1963): 371–78.
44. Rosenhan, D. L. "On Being Sane in Insane Places," *Science* (January 1973): 250–58.
45. Hofling, C., Brotzman, E., Dalrymple, S., Graves, N., and Pierce, D. "An Experimental Study in Nurse-Physician Relationships," *Journal of Nervous and Mental Diseases* 143 (1960): 171–80.
46. Bracht, N. and Gleason, J. "Strategies and Structures for Citizen Partnerships." In *Health Promotion at the Community Level*, ed. N. Bracht. Newbury Park: Sage Publications, 1990: 109–24.
47. Green, L. W. and Raeburn, J. "Contemporary Developments in Health Promotion: Definitions and Challenges." In *Health Promotion at the Community Level*, ed. N. Bracht. Newbury Park: Sage Publications, 1990: 29–44.
48. Hatch, J., Moss, N., Saran, A., Presley-Cantrell, L., and Mallory, C. "Community

Research: Partnerships in Black Communities," *American Journal of Preventive Medicine* 9 (1993): 27–31.

49. DeCambra, H., Enos, R., Matsunaga, D. S., and Hammond, O. W. "Community Involvement in Minority Health Research: Participatory Research in a Native Hawaiian Community." *Cancer Control Research Reports for Public Health*, NCI (October 1992): 2–9.

50. Peters, M. and Robinson, V. "The Origins and Status of Action Research," *Journal of Applied Behavioral Science* 20 (1984): 113–24.

51. Elden, M. "Sharing the Research Work: Participative Research and its Role Demands." In *Human Inquiry*, ed. P. Reason and J. Rowan. Chicester: John Wiley, 1986.

52. Susman, G. and Evered, R. "An Assessment of the Scientific Merits of Action Research," *Administrative Science Quarterly* 23 (1978): 582–603.

53. Rimer, B. K., Keintz, M., Fleisher, L., Davis, S. A., and Engstrom, P. F. "Planning a Cancer Control Program for Older Citizens," *Gerontologist* 23 (1983): 384–89.

54. Lefebvre, R. C. "Strategies to Maintain and Institutionalize Successful Programs." In: *Health Promotion at the Community Level*, ed. N. Bracht. Newbury Park: Sage Publications, 1990: 209–28.

55. Michels, R. and Eth, S. "Ethical Issues in Psychiatric Research on Communities: A Case Study of the Community Mental Health Center Program." In *Ethical Issues in Epidemiologic Research*, ed. L. Tancredi. New Brunswick, NJ: Rutgers University Press, 1981: 71–97.

56. Schulte, P. A. "The Epidemiologic Basis for the Notification of Subjects of Cohort Studies," *American Journal of Epidemiology* 121 (1985): 351–61.

57. Gamble, V. N. "A Legacy of Distrust: African Americans and Medical Research," *American Journal of Preventive Medicine* 9 (1993): 35–38.

58. Dressler, W. W. "Commentary on Community Research: Partnership in Black Communities," *American Journal of Preventive Medicine* 9 (1993): 32–34.

59. Raczynski, J. M. and Lewis, C. M. "Reconciling the Multiple Scientific and Community Needs." In *Health Behavior Research in Minority Populations: Access, Design and Implementation*, ed. D. M. Becker, D. R. Hill, J. S. Jackson, D. M. Levine, F. A. Stillman, and S. M. Weiss. Bethesda: NIH, NHLBI, DHHS (NIH Publ. No. 92-2965), 1992: 216–28.

60. Taub, A., Kreuter, M., Parcel, G., and Vitello, E. "Report from the SOPHE/AAHE Joint Committee on Ethics," *Health Education Quarterly* 14 (1987): 79–90.

61. Greider, T. "Ethical Dilemmas and Publishing Constraints of Client-based Applied Practitioners," *Human Organization* 52 (1993): 432–33.

62. Strasser, T., Jeanneret, O., and Raymond, L. "Ethical Aspects of Prevention Trials." In *Ethical Dilemmas in Health Promotion*, ed. S. Doxiadis. Chichester: John Wiley and Sons, 1987: 183–93.

63. Farquhar, J. W., Fortmann, S. P., Maccoby, N., et al. "The Stanford Five City Project: An Overview." In *Behavioral Health: A Handbook of Health Enhancement and Disease Prevention*, ed. J.D. Matarazzo, S.M. Weiss, J.A. Herd, N.E. Miller, and S.M. Weiss. New York: John Wiley and Sons, 1984: 1154–65.

64. Farquhar, J. W., Fortmann, S. P., Flora, J. A., et al. "Effects of Community-wide Education on Cardiovascular Disease Risk Factors: The Stanford Five City Project," *Journal of the American Medical Association* 264 (1990): 359–65.

65. Weed, D. L. "Science, Ethics Guidelines, and Advocacy in Epidemiology," *Annals of Epidemiology* 4 (1994): 166–71.

66. Lerman, C. and Croyle, R. "Genetic Testing for Breast-ovarian Cancer Susceptibility," *Archives of Internal Medicine* 154 (1994): 609–16.
67. Nuffield Council on Bioethics. *Genetic Screening: Ethical Issues.* Published by London: Nuffield Foundation, December 1993.
68. Oster, H., Allen, W., Crandall, L., Moseley, R. E., Dewar, M. A., Nye, D., and McCrary, S. "Insurance and Genetic Testing: Where Are We Now?" *American Journal of Human Genetics* 52 (1993): 565–77.

9

Ethical Issues in the Interaction with Subjects and Disclosure of Results

PAUL A. SCHULTE
MITCHELL SINGAL

Full disclosure of research results to study participants is now standard practice by some, but not all, epidemiologic and medical practitioners.[1–6] This practice has been influenced by historical events, especially the Nuremburg Code and the Helsinki Declaration,[7] that attest to patients' and research subjects' rights to relevant disclosure about potential risks and benefits of experimental biomedical procedures, as well as to refuse involvement. The practice has further been brought into focus by separate though related developments such as the 1978 Belmont Report on human subjects in research,[1] the right-to-know [8] and worker notification [9] movements, and various efforts by professional organizations to formulate codes of ethics for epidemiologists [10–12] and other health professionals. These efforts embody a respect for autonomy that is a fundamental moral principle widely accepted in democratic societies.[13–15] Based on this principle, individuals are considered to be in the best position to protect their lives and interests if they are informed about a known risk or other pertinent factors.

Although the standard of full disclosure of research results is now adhered to by some epidemiologists, there is still a need for an overview of the elements involved and the ethical issues inherent in each component in order to provide a basis for wider acceptance. The elements of disclosure and communication discussed in this chapter require resource allocations that investigators and funding agencies are not used to considering. Supporting appropriate forms of communication without providing adequate resources also can have ethical implications for investigators and their institutions. In general, the issue of disclosure has been discussed in the context of clinical, rather than epidemiologic, research.[16] This

chapter will address the components of epidemiologic studies that affect the reporting of results. These include (1) subject recruitment and informed consent,
(2) privacy and confidentiality, (3) interpretation of test and study results, (4)
communication of test results, and (5) communication of study results. We begin
by defining a few important terms.

Definitions

Our topic is disclosure of results. By *results*, we mean not only the epidemiologic findings of studies, but also each individual's medical or biological test
data. By *results*, we also mean not only the group comparison values such as incidence rates and risk ratios, but also the interpretation of those summary statistics in terms of subsequent risk to members of the studied population—that is,
the extent to which the group or individual is at risk of disease. Individual-spe-
cific results indicate that, in general, the individual's risk will be greater, less, or
the same as a particular group's risk, depending on his or her specific risk-factor histories. Quantitatively, an individual risk-function may be calculated when
individual risk information is available to be incorporated into statistical models.[17,18]

By *disclosure*, we mean the act of informing or notifying study subjects (as a
group or individually) of the test or study results and the risks implied by those
results.[18,19] Such disclosure is a form of risk communication. We also include in
this disclosure all risks attendant to participating in a study. Therefore, we discuss subject recruitment and informed consent and the ethical issues related to
communication in those efforts. Disclosure also includes broad dissemination of
research results and information through relevant forms of publication and news
reports.

Disclosure can be a simple task but it can also be part of a complex commu-
nicative process. What one person says is not always what another person hears,
since beliefs and opinions can polarize the deliverer and recipient of a communication. Thus, a disclosure may be adequate, but the subject's understanding inadequate. The recipient may accept or reject what is consistent or inconsistent
with his or her beliefs,[20] and may do so with or without reflection. Hence, when
communicating, it is critical to anticipate how the communication will be received and to select appropriate channels and methods.[21]

Subject Recruitment and Informed Consent

Provision of test or study results is not always the first communication between
investigators and study participants, unless the investigation only centers on

linked records obtained through legislative or other authority. When a study involves participation of subjects or permission to use their records, the participants need to be recruited, and the principle of respect for autonomy dictates that they be told of the purpose, risks, and benefits of the study. This is done (however effectively or ineffectively) through the process of administering the informed consent document. There is an extensive body of literature on the meaning and justification of informed consent. The focus has evolved from the researcher's obligation to disclose information to an emphasis on the subjects' understanding and consent.[22-24] In theory, before a participant is asked to sign the document, an oral explanation is given and any questions the participant has are answered. The document describes the tests to be done, although this may be categorical (for example, "tests of kidney function or damage") rather than a detailed list. Limitations of tests and their meaning for individual participants or for general research are discussed.[19] Maximizing the understanding of potential study subjects through this process can increase subject refusals, thereby contributing to response bias. However, this is one of the costs of epidemiologic research in a democratic society.[21] The effect on validity of informing participants of the study's purposes should be assessed on a case-by-case basis.

Coercion and manipulation of subjects is an important ethical issue to consider in the consent process. Researchers must depend on subjects' voluntary participation, free of both threats and undue inducements. Also important is the accurate portrayal of risks and benefits to potential study subjects. Researchers need to use clear language and to avoid inadvertent misrepresentation. A recent review of informed consent given by hospital patients who participated in research demonstrated that they had low levels of recall, understanding, and knowledge subsequent to requests for consent.[25] The reasons cited for this lack of comprehension involved clarity, language, and the formats used. The ethical consideration underlying subject recruitment into research studies is that the participants should gain a genuine understanding of the study purpose, the benefits to be derived, and the risks involved.

Researchers can directly coerce subjects by threatening unwanted outcomes for noncooperation, such as loss of job. But more commonly, they can indirectly manipulate subjects by inadvertently (or even intentionally) overstating the personal benefits of participation or general significance of the study. It is important that researchers affirm that no penalty attaches to nonparticipation, and that they acknowledge their own interest in obtaining a high participation rate. Though the former may be standard practice for government agencies, universities, and others, the latter is typically not made explicit.

In recruiting subjects for studies and adequately informing them of the risks and benefits of participation, researchers should detail the study activities and also describe envisaged uses of the data. Nevertheless, questions will remain about unspecified and even unknown future uses. For example, the limitations of conducting additional analyses that are unrelated to the original study purpose are uncertain.[26] Sometimes epidemiologic studies involve collection and banking of biological specimens. A number of questions have arisen about the extent to which investigators, during recruitment, must make participants aware that specimens could be used in future research, as yet unknown or unplanned.[26] Another important question is whether specimens collected for one purpose can be used for related or distinctly different research. For example, during a study of premalignant effects of a carcinogen, what if a new assay is developed that will allow for assessment of a different mutation than the one stipulated in consent forms? Does this closely related endeavor require new consent? As a further example, may blood specimens banked in a cardiovascular study be used to look for cancer markers? Or, may they be used to determine the prevalence of antibodies to a newly discovered infectious agent not suspected of being related to cardiovascular disease? Similar concerns may also pertain to records (such as employment and hospital medical files) that are collected for one purpose but used for other purposes. A solution that some investigators have adopted is to include in informed consent documents a statement that the data or specimens might be used in other, as yet unspecified, analyses. This catch-all can be useful but it is arguably too broad in certain contexts.

Some researchers may feel constrained by human subjects requirements that prohibit performance of additional assays on banked specimens. They may reasonably question whether the rights of subjects are disregarded when initially unspecified assays are conducted on specimens collected for another purpose. Different and even opposing answers to this question may be ethically defensible.

The banking and use of specimens also raise the question of ownership of specimens. In one instance, a clinician used a patient's specimens to develop, patent, and profit from a cell line, and was sued by the patient. This is a clear illustration of how unresolved these matters are.[27,28] Related questions of access involve whether other scientists, or even nonscientific interests such as insurance companies or employers, can make use of banked specimens.

A further issue, which has received less attention, concerns what should be done when results are obtained from such additional assays.[26] Does the investigator have a responsibility to communicate these new or additional findings to the subjects? This is akin to the responsibility to communicate test results, which is discussed in a subsequent section.

Another aspect of informed consent is the situation in which the group is the unit of study or intervention, rather than the individual.[29] There is virtually no literature concerning consent for epidemiologic studies or interventions focused on groups of people or communities. Clearly, if individuals within these groups are actual participants, then the above discussion applies. However, when the study involves only linkage of records requiring no individual permissions, or when it involves only comparisons between a community with an intervention and one without it, the issues of informed consent are not widely discussed.

Is the concept of "group consent" an important one? Often in the past, consents in such situations have been obtained from representatives or proxies of the affected group (for example, Congress, a health commissioner, company officials, or union representatives). The principle of respect for autonomy applies to individuals as group members as well as separately, but the application of the principle to the group is more complicated since different people in a group may have conflicting opinions. In such cases, the interests of the common good may override the preferences of individuals. Historically, citizens opposed to a public project (such as an immunization program or a nuclear power plant) that involves shared risks have no right to stop the project once due process is completed. Whether the same rationale holds for participation in epidemiologic research in which the *group* is the unit of interest is arguable, but perhaps likely.

Privacy and Confidentiality

When a person agrees to participate in research, he or she expects that the information or biological specimens that are provided will be used only for the espoused purposes of the study. The subject consents to provide the specimens and various demographic and risk-factor information, and, hence, cooperates in the specified research. The subject generally does not consent or imply consent to distribution of the data in a way that identifies him or her individually to any other parties, such as employers, unions, insurers, credit agencies, or lawyers.[26]

Unwarranted disclosure of personal information violates both privacy and confidentiality. Privacy is the condition of limited access by others in terms of either physical access, personal information, or attention.[22,30] Claims to privacy are claims to control access to what one takes to be his or her restricted personal domain. Confidentiality arises from a pledge or obligation to hold a confidence. The maintenance of confidentiality requires the protection of confidences from third parties under certain circumstances.[30] This obligation is not absolute, and investigators should (as is required of federal and federally funded investigators) inform research participants of the types of situations in which apparently "confidential" data will be released.

In the United States, there is a stipulation that records in government-sponsored studies will be maintained according to the Privacy Act of 1974 (PL 93–579). Researchers have an obligation to inform participants of methods of protection and of the circumstances under which records will be disclosed. Title 5 of the Code of Federal Regulations (5 CFR 297.401) describes the conditions under which records held by the federal government can be disclosed. These are shown in Table 9–1, which lists the twelve situations under the Privacy Act in

Table 9–1. Conditions under which a Federal Agency Can Release an Individual's Records to Another Party (5 CFR 297.401).

1. They are necessary for protecting the health and safety of other persons.
2. A researcher uses them only for statistical research.
3. Agency officials, or groups working with an agency, need the records for uses compatible with the purpose for which the information was collected.
4. They are needed by agency personnel, who use the records in performance of their duties.
5. The release is required by law.
6. The Bureau of Census needs them for census or survey work.
7. The National Archives requires them for historical purposes.
8. Either House of Congress requests an individual's records.
9. The Comptroller General needs them for the General Accounting Office.
10. A court orders them.
11. A consumer reporting agency requires them to assist the federal government in collecting a claim owed the government.
12. The records are requested under the terms and conditions of the Freedom of Information Act, and their release would not invade an individual's privacy.

which it is permissible to release information in identifiable form. These conditions pertain to almost all federal record systems (although, depending on the particular system, one or more of the conditions may not be relevant). Confidentiality can be more assertively protected in studies sponsored by agencies within the Public Health Service if the investigator obtains a special clearance, provided by Section 308(d) of the Public Health Service Act [42 U.S.C., 242m(d)], which bars disclosure to any party other than the subject.

Standard practices to maintain privacy and confidentiality are generally followed in research, particularly federally funded research, and are usually observed in academic, business, and labor settings.[10–12] However, if disclosed, personally identifiable data collected for epidemiologic and medical studies can be misused in ways detrimental to participants. Such misuses can include discrimination, stigmatization, or denial of opportunity, or all of these in regard to obtaining or keeping insurance, employment, or financial credit.

Researchers may violate privacy and confidentiality unwittingly by publishing data sets with enough covariate information to allow identification of particular subjects. This is not generally the case, but may occur in small or pilot studies or studies in which subjects have unique characteristics. Confidentiality may also be breached during the data-collection period. This is often inadvertent or because inadequately trained researchers have caused the identity of subjects to be linked to other identifiers, resulting in unwarranted disclosures.[31]

Dissemination or revelation of personal results beyond the explicit purposes for which data or specimens were collected intrudes on subjects' privacy and likely violates obligations of confidentiality. Inadvertent labeling of a subject as "abnormal," or distribution of his or her questionnaire or test results, could adversely affect a person's ability to obtain insurance, employment, or credit, or to interact socially.[32] There has been little study of the psychological impact of such disclosure. Thus, as Nelkin and Tancredi [32] note, some union leaders are concerned that if workers' genetic test data are released, some of them will bear a "genetic scarlet letter" and become "lepers" or "genetic untouchables." By extension, groups and communities may suffer this same type of stigmatization.

Groups may have a right to confidentiality of unlinked epidemiologic data (that is, data without identifiers). Just as an individual can be stigmatized by disclosure of personal information, so theoretically can a group or community. Epidemiologists have a responsibility not to inadvertently disclose information about a group that could harm that group for no overriding public good. Again, as with confidentiality of an individual's information, public health needs may override a breach of confidentiality. In general, a group's right to privacy is less than an individual's because society has a greater claim to know about risks to communities.

Interpretation of Test and Study Results

The communication of epidemiologic and medical research findings requires correct interpretation of the findings, in part because individual test and epidemiologic study results can have social, political, and economic implications. Correct interpretation is also an issue in distinguishing the meaning of an epidemiologic finding from an individual clinical result. With each study, investigators are confronted with the question of what to tell study participants. The participants may want a clinical interpretation when study results have only an epidemiologic significance.[18,33] Or participants may want action: recommendations to ban or promote a drug, eliminate an environmental hazard, or blame a particular risk factor. Researchers may not have complete and conclusive data to support calls for such action. While researchers need to resist overselling or underselling their findings, they also have a responsibility to provide the most definitive conclusion possible.[34,35]

The interpretive issues that impinge on individual notification of a study's results include: (1) whether surviving subjects are at the same risk as the overall study population from which the risk information was computed; (2) whether group data can be used as the basis of individual risk notifications; and (3) whether the assessment of many outcomes requires a greater threshold for statistical significance for any single disease or cause of death before such a finding would merit inclusion in a notification effort.[18]

Inappropriate interpretation of epidemiologic results can have ethical implications because a researcher has a responsibility to provide an accurate interpretation of data. Thus, it is incumbent upon a researcher disclosing results to indicate that epidemiologic risk information is group-specific, that is, the experience of one group is compared with that of another group. Such data do not necessarily address the experience of an individual within the group. A determination cannot be made about whether the risk information that is derived from the study population is applicable to each individual member. From a public health point of view, members of a group may be at high risk. Individuals who have had the exposure or risk factor in question are likely to have some increased risk, but researchers cannot predict the exact rate of increase.[36] Also, the researcher should explain that in many epidemiologic studies those with the outcome of interest may have been those who had the highest exposures or were the most susceptible. Therefore, the survivors are not necessarily at the same risk, yet the researchers would be sending these individuals notification that they are at risk. To avoid this problem, each study needs to be carefully and individually evaluated.[18] Finally, when a study involves multiple comparisons, it might be important for researchers to distinguish findings based on *a priori* hypotheses from those based on *a posteriori* hypotheses. In the latter case, a stricter test of significance might be warranted.

Data derived from studies using biological specimens is another area in which interpretation is problematic. Researchers have a responsibility to choose appropriate study designs, and to interpret biomarker tests correctly. Investigators cannot allow themselves to be misled by the extensive variation in genetic and biochemical individuality depicted by such test results.[37] Otherwise, the inherent variability among individuals will influence the interpretation and communication of biomarker data.

This natural variability makes it essential to know the range of biomarker values in the general population. Depending on the biomarker, the range of normality can be quite extensive. A healthy level for some individuals may indicate a health risk for others.

Many studies involve biomarkers for which a "normal" range has not been established. Nonetheless, the researcher should provide each subject with some perspective on results, even if the meaning of the results is not known. This could be accomplished by providing subjects not only with their own results, but also with an indication of the study group's mean and range, as well as those for any comparison group.

Interpreting studies that involve biological markers and relaying the results to the study group pose several dilemmas. As discussed above, one conflict arises because interpretation of results is often influenced by the tension between group effects and individual effects.[33] Research data may yield information on group risks but not indicate individual risk. This dilemma is a general feature of epidemiologic research and is not limited to studies using biological markers, which are referred to as "molecular epidemiology." Biological markers can indicate exposure, effect, or susceptibility. Each of these may have their own disclosure requirements and issues. For example, not all markers of effect will be diseases; they may, in some cases, represent homeostatic changes. Or markers of susceptibility may only be relevant in the presence of a specific type of exposure. These distinctions must be explained when communicating test results to subjects.

One of the major potential advantages of molecular epidemiology is the ability to obtain specific information that may be predictive of some risks to some individuals.[33,38,39] The exquisite sensitivity of individual risk determinations based on gene assessments puts researchers and society in difficult positions with respect to interpretation of results when markers are not yet validated, but are suspected indicators of risk or susceptibility.

Communication of Individual Test Results

The responsibility to communicate both individual test results and overall study results to each individual is not universally recognized, although it is acknowledged by some federal agencies. Test results include the findings from any physical measurement, medical procedure, or analysis of a biological specimen. An explanation of the meaning or uncertainty of such results may be considered an essential part of the communication.[19,33] This communication and explanation is consistent with the principle of autonomy. Subjects can provide the information to their physicians or use it to advocate for controls on exposure.

The goal of communicating test results is not only to provide information to the study subjects, but to do it in a way that is informative and understandable. A few years ago, we reviewed a series of studies conducted by the National Institute for Occupational Safety and Health (NIOSH) to evaluate communication issues.[19] In most of the studies reviewed, the language in results notification letters appeared to be relatively clear. The process of letter development, however, involved no field testing, even among participants or surrogates with low educational levels. Whether the information was entirely understandable to participants who received the letters has not been studied. In general, the letters did not result in an extensive response from the recipients, either through the telephone number provided or by mail. Although no letter can speak completely to the diverse educational, literacy, or comprehension levels of heterogenous groups of workers, the results notifications reviewed appeared to be generally intelligible by study participants and other nonprofessional persons. The letters illustrated a variety of efforts to express and explain technical information. Further, they were reviewed and evaluated by an Institutional Review Board, which may have contributed to their effectiveness and clarity.

Another ethical issue in communicating results is whether the notifier has an obligation to ensure that medical follow-up is available for test subjects. This service is not ordinarily considered a primary responsibility of an epidemiologic investigator. Still, health researchers may have an ethical obligation not only to recommend appropriate follow-up but also to motivate, encourage, or even require (in the case of some government agencies) third parties such as employers, other government agencies, and unions to provide or arrange for follow-up.

A special example of informing subjects of test results is the United States Public Health Service (PHS) policy on notifying those tested of their HIV seropositivity status. The policy, signed in 1988 and based on guidelines developed in 1984,[40,41] applies to all intramural and extramural PHS activities, including domestic and foreign research and health services activities. It requires that in HIV testing conducted or supported by PHS, individuals whose results are associated with personal identifiers must be informed of their results and provided with the opportunity to receive appropriate counseling. Exceptions are made under special circumstances set forth in the policy.

Despite an ethical basis for disclosure, there is the possibility that even warranted disclosures could have harmful effects. Concerns have been raised about illness behaviors, such as workplace absenteeism, of individuals notified of risk.[42] These kinds of effects have also been mentioned as a reason for not supporting disclosure of study results. The question arises, who should decide if information that pertains to a person is too fear-inducing and that disclosure should be avoided? This, in turn, raises the issue of paternalism in conflict with subjects' rights of self-determination. There does not appear to be a strong argument for limiting disclosure. Nonetheless, it is incumbent on those disclosing information to anticipate the needs of the recipient and to provide or encourage supportive measures such as counseling.

Communicating Study Results

To Study Participants

An essential question is: To what extent should a research agency, a corporation, or a university use its resources to find and notify study subjects?[21] This is illustrated by the problem of disclosing study results to surviving members of retrospective occupational cohort mortality studies, a challenge that occupational epidemiologists faced in the early 1980s. Prior to that time, epidemiologists did not routinely notify subjects of epidemiologic study results, particularly surviving members of populations evaluated by retrospective cohort mortality studies.[9,43] This type of investigation involves identifying a cohort of workers, following that cohort of workers, and evaluating the mortality experience of the cohort by comparing it with reference mortality rates. A measure of that comparison is the standardized mortality ratio.

Retrospective cohort mortality studies usually involve a records search with no direct contact with living members or next of kin of deceased members of the cohorts. In the 1970s and early 1980s, the prevailing belief was that sufficient dissemination entailed reporting results to companies and unions and publishing the study in a scientific journal. The ethical basis for informing surviving cohort members of study results, as Bayer[43] noted in reviewing the issues, was the following:

- Respect for the autonomy of persons required notification because it would permit individual workers to choose appropriate courses of action on the basis of relevant information.
- Beneficence required individual notification, not only because on balance it would produce more benefits than harm for those informed, but because it might well produce altered social policy.
- Justice required that those who had already been burdened by toxic exposure be given an opportunity to seek redress. Failure to provide notification would represent a compounding of an unfair deprivation.

Other questions parallel those issues considered in the above discussion of communication of individual test results: uncertainty, clarity, perspective, and follow-up. However, study results differ from individual test results in ways that may have ethical implications. Epidemiologic studies yield *group* results. Hence, the meaning for each individual subject is only on a group basis (unless individual risk functions have been calculated). Investigators face ethical complexities in trying to communicate accurately this characteristic of epidemiologic studies, and their attempts to do so can have opposing effects. They can underestimate the risks to group members by attributing them to a few highly exposed or genetically susceptible individuals, and thus discount the risk to the majority of the cohort. Or, there is the possibility that investigators can overestimate the risk by failing either to evaluate potential risk factors related to individual differences in susceptibility, or to note characteristics such as the exposure period, duration, and latency that would indicate that only a subset of the cohort was actually at risk.

Another difficult aspect of communication involves the failure to distinguish between relative, absolute, and attributable risk, and then not to consider which are important for the population.[21,44] A high relative risk of a very rare disease may trigger different communications and follow-up recommendations than a lower relative risk of a more common disease. Ethical issues might be involved when researchers or officials exaggerate or minimize a risk by selectively emphasizing one type of risk over another. The nature of health risks in terms of probability is often not understood by the general public, and risk communicators may have to make extra efforts to address this issue.

The communication of study results indicating risk to a cohort may create a "high-risk group" in society.[21,45] This label has various meanings to different sectors of society. To the subjects it can have the exaggerated meaning that they are entered into a lottery involving their health. Some may be able to put their risk into perspective; others may need counseling or support. All may need certain periodic medical screening to determine whether they have developed signs of the disease for which they are at risk, and whether institution of secondary or tertiary preventive measures is appropriate. The ethical responsibilities of researchers and research institutions (including corporate research groups) to high-risk subjects have not been well delineated. One might argue, however, that research entities do have a responsibility to consider these questions and be forces in fostering the implementation of appropriate support and surveillance.

In the past, such individual notification activities were nonexistent or minimal. Some may wonder whether the obligation to use these resources may serve as a disincentive to the initiation of new research. However, we suspect that a similar argument was also made during debate on implementing informed consent, and there is no evidence that research has been hindered by that ethical obligation. A basic, but far from the only, ethical question is: What is the acceptable minimum effort that should be considered for notification and assistance?

Once notified, cohort members, individually or collectively, may seek legal redress for real or perceived damage, including anxiety attendant to risk status.[21] The ethical issue here, as well as that underlying all of the discussion thus far, is the presumption that the results are reliable because they are derived from research that is based on a firm scientific foundation.[46] That is, the research incorporates a good rationale, study design, execution, and analysis, and the investigators have attended to the details of the study. Irresponsible conduct in research includes both intentional and unintentional mistakes. These range from fraud, conflict of interest, and malfeasance to self-deception and gullibility.[47–49] The importance of responsible conduct of research can be seen in the extent to which the results of an epidemiologic study can trigger untoward effects.

Scientists in general, and epidemiologists in particular, are recipients of the public's trust because of a tradition of personal honor and integrity and the practice of self-regulation (such as by peer review). Thus, when an epidemiologic finding is disclosed, at the very least the subjects and the public should have confidence that all efforts were made to ensure that the finding is valid given the state of knowledge. Subjects' next concern is what a study says about their risk or harm and what they can do about it. Investigators are accountable for the impact of studies that have not been conducted responsibly. Even with conscientiously conducted studies, the investigator has an obligation to be aware of the effects that research may have and the needs of study subjects (counseling, preventive action, or medical surveillance and follow-up). The investigator, however, does not bear the entire weight of the ethical responsibilities of research. The institution supporting the researchers may share these duties. As Samuels[50] noted, "There is a lesson in Greek Philosophy lost in the modern quest for understanding what is and what is not ethical. In the *Republic*, Plato reminds us that there is an organic relationship between individual behavior and the character of the institution or social structure in which the behavior takes place." Hence, the institution funding or conducting research, be it a corporation, university, or labor union, may be ultimately responsible for ensuring appropriate notification and, in some cases, follow-up.

The conclusions reached in this chapter regarding the ethical communication of results are unlikely to be universally adopted. However, these conclusions have been presented by us and others to various groups, and in a variety of forms. Though not always accepted, they appear now to represent a consensus on the ethics of risk communications.[10,11] Sandman[51] has identified communication responsibilities of epidemiologists:

1. Tell the people who are most affected what you have found—and tell them first.
2. Make sure people understand what you are telling them, and what you think the implications are.
3. Develop mechanisms to bolster the credibility of your study and your findings.
4. Acknowledge uncertainty promptly and thoroughly.
5. Show respect for public concerns even when they are not scientific.
6. Involve people in the design, implementation, and interpretation of the study.
7. Decide that communication is part of your job, and learn the rudiments.

These recommendations are consistent with the responsibility to disclose risks and the principle of respect for autonomy of subjects in epidemiologic studies.

To the Scientific Community and Society

In addition to issues involving the dissemination of study results to participants and other cohort members, there are ethical issues involved in the process of disseminating results to the scientific community (and, ultimately, the general public). In general, that process is publication in peer-reviewed scientific journals. Other mechanisms include official government reports; publications by nongovernmental research institutions; and unpublished reports such as post-graduate theses, and letters and memoranda conveying results of government agency investigations. In addition, *ad hoc* methods, such as "whistle-blowing," may represent a socially responsible means of disclosure.[52]

Publication bias[53] may be an ethical issue for the investigator if it involves an intentional decision not to publish. This decision might be reached by either the study's sponsor or the investigator, based on the study's outcome (unfavorable or otherwise unwanted results), or by the investigator because of decreased interest or competing demands on his or her time. The former has ethical implications; the latter typically does not.

Lack of timely publication was claimed, for example, when the asbestos industry allegedly prevented publication of industry-sponsored animal experimental data that reportedly documented the carcinogenicity of asbestos,[48] and when the results of animal experiments demonstrating vinyl chloride's carcinogenicity were reportedly initially suppressed by the study's chemical industry sponsors.[52,54] These examples illustrate the ethical dilemma that may arise if the party with financial or institutional control over a study has different interests than those of the scientists who conduct the study. The latter presumably have not only a personal and professional interest in publishing results, especially new findings, but may also feel a societal obligation to disseminate results that have public health ramifications.

Nonpublication of "negative" studies has been said to occur because they are perceived as less scientifically newsworthy by journal editors and reviewers[53] and the general public. But perhaps more important, a study may not be published because it is never *submitted* to a journal, investigator loss of interest being a commonly cited reason in one study of the problem.[55] Although the investigator's choice to abandon (not prepare a manuscript for) a seemingly unfruitful study may not involve the same *personal* ethical dilemma as the examples cited in the previous paragraph, the resulting publication bias may nonetheless have an adverse effect on subsequent interpretation of the available data,[56] including meta-analyses, and possibly (depending on the subject) on medical care[57] or public health policy decisions.

Suggestions to address publication bias and the accompanying ethical issues include registration of studies at the time they are undertaken, publication of protocols, requiring publication as a condition of funding, and making institutional review boards responsible for ensuring that studies are submitted for publication.[56,57] The last two proposals would establish the commitment to attempt to publish the study as both an ethical and an institutional obligation.[56,58] This would have at least two beneficial effects for the investigator. First, it would legitimize the notion that a well-designed, well-conducted study is worthy of publication, regardless of whether the results are "positive," "negative," or inconclusive.[59] Second, such a policy would effectively end the ability of private-sector sponsors to restrict the right of institutionally based investigators to publish. Further, although the proposals might not have direct applicability to research by private consultants or companies, their adoption by academic institutions, government agencies, and other research organizations might make the proposals the standard of practice and thereby pressure private researchers to adopt them too.

An investigator's potential conflicts of interest clearly have ethical implications. Disclosure requirements have been proposed for, and adopted by some, medical journals, particularly with regard to financial conflicts.[60,61] However, such requirements have been criticized as "the new McCarthyism in science" on the grounds that they result in work being judged by its source rather than on its merits.[61] An alternative that seems to accommodate the concerns of advocates on both sides of the debate would be not to disclose such source information to reviewers (much as some journals don't identify authors to reviewers), but to do so for readers.[61] Even so, according to the International Committee of Medical Journal Editors, "Because readers may be less able to detect bias in review articles and editorials than in reports of original research, some journals do not accept reviews and editorials from authors with a conflict of interest."[60]

Disclosure from a Multicultural Perspective

The ethical conduct of research, particularly pertaining to disclosure of results, has been discussed in this chapter from a United States perspective for research conducted in the United States. Researchers may face issues of disclosure, however, in different cultural contexts. For example, in some European countries, constraints on data management have made it difficult or impossible to notify populations at risk of various diseases. Are the principles discussed in this chapter universal, or can accommodations be made for cultural differences?[62,63] Conduct of epidemiologic research in developing countries is often attractive because of unique exposure situations, low costs, and fewer, less complex administrative rules and requirements.[64] In many developing countries, legal provisions for ethical oversight of biomedical research on human subjects have not yet been written. As LaVerta and Linares[64] note:

From a multicultural perspective, the increasing volume of biomedical research on human subjects conducted in developing countries by investigators from developed nations gives rise to sensitive ethical problems. In principle, ethical considerations applying to human subjects are the same everywhere in the world. One must admit that the uniform application of these considerations in different areas is extremely difficult.[64]

This may be especially true in obtaining informed consent and disclosing results. Nonetheless, if the principles discussed in this chapter do express fundamental moral obligations, it is hard to imagine a justification for dispatching those obligations merely because they are not explicitly recognized in local customs. Scarce resources, cultural relevance, and local reality will affect the exact application of such practices.

Conclusion

Some commentators claim that in the last twenty-five years respect for autonomy has superseded beneficence as the first principle of biomedical ethics.[65] This has coincided with or possibly has been the underlying cause for the equalization of the physician-patient relationship, and, more to the point of this discussion, of the researcher-participant relationship. Research participants can now expect that they will be told of risks and benefits of studies and of the findings that derive from them.

Pellegrino,[65] however, argues that respect for autonomy, as it is often construed and as its demands are understood in institutions, has certain moral and practical limitations that can be eased by linking autonomy to respect for the integrity of persons. Thus, the relationship between the researcher and the participant should not be seen in terms of a one-way process of communication, but rather as an equal partnership built on a view of the dignity of both the researcher and the participant and the respect that should be accorded to each. In this scenario, the researcher not only acts in a way that lets subjects decide whether to participate in a study, but also disseminates results fully and honestly, in a manner that presents minimal risk to the participants. Further, the researcher considers the subject's needs resulting from participation in the study and receipt of results, and makes some effort to address those needs.

Several important questions remain. If all of the proposed ethical obligations we discussed were fulfilled as standard practice, would the resultant burden on an epidemiologic researcher be great enough to discourage important work? Would the research subjects benefit, or would they merely be inundated with information (consent forms, individual results, overall study results) that, even if understandable, would be of uncertain value to them? Are ethical lapses related to inadequate disclosure common in epidemiologic research, and resultant adverse effects consequential? Or does this concern about ethics represent nothing more than institutional and societal overreaction to isolated past lapses, highly publicized lawsuits, and demands of special-interest groups? These questions characterize the continuing debate over both the nature of the ideal state of affairs and the practical problems involved in attaining it.

References

1. National Commission for the Protection of Human Subjects of Biomedical and Behavioral Research. *The Belmont Report: Ethical Principles and Guidelines for the Protection of Human Subjects of Research.* Washington, D.C.: U.S. Government Printing Office, 1978. Dept. of Health, Education, and Welfare Publication No. (05)78-0012.
2. U.S. Department of Health, Education and Welfare. "Protection of Human Subjects," *Federal Register* 43 (November 30, 1978): 56174–198.
3. Department of Health and Human Services. "Regulations for the Protection of Human Subjects." 45 CFR 46.
4. Fayerweather, W. E., Higginson, J., and Beauchamp, T. L., eds. "Ethics in Epidemiology," *Journal of Clinical Epidemiology* 44 (suppl. 1) (1991).
5. Baker, E. L., Schulte, P. A., and French, J. G. "Worker Notification Activities at the National Institute for Occupational Safety and Health: Past and Present." In *Occupational Health in the 1990s; Developing a Platform for Disease Prevention,* ed. P. J. Landrigan and I. J. Selikoff. *Annals of the New York Academy of Science* 572 (1989): 144–150.

6. Zahm, S. H. "On Epidemiology and the Obligation to Notify Study Subjects," *Epidemiology Monitor* 13 (1992): 5.
7. Duncan, A. S., Dunstan, G. R., and Welbourn, R. B., eds. *The Dictionary of Medical Ethics.* London: Darton, Longman and Dodd, 1977.
8. Baram, M. S. "The Right-To-Know and the Duty to Disclose Hazard Information," *American Journal of Public Health* 74 (1984): 385–90.
9. Schulte, P. A. and Ringen, K. "Notification of Workers at High Risk: an Emerging Public Health Problem," *American Journal of Public Health* 74 (1984): 485–91.
10. "Guidelines for Good Epidemiology Practices for Occupational and Environmental Research," Washington, D.C.: Chemical Manufacturers' Assn, 1991.
11. Beauchamp, T. L., Cook, R. R., Fayerweather, W. E., Raabe, G. K., Thar, W. E., Cowles, S. R., and Spivey, G. H. "Ethical Guidelines of Epidemologists," *Journal of Clinical Epidemiology* 44 (suppl. 1) (1991): 151S–69S.
12. Report of the Society for Epidemiologic Research Committee on Ethical Guidelines (Stolley, P., Rothman, K., Shapiro, S., Stein, Z., Szklo, M.), May 12, 1989.
13. Richter, E. D. "The Worker's Right-To-Know: Obstacles, Ambiguities and Loopholes," *Journal of Health Politics* 6 (1981): 339–46.
14. "Informing Workers and Employees about Occupational Cancer," *National Academy of Sciences: Committee on Public Information in the Prevention of Occupational Cancer.* Washington, D.C.: U.S. Department of Labor, 1977.
15. Gewirth, A. "Human Rights and the Prevention of Cancer," *American Philosophical Quarterly* 17 (1980): 117–25.
16. Jones, J. H. *Bad Blood.* New York: The Free Press (Macmillan), 1981.
17. Truett, J., Cornfield, J., and Kannel, W. "Multivariate Analysis of Coronary Heart Disease in Framingham," *Journal of Chronic Diseases* 20 (1967): 511–24.
18. Schulte, P. A. "Epidemiologic Basis for the Notification of Subjects of Cohort Studies," *American Journal of Epidemiology* 121 (1985): 351–61.
19. Schulte, P. A. and Singal, M. "Interpretation and Communication of the Results of Medical Field Investigations," *Journal of Occupational Medicine* 31 (1989): 589–94.
20. Samuels, S. W. "Communicating with Workers (And Everyone Else)," *American Industrial Hygiene Association Journal* 40 (1979): 1159–63.
21. Schulte, P. A. "Ethical Issues in the Communication of Results," *Journal of Clinical Epidemiology* 44 (1991): 575–615.
22. Beauchamp, T. L. and Childress, J. F. *Principles of Biomedical Ethics.* 4th ed. New York: Oxford University Press, 1994.
23. Faden, R. R. and Beauchamp, T. L. *A History and Theory of Informed Consent.* New York: Oxford University Press, 1986.
24. Katz, J. "Disclosure and Consent." In *Genetics and the Law II*, ed. A. Milunsky and G. Annas. New York: Plenum Press, 1980.
25. Silva, M. C. and Sorrell, J. M. "Enhancing Comprehension of Information for Informed Consent: A Review of Empirical Research," *Institutional Review Board: Review of Human Subject Research* 10 (1988): 10–15.
26. Schulte, P. A. and Sweeney, M. H. "Ethical Considerations, Confidentiality Issues, Rights of Human Subjects and Uses of Monitoring Data in Research and Regulation." Proceedings of the Symposium on Human Tissue Monitoring and Specimen Banking: Opportunities for Exposure Assessment, Risk Assessment and Epidemiologic Research. *Environmental Health Perspectives* vol. 103, Supp. 3, 1995: 69–74.

27. Office of Technology Assessment. "New Developments in Biotechnology." 1. Ownership of Human Tissues and Cells. OTA-BA-337. Washington D.C.: U.S. Government Printing Office, 1987.
28. Cooper, J. P. *Biotechnology and the Law*. New York: Clark Boardman Co., Ltd., 1985.
29. Michels, R. and Eth, S. "Ethical Issues in Psychiatric Research on Communities: A Case Study of a Community Mental Health Center Program." In *Ethical Issues in Epidemiological Research*, ed. L. Tancredi. New Brunswick: Rutgers University Press, 1986: 71–98.
30. Bok, S. *Secrets: On the Ethics of Concealment and Revelation*. New York: Pantheon Books, 1982.
31. Robbins, L. N. "Consequences of the Recommendations of the Privacy Protection Study Commission for Longitudinal Studies." In *Ethical Issues In Epidemiological Research*, ed. L. Tancredi. New Brunswick: Rutgers University Press, 1986: 99–114.
32. Nelkin, D. and Tancredi, L. *Dangerous Diagnostics. The Social Power of Biological Information*. New York: Basic Books, Inc., 1989.
33. Schulte, P. A. "Interpretation and Communication of Molecular Epidemiologic Data." In *Molecular Epidemiology: Principles and Practices*, ed. P. A. Schulte and F. P. Perera. San Diego: Academic Press: 233–50.
34. Committee on the Conduct of Science, National Academy of Sciences. *On Being a Scientist*. Washington, D.C.: National Academy Press, 1989.
35. Smith, M. L. "On Being an Authentic Scientist," *Institutional Review Board* 14 (1992): 1–4.
36. Schulte, P. A. "Individual Notification of Workers Exposed to 2–Naphthylamine." In *Effective Risk Communication*, ed. V. T. Covello, D. B. McCallumn, and M. T. Pavlova. New York: Plenum Press, 1989: 105–08.
37. Motulsky, A. G. "Human Genetic Individuality and Risk Assessment." In *Phenotypic Variation in Populations: Relevance to Risk Assessment*, ed. A. D. Woodhead, M. A. Bender, and R. C. Leonard. New York: Plenum Press, 1988: 7–9.
38. Shields, P. G., and Harris C. C. "Molecular Epidemiology and the Genetics of Environmental Cancer," *Journal of the American Medical Association* 246 (1991): 682–87.
39. Thilly, W. G. "Mutational Spectrometry: Opportunity and Limitations in Human Risk Assessment." In *Human Carcinogen Exposure, Biomonitoring and Risk Assessment*, ed. R. C. Garner, P. B. Farmer, G. T. Steel, and A. S. Wright. New York: Oxford University Press, 1991: 127–34.40. OPRR Reports: Policy on informing those tested about HIV status, 1988.
40. OPRR Reports: Policy on informing those tested about HIV status, 1988.
41. OPRR Reports: Guidelines for Institutional Review Boards for AIDS Studies. December 26, 1984.
42. Sands, R. G., Newby, L. G., and Greenberg, R. A. "Labeling of Health Risks in Industrial Settings," *Journal of Applied Behavioral Sciences* 17 (1985): 359–74.
43. Bayer, R. "Notifying Workers at Risk. The Politics of the Right-to-Know," *American Journal of Public Health* 76 (1986): 1352–56.
44. Higginson, J. and Chu, F. "Ethical Considerations and Responsibilities in Communicating Health Risk Information," *Journal of Clinical Epidemiology* 44 (suppl. 1) (1991): 51S–56S.
45. Schulte, P. A. "Problems in Notification and Screening of Workers at High Risk of Disease," *Journal of Occupational Medicine* 28 (1986): 951–57.

46. *National Academy of Sciences.* "Responsible Science: Ensuring the Integrity of the Research Process." Vol 1. Washington, D.C.: National Academy Press, 1992.
47. Bailar, J. C. "Science, Statistics, Deception." In *The Ethical Dimensions of the Biological Sciences*, ed. R. E. Bulge, E. Heitman, S. J. Reiser. Cambridge: Cambridge University Press, 1993: 103–05.
48. Hardy, H. and Egilman, D. "Corruption of Occupational Medical Literature: The Asbestos Example" (Letter), *American Journal of Industrial Medicine* 20 (1991): 127–29.
49. Broad, W. and Wade, N. "Self-Deception and Gullibility." In *The Ethical Dimensions of the Biological Sciences*, ed. R. E. Bulger, E. Heitman, and S. J. Reiser. New York: Cambridge University Press, 1993: 80–92.
50. Samuels, S.W. "Ethics and Ethical Codes in Occupational Medicine." In *Environmental and Occupational Medicine*, ed. W. N. Rom. Boston: Little, Brown & Co., 1982.
51. Sandman, P. M. "Emerging Communication Responsibilities of Epidemiologists," *Journal of Clinical Epidemiology* 49 (1991): 541–50.
52. Nelkin, D. "Whistle Blowing and Social Responsibility," *Progress in Clinical Biological Research* 128 (1983): 351–57.
53. Dickersin, K. "The Existence of Publication Bias and Risk Factors for Its Occurrence," *Journal of the American Medical Association* 263 (1990): 1385–89.
54. Epstein, S. S. *The Politics of Cancer.* San Francisco: Sierra Club Books, 1978: 102–04.
55. Dickersin, K., Min, Y. I., and Meinert, C. L. "Factors Influencing Publication of Results," *Journal of the American Medical Association* 267 (1992): 374–78.
56. Szklo, M. "Issues in Publication and Interpretation of Research Findings," *Journal of Clinical Epidemiology* 44 (suppl. 1), (1991): 109S–13S.
57. Chalmers, I. "Underreporting Research is Scientific Misconduct," *Journal of the American Medical Association* 263 (1990): 1405–08.
58. Rennie, D. and Flanagin, A. "Publication Bias. The Triumph of Hope Over Experience" (Editorial), *Journal of the American Medical Association* 267 (1992): 411–12.
59. Chalmers, T. C., Frank, C. S., and Reitman, D. "Minimizing the Three Stages of Publication Bias," *Journal of the American Medical Association* 263 (1990): 1392–95.
60. International Committee of Medical Editors. "Conflict of Interest," *Lancet* 341 (1993): 742–43.
61. Rothman, K. J. "Conflict of Interest: The New McCarthyism in Science," *Journal of the American Medical Association* 269 (1993): 2782–84.
62. Veatch, R. M., ed. *Cross Cultural Perspectives in Medical Ethics: Readings.* Boston: Jones and Bartlett Publishers, 1989.
63. Tranoy, K. C. "Is There a Universal Research Ethics?" *Progress in Clinical Biological Research Research* 128 (1983): 2–12.
64. LaVerta, D. S., and Linares, A. M. "Ethical Principles of Biomedical Research on Human Subjects: Their Application and Limitations in Latin America and the Caribbean." In *Bioethics: Issues and Perspectives*, ed. S. S. Connor and H. L. Fuenzalida-Puelma. Washington, D.C.: Pan American Health Organization, 1990: 107–15.
65. Pellegrino, E. D. "The Relationship of Autonomy and Integrity in Medical Ethics." In *Bioethics: Issues and Perspectives*, ed. S. S. Connor and H. L. Fuenzalida-Puelma. Washington, D.C.: Pan American Health Organization, 1990: 8–17.

IV

THE STUDY OF VULNERABLE POPULATIONS

10

Ethical Issues in Epidemiologic Research with Children

SANFORD LEIKIN

The epidemic diseases of childhood have been monitored since ancient times. In the Hebrew Talmud, for instance, Rabbi Ismael ben R. Jose describes *askara*, or diphtheria, as follows: "Askara is a much-dreaded epidemic disease which usually attacks children, is located in the throat, and kills the patient by a painful death from suffocation."[1] So much was this disease feared by the Hebrews that the first case to manifest in a community was heralded by a warning blast of the *shofar* (ram's horn trumpet), although under ordinary circumstances it was sounded only after the third case of an epidemic disease.

Serious inquiry into outbreaks of childhood diseases has continued to the present. In fact, the origin of pediatrics as a specialty is associated with scholarly dissertations on communicable diseases such as infectious diarrhea, scarlet fever, diphtheria, measles, and tuberculosis.[1] These illnesses were rampant in foundling homes, orphanages, and among the poor where the early pediatricians began their practices. Studies were performed to determine their causes and modes of transmission. Many improvements in child health resulted from these efforts.

Nevertheless, children's diseases of an epidemic nature persist as a major world health problem. The total number of child deaths under five years of age in developing countries alone is 12.9 million annually.[2] Of this number, more than sixty percent result from pneumonia, diarrheal disease, or vaccine preventable diseases. Other common causes are measles, pertussis, neonatal tetanus, tuberculosis, and malaria. Epidemiologic studies continue to be important in learning about outbreaks of childhood diseases, and evaluating efforts that are taken to eliminate or control them.

Before the second half of this century, little attention was paid to the ethical propriety of performing epidemiologic studies on children,[3] but the conduct of research with vulnerable populations has since come under scrutiny.[4,5] A number of striking events stimulated this concern and the subsequent regulation of the performance of research in the United States. The grotesque experimentation of the Nazis revealed during the Nuremberg trials led to the Nuremberg Code.[6] The vital provision of the code was the informed, voluntary consent of the subject. If accepted literally, this crucial requirement of first-party consent of the subject would eliminate children as research subjects. However, the Declaration of Helsinki issued in 1964 by the World Medical Association stated that individuals with limited capacity to consent can participate in research if they are provided with special protections and adequate surrogate decision makers.[7]

In the United States, Congress established the National Commission for the Protection of Human Subjects of Biomedical and Behavioral Research to examine the ethical conduct of human research. The commission identified three ethical principles underlying the conduct of research and developed guidelines for the protection of human subjects of research.[8] In this chapter, an outline of the guidelines is provided as a preface to the subsequent discussion. Another of the commission's major accomplishments was its report and recommendations on research involving children.[9] They recognize children's vulnerability and diminished decisional competence and the need for parental involvement. The recommendations undergird the ethical conduct of research with children in the United States. Therefore, the report and its recommendations are discussed below in detail, along with a description of similar guidelines from other national and international organizations.

The risk of harms to children involved in epidemiologic research are also important to consider in order to determine whether the research is justified and to obtain adequate informed consent or permission for their participation. These risks are described in this chapter. Besides the tragic outcomes in mortality and morbidity caused by the HIV/AIDS epidemic, striking ethical problems can also arise when epidemiologic studies of this disease include children. The final section of this chapter is devoted to a discussion of these issues.

The National Commission's Reports

In the 1950s and 1960s, the American public became aware of several apparently egregious research projects that resulted in public criticism.[10] Responding to the public's increasing disquiet over the ethical conduct of human research, in 1974 Congress passed PL 93–348, creating the National Commission for the Protection of Human Subjects of Biomedical and Behavioral Research.[11]

The Commission considered the matter of the ethical conduct of research during the next four years. It then published its Belmont Report: Ethical Principles and Guidelines for the Protection of Human Subjects of Research.[8] The report distinguishes between research, on the one hand, and the practice of accepted therapy, on the other. It also identifies three basic principles that govern the conduct of all human research: respect for persons, beneficence, and justice. Respect for persons incorporates at least two ethical convictions: first, that individuals should be treated as autonomous agents; and second, that persons with diminished autonomy should be protected. The principle of beneficence requires that we maximize possible benefits and eliminate or minimize possible harms. Justice in the research context concerns equitable distribution of the benefits and burdens of research.

In addition to presenting these principles, the report describes their applications in the conduct of research: informed consent and the assessment of risks and benefits. Informed consent, based on the principle of respect for persons, requires that subjects, to the degree they are capable, be given the opportunity to choose what shall or shall not happen to them. The requirement that risks and benefits be assessed derives from the principle of beneficence. The term *risk* refers to a possibility that harm may occur. When risk is expressed quantitatively, it usually indicates the probability of being harmed and the magnitude of the conceived harm. The word *benefit*, used in the research context, refers to something of positive value related to health or welfare. In contrast to risk, benefit is not a term that expresses probabilities. Thus, risk/benefit assessments are concerned with the probabilities and magnitude of the possible harms and anticipated benefits of research. Risks and benefits are of different kinds. The risks can be psychological, physical, legal, social, and economic, with corresponding benefits. These research risks and benefits may affect individual subjects, their families, and particular groups within society.

The National Commission's Report on Research Involving Children

In addition to providing an ethical framework for the conduct of research, the National Commission deliberated on the ethics of research related to vulnerable populations, such as fetuses, prisoners, and children. A major controversy it confronted was whether research, particularly nontherapeutic research, should be performed on children, and, if so, under which conditions. The most restrictive position on this matter is that of Ramsey, who argued that research that does not directly benefit individual children is always ethically impermissible.[12,13] According to him, consent is the key ethical problem. Because the young are not capable of giving full and informed consent, no research ought to be performed on them unless it holds out the possibility of direct benefit. Ramsey was also concerned with the risk of harm as well as the violation of autonomy. Despite the fact that research may promote knowledge generalizable to children as a group, such good can never outweigh the risk to the individual child. For Ramsey, the ends of research do not justify using children as the means.

In contrast, McCormick contended that children can be involved in research, even if it will not directly benefit them, as long as the research poses no discernible risk and will benefit them as a group.[14]

But Ramsey countered that there is an important difference between *no discernible risk* and *discernibly no risk*; the latter standard presumes empirical evidence of safety, while the former does not. Because research procedures always involve some intrusion, not incurring any discernible risk seems fundamentally impossible. Hence, the definition of *minimal risk* was designated by the commission as the quantity that would be permissible without additional justification.

McCormick further asserted that children are social beings who have a moral obligation to help others when there is little cost to themselves. Thus, according to his view, children are morally obligated to participate in research for the good of all. Moreover, parental consent is said to be morally valid for both therapeutic and nontherapeutic research, because it accepts a reasonable presumption of the child's obligations. According to McCormick, the parent is the vehicle for choosing what the child should rightly choose if he were so situated that he knew what he ought to do. Bartholme further advanced the argument by suggesting that children's involvement in research might benefit them, because it could encourage their moral development and stimulate altruism.[15]

The commission considered all of these opinions but ultimately sided with none of them. Among its major concerns was why it is necessary to do research on children at all. Two factors were the absence, in numerous instances, of suitable alternative populations of research subjects, and the negative consequences of not conducting research on children in those instances. Such consequences might include the perpetuation of harmful practices, the introduction of untested practices, and the failure to develop new treatments for disease.[9]

Possible alternative populations for research involving children are animals and adult humans, but limitations exist for both. In the study of epidemic diseases their drawbacks are especially relevant. Most epidemic diseases cannot be replicated in animals. Some occur only in children. Moreover, the pathologic changes and the clinical manifestations of these diseases, as well as their mortality rates, differ substantially between adults and children. The results of immunizations or other efforts to prevent their occurrence or their outcome in these two populations may also vary significantly.

Prohibiting children's participation in research would have a profound effect on the welfare of many children. It would impede innovative efforts to develop new prophylactic methods or treatments for diseases that affect them, while research to prevent or treat adult disease would continue. Even research efforts on adult disease would be hampered, as many common and serious diseases that affect adults probably have their origins in childhood. For example, the development of atherosclerosis and essential hypertension of adulthood is associated with risk factors found in children.[16] Not allowing children's participation in research would also lead to the introduction of innovative practices without the advantage of sound evidence and sober evaluation. Taking all of the above matters into account, the commission concluded that research involving children is important for the health and well-being of all children and can be conducted in an ethical manner. This conclusion became the commission's first recommendation. It further recognized that the vulnerability of children, which arises from their dependence and immaturity, raises questions about the ethical acceptability of involving them in research. "Such ethical problems can be offset," the commission stated, "by establishing conditions that research must satisfy to be appropriate for the involvement of children."[9] Such conditions are set forth in its subsequent recommendations.

The National Commission's Recommendations

As part of its section on recommendation, the Commission offered several definitions. *Children* are defined as "persons who have not attained the legal age of consent to general medical care as determined under the applicable law of the jurisdiction in which the research will be conducted."[9] Using the age of consent for general medical treatment distinguished it from age of consent for treatment of specific conditions, such as pregnancy, drug addiction, or venereal disease.

In addition, minimal risk is defined as the probability and magnitude of physical or psychological harm that is normally encountered in the daily lives, or in the routine medical or psychological examination of, healthy children. Assessment of the degree of risk should take into account the age of the prospective subject. Besides the more obvious physical or psychological harm, the possible effects of disruption, separation from parents, or unusual discomfort should also be considered. Examples of medical procedures presenting no more than minimal risk cited by the Commission are routine immunization, modest change in diet or schedule, physical examination, obtaining blood and urine specimens, and developmental assessments. Similarly, many routine tools of behavioral research, such as most questionnaires, observational techniques, noninvasive physiological monitoring, and psychological tests and puzzles, may be accepted as presenting no more than minimal risk.

The Commission also commented on three other factors concerning risk: (1) the possibility that questions about some topics may generate such anxiety or stress as to involve more than minimal risk; (2) research in which information is gathered that could be harmful if disclosed should not be considered minimal risk unless adequate provisions are made to preserve confidentiality; and (3) research in which information will be shared with persons or institutions that may use such information against the subjects should be considered more than minimal risk.

In its second recommendation, the Commission described the conditions under which research with children should proceed: (1) the research is scientifically sound and significant; (2) where appropriate, studies have been conducted first on animals and adult humans, then on older children, prior to involving infants; (3) risks are minimized by using the safest procedures consistent with sound research and by using procedures performed for diagnostic or treatment purposes whenever feasible; (4) adequate provisions are made to protect the privacy of children and their parents, and to maintain confidentiality of the data; and (5) subjects are selected in an equitable manner.

Parental Permission and Children's Assent

Recognizing that children cannot give legal consent, the commission further recommended that prior to the child's participation the parents' or guardian's permission should be obtained, and that assent be obtained from those children whom the institutional review board (IRB) judges are capable of assenting. Soliciting parental permission (as distinguished from consent) satisfies the principle of respect for persons by respecting the child's need for care and protection; and by respecting the authority of parents to make decisions regarding their children's lives and activities (as long as that authority is not abused). This position reflects the traditional view that parents have general responsibility for the care and custody of their children and correlative rights with respect to that responsibility. However, the Commission also recommended that if the IRB determines that a research protocol is designed for conditions or for a subject population for which parental or guardian permission is not a reasonable requirement to protect the subjects (for example, in the case of neglected or abused children), it may waive the permission requirement.

Obtaining the child's assent accords with the ethical principle of respect for persons. That principle not only requires respecting the decisions of autonomous persons, but it also compels honoring the choices of individuals with diminished autonomy to the extent that they have developed the capacity to make choices. In determining whether to seek assent, the Commission recommended that the IRB consider the "age, psychologic state, and the maturity of the children involved." These criteria imply that the child is able to conduct certain cognitive functions: (1) to understand what is being asked immediately and generally; (2) to have a notion that permission is being sought independently; and (3) to make choices free from outside constraints. While these are general gauges of decisionmaking ability, they fail to reflect certain important aspects of children's decision making.[17] These include current knowledge about the development of children's cognitive capacities and their understanding and reasoning about health care research. Other considerations are young persons' ability to recognize and express fulfillment of their rights, their conformity or nonconformity to authority figures, and their perception of their obligation to others.

The recommendations for parental permission and children's assent were subsequently incorporated into federal regulations on children's research.[18] The regulations define assent as "a child's affirmative agreement to participate in research." But, according to the regulations, if "the research holds out a prospect of direct benefit that is important to the health or well-being of the children and is available only in the context of the research, the assent of the children is not a necessary condition for proceeding with the research."[18] This statement indicates that either not seeking assent or overriding the child's veto is allowable in the conduct of therapeutic research. The National Commission specifically recommended that in the conduct of nontherapeutic research, "A child's objection to participation should be binding, . . ." but the Federal regulations make no comment on the question of dissent to nontherapeutic research.[9,18] This is unfortunate because it leaves unclear the weight of a minor's dissent in research that does not offer direct benefit to him or her.

Research Risk Categories

Also identified by the commission and included in the regulations are four research risk categories:[9,18] (1) research not involving greater than minimal risk; (2) research involving greater than minimal risk but presenting the prospect of direct benefit to the individual subjects; (3) research involving a minor increase over minimal risk and holding out no prospect of direct benefit to the individual subjects, but likely to yield generalizable information concerning the individual's condition; (4) research (not included in the previous three categories) that presents an opportunity to understand, prevent, or alleviate a serious problem affecting the health or welfare of children.

If the IRB determines that the research falls into the first three categories, the research may be approved by the IRB provided that it meets the general conditions concerning the conduct of children's research, and appropriate provisions are made for parental permission and children's assent. If the IRB determines that the research falls into category four, the Secretary of the Department of Health and Human Services must approve the research after consultation with a panel of experts in pertinent disciplines and following public review and comment. On two occasions, panels have reviewed and commented on category-four research.[19,20]

Wards

Children who are wards of the state or any other agency or institution can participate in research categories one and two (see above).[18] But federal regulations allow these children to participate in categories three and four only if the research relates to their status as orphans, abandoned children, and the like; or if the research is conducted in a school or similar group setting in which the majority of the children involved as subjects are not wards of the state. Further, an advocate must be appointed for each child who is a ward. The advocate should not be associated in any way with the research or the guardian organization, and he or she should act to promote the best interests of the child during participation in the research. These limitations on research are intended to allow us to learn more about the effects of various settings in which children who are wards of the state may be placed, and about the circumstances surrounding child abuse and neglect. Yet they avoid embarrassment or psychological harm that might result from excluding these children from research projects in which their peers in a school, camp, or other group setting will be participating.

Ethical Guidelines of Other Countries

Developed Countries

In addition to the United States, other countries have deliberated on the ethical conduct of children's research. Guidelines of the British Paediatric Association's Ethics Committee and of the Australian College of Paediatrics are similar to the recommendations made by the National Commission in their affirmations that: (1) the conduct of research on children is important; (2) research should be done on older individuals before it is done on younger ones; (3) research should be well designed, well conducted, and should involve a statistically appropriate number of subjects; and (4) all research proposals should be submitted to a local research ethics committee for review.[21,22] These two sets of guidelines also require parental or guardian consent, and the child's assent, before proceeding with the research. The British guidelines have a "minimal" risk category, but they stipulate that blood sampling can be done for research purposes only if the sample is taken as part of treatment. Further, they state that it would be unethical to submit child subjects to more than minimal risk when the procedure offers no benefit to them.

In Canada, the extent to which research on children can be conducted is unclear. The Medical Research Council of Canada's guidelines on research involving human subjects state that parents "may permit others to handle their children in ways that would otherwise constitute a technical or minor legal assault, but not where pain or discomfort beyond carefully defined limits would be liable to occur."[23] Some commentators have interpreted this section of the guidelines to mean that parents cannot consent to nontherapeutic research involving venipuncture. Reports from other developed countries consider the ethical implications of research on children, but formal statements from government or national organizations have not been issued.[24,25]

Developing Countries

Because the Nuremberg Code and the Declaration of Helsinki have a Western cultural orientation, they may not be applicable to developing countries. The Council for International Organizations of Medical Sciences (CIOMS) and the World Health Organization (WHO) examined this matter, and issued *International Ethical Guidelines for Biomedical Research Involving Human Subjects*.[26] They are designed to be of use in defining national policies on the ethics of biomedical research, applying ethical standards in local circumstances, and establishing or redefining adequate mechanisms for ethical review of research involving human subjects. Owing to the importance of epidemiology, particularly for public health, and to the need for international policy for ethical review of such studies, the CIOMS guidelines were prepared with special attention to epidemiologic studies.

A section of the guidelines concerns research with children. It states that in order to justify any research on children, the investigation must be relevant to their health needs as a group. Before undertaking research with children, the guidelines also require the investigator to ensure that: (1) children not be involved, if the research question can be answered by using adults; (2) a parent or legal guardian has given proxy consent; (3) "consent" of each child has been obtained to the extent of the child's capabilities; (4) the child's dissent to participation should be honored, unless according to the research protocol the child would receive therapy for which there is no medically acceptable alternative; and (5) the risk presented by interventions not intended to benefit the individual child-subject is low and commensurate with the importance of the knowledge to be gained. The CIOMS guidelines also state, "When an ethical review committee is persuaded that the object of the research is sufficiently important, slight increases above minimal risk may be permitted."[26] Review of the various national guidelines as well as those by CIOMS indicates that, with a few exceptions, there is a striking agreement about what is ethically required in order to perform research on children.

In the CIOMS guidelines, requesting the child's "consent" and honoring his or her dissent to research involvement indicate that each child's personhood is to be respected. However, in many developing societies the concepts of personhood and autonomy differ significantly from the Western view. For example, in certain African societies selfhood cannot be extricated from a dynamic system of social relationships, both of kinship and of community as defined by the village.[27] Even adults in these societies may not have the necessary awareness of the implication of participation in an experiment to give adequately informed consent directly to investigators. Moreover, many of these countries are in a preindustrial, agricultural stage where the orientation is toward a strong family unit with a more authoritarian parental attitude than in developed countries. As a result, children's personhood and autonomy may not be perceived as they might be in other cultures. When children are recruited for epidemiologic research, their assent may not be sought nor their dissent honored. Recognizing that in foreign countries procedures followed to protect human subjects may differ, the U.S. federal regulations were recently revised regarding collaborative studies conducted between U.S. departments or agencies and investigators in other countries. The regulations now require the assurance that protections afforded to subjects in those countries are "at least equivalent" to those provided by U.S. federal regulations.[28] What impact this policy will have on children's research in foreign countries remains to be determined.

Epidemiologic Research Procedures Performed on Children

Conducting epidemiologic research on children may require the use of a number of different methodologies. These include examining subjects' medical or school records; interviewing older children, and interviewing the parents or other caretakers of younger children; requesting youth to complete questionnaires and other survey instruments; performing physical examinations; obtaining bodily tissues or fluids; and collecting excreta for laboratory examination.

These interventions can include different kinds and levels of harm to the subjects or their families. The harms include physical distress or impairment, emotional distress, invasion of privacy, and breach of confidentiality. In epidemiologic research, the risk of harm of many of the procedures employed usually does not exceed the probability and magnitude of physical or psychological harm that is normally encountered in children's daily lives, or in routine medical or psychological examination. Thus, the procedures can be considered to present no more than minimal risk. However, sometimes they impose greater than minimal risk, as discussed below.

Risk of Physical Harm

Most epidemiologic research in children that requires blood specimens drawn from an antecubital vein is accepted as minimal-risk research, unless frequent venipunctures are to be performed or an excessive volume of blood is to be taken. The assessment of antecubital venipuncture as minimal risk is supported by the perceptions of parents of preschool children who participated in nontherapeutic research.[29]

Nonetheless, other medical procedures may be performed in which specimens are obtained for nontherapeutic purposes; for example, spinal taps, tympanocentesis, or venous blood specimens from the femoral or jugular region. These are often more painful than antecubital venipunctures or may result in significant harmful sequelae. Despite the frequent use of many of these procedures for clinical purposes, conceptual and empirical difficulties still exist in estimating their riskiness for research. Providing a minimal risk category requires that IRBs define "an increase over minimal risk" and "no more than minimal risk." However, Kopelman contends that the key concept of minimal risk is problematic because of the different interpretations it permits for the risks of everyday life.[30] Moreover, a survey shows inconsistencies in the understanding of these risk categories among chairpersons of pediatric departments and directors of pediatric clinical research units in the United States.[31] These difficulties suggest that investigators and IRBs need better standards for risk assessment in children's research.[32,50]

Risk of Psychologic Harm

Although completing questionnaires or answering questions about one's conduct or personal relationships may not be disturbing, answering some questions, particularly for adolescents, may cause emotional distress. Interviews or survey instruments with queries that remind the young person of physically or emotionally traumatic episodes in their lives or about personal actions that are morally or socially questionable may produce anxiety or feelings of guilt. These emotional reactions may be of a temporary or prolonged duration.

Invasion of Privacy and Breach of Confidentiality

Inquiry about matters related to health clearly intrude on one's privacy. Control over knowledge about oneself and particularly about one's body is basic to respect for the person and is often constitutionally protected. Young people, with their growing wish for self-determination, are particularly sensitive to infringements of privacy, and may strongly object to others learning particulars about their personal lives or behavior. Loss of control over such information, whether through compelled disclosure or breach of confidentiality, subjects many young individuals to embarrassment and degradation.

In addition, a breach in confidentiality could result in more serious harms for minors. Denial of educational, employment, or economic opportunities could occur. Social rejections could result, and in some instances even their lives or property could be threatened.[33] Of particular relevance are breaches of confidentiality in which parents learn of their teenager's sexual activities or of other behaviors that the parents oppose. Serious recriminations, including parental rejection or even physical abuse, may result in such instances. Hence, investigators must always maintain confidentiality of all records associated with epidemiologic research on youth, unless otherwise required by law.

Risk-Benefit Assessment

A normative statement in all codes and regulations concerning the ethics of research is that there must be a favorable balance between harm and benefit. Without a favorable balance there is no justification for beginning the research. The performance of most epidemiologic research studies offers no direct benefit to the subject. Nevertheless, the results of much epidemiologic research have the possibility of benefit to society or to certain societal groups. If the research offers trivial or no benefit to society, it should not be conducted, even though it poses no more than minimal risk. But in considering his or her research, the epidemiologic investigator should identify the nature and estimate the probability and magnitude of any expected harm. Jonas suggests one test that can lend credibility to a pediatric investigator's claim that the expected benefits merit the taking of the risks.[34] This is the investigator's willingness to allow his or her own children to participate in the research.

Pediatric HIV/AIDS Research

In the United States, only 2% of reported cases of AIDS occur in children under thirteen years of age and another 1% of cases occur in adolescents thirteen to twenty-one years of age.[35] Yet HIV infection and AIDS represent major health problems in the young. There are 6,000 to 30,000 children with HIV infection in the United States.[36] Moreover, the United Nations Development Program reports that among sexually active people, young women in their teens and early twenties have the highest rate of HIV infections. As one adolescent medicine specialist recently said, "Adolescents are the leading edge of the next wave of the epidemic."[37] Because of the extremely long latency period between HIV infection and the onset of illness, many individuals infected as adolescents will not manifest AIDS until they are older. The tragic outcome of this observation already shows in the rising HIV-related mortality in young Americans between twenty-five and forty-four years of age.[38]

Some have suggested that our efforts to control the epidemic should be targeted at individuals in a relative handful of socially "marginalized" communities (inner city drug abusers and prostitutes).[39] While it is important to include those individuals in epidemiologic studies, it is erroneous to believe that HIV/AIDS will disappear if our efforts are limited to these groups. HIV infection is spreading slowly, but relentlessly, into all sectors of our society.[39] Our epidemiologic studies, therefore, must cover a wide segment of the population rather than just particular groups. Such efforts in pediatric research can lead to better information about the transmission of HIV infection to neonates, and investigations about the factors affecting morbidity and mortality in children and adolescents.

Ethical Issues in AIDS Epidemiologic Research in Children

The ethical problems that arise in conducting AIDS epidemiologic research in children are not dissimilar to those that occur in other epidemiologic research, but the medical, social, and familial complexities of HIV infection make the ethical issues more difficult to address. The nature of HIV transmission and the fact that individual behavior plays a large part in the transmission are principal factors in these ethical concerns. Children can acquire HIV infection through one of several routes: receipt of infected blood or blood products; vertical (perinatal) transmission from mothers who are drug users or whose sexual partners are infected; breast-feeding; or sexual abuse.

HIV transmission in adolescents occurs much as in adults: receiving infected blood or blood products; sharing drug-injection paraphernalia; unprotected anal sexual intercourse; or heterosexual spread to female partners of infected males. The rate of heterosexual transmission is increasing rapidly among adolescents, although homosexual-bisexual spread predominates in young men.

Societal reaction to individuals exhibiting homosexual-bisexual behaviors or intravenous drug abuse, and to women with HIV infection who bear children, often results in social stigma and economic ostracism. The ethical issues often arise: (1) when conducting epidemiologic perinatal screening for HIV infection; (2) in obtaining parental permission for the child's participation in research; and (3) in considering the role of adolescents in decision making about their participation in epidemiologic research.

Neonatal Screening

Detecting possible HIV infection in newborns is an active target of epidemiologic inquiry. In fact, the United States Centers for Disease Control and Prevention has sponsored anonymous HIV antibody testing in neonatal blood taken for metabolic testing on more than two million women in several states and cities. Screening for a variety of other medical conditions that require early treatment is now being conducted on identified neonates in all states and the District of Columbia. One could ask, why not include HIV infection in this routine testing, or treat HIV just like any other disease? But HIV infection is not comparable to genetic neonatal conditions. Identifying infants at risk for HIV infection carries the potential for special harms, as the tragic phenomenon of boarder babies (those well enough to leave the hospitals but unwanted because of their HIV status) dramatically attests.[40]

Testing newborns for HIV antibody also raises the issue of invasion of the mother's privacy. Such testing imposes HIV screening on mothers, in effect, because HIV antibody detected in the neonate's blood is maternally derived.[39,41] Moreover, if the infant is found to have HIV antibodies and the mother did not previously know that she had HIV infection, the possibility exists that the mother will have to face her own illness and its consequences, as well as concerns about her child.

If neonatal screening is to be conducted that would identify specific infants, the permission of the child's parents or guardian is required. To obtain permission, the investigator must provide information to the infant's surrogate about the benefits, if any, of participation in the research, and also about its attendant risks. As indicated above, testing newborns for HIV raises the issue of invasion of the mother's privacy in addition to the harms to the babies. As a consequence, the mother may suffer discrimination, including loss of housing, employment or educational opportunities, and child care services. She may also be socially ostracized, or be emotionally or physically abused. Besides these harmful effects, and having to deal with her own illness and its consequences, she may receive coercive counseling to abort her fetus or to be sterilized if she undergoes prenatal testing and is found to be infected.[38,40] Thus, if the testing is *not* anonymous, the investigators conducting HIV epidemiologic screening protocols must obtain permission to perform their research and must give assurances that strict confidentiality will be maintained.

A further diagnostic factor also presents a major problem in neonatal screening for HIV infection. Current methodology only allows for the detection of passively transferred maternal antibodies, indicating maternal infection, and does not specifically identify infection in the infant. The detection of passively transferred antibody, which can persist for several months, only indicates that the infant is at risk for infection because of intrauterine exposure. Only 20% to 30% of infants who are at risk of perinatal exposure will actually turn out to be infected.

If an accurate diagnostic test were available for use in the newborn period or during early infancy, would screening be justified in order to benefit the child? Until recently, the arguments in favor of screening to treat or protect HIV-identified infants have not been compelling.[40] However, a number of virologic tests have now become available that permit early diagnosis of HIV infection in infants in the first months of life. Approximately 50% of infected infants can be identified at or near birth with these techniques, and more than 95% can be diagnosed by three to six months of life.[42] Based on current knowledge, there is not enough information available to recommend routine antiretroviral therapy for HIV-infected asymptomatic children with normal immune status. However, using the CD4 lymphocyte count as a criterion for initiating therapy, antiretroviral clinical trials are now being conducted in asymptomatic children. Further, epidemiologic investigation shows that young infants with HIV infection who are three to six months of age are particularly prone to *Pneumocystis carinii* (PCP) infection.[43] Effective prevention of PCP is available for these infants. These facts argue strongly for identifying the infant at risk for infection as early in life as possible. Thus, in requesting consent for prenatal screening or permission for neonatal screening, the epidemiologic investigator must inform the pregnant women or mothers of neonates about the possible benefits to the child, as well as about the risks of the research to themselves and to their offspring.

Parental Permission for Research

Because parents are available to act as advocates for their child under ordinary circumstances, seeking parental permission for research is relatively uncomplicated. But, as a result of factors such as drug abuse, marital discord, and parental discord, Ackerman has argued that "there are many cases in which an HIV-infected child's biological parent provides inadequate and discontinuous advocacy."[44] In such cases, the child may be well served by the use of third-party advocates who can oversee decisionmaking for research purposes.

More extreme than these cases are circumstances in which requiring parental or guardian permission for research may be unreasonable on either practical or theoretic grounds. In these situations federal regulations provide for waiving the permission requirement, on the condition that an appropriate mechanism for protecting the subjects can be substituted. The children who are most likely to generate consideration of this waiver are those who lack parental guardians: children in foster care, those living with relatives other than parents, or those who are wards of the state or of an agency. Suggested mechanisms for appropriate substitutions include expanding the range of foster parents' discretion, improving the decision-making process within child welfare agencies, and using special processes of research review.[40,50] Whatever form the mechanism takes, it must be consistent with federal, state, or local law.

Adolescents

It is generally accepted that the counsel, guidance, and support of concerned family members is important to the adolescent. But attempts to force their involvement on the adolescent may alienate the young person who is seeking care for sensitive or personal health issues. If the parents are informed about their son's or daughter's condition, the teenager may not seek help and possibly be exposed to serious health hazards. For this reason, state laws have been enacted that allow minors to seek medical treatment and to give consent on their own account for venereal disease, alcohol and drug abuse, and mental health and contraceptive counseling. The courts have also determined that when a medical intervention entails only a small risk, mature minors (that is, those over fourteen years of age) can decide whether to accept treatment without parental consent.[45] Further, the federal regulations define "children" as "persons who have not attained a legal age for consent to treatment or procedures involved in the research under the applicable law of the jurisdiction in which the research will be conducted" (45 CFR 46.402). This definition appears to extend to those who have the legal right to consent to treatment or a complementary authority to consent to related research procedures.[46,50]

Nevertheless, several arguments have been offered against a permissive interpretation of the law and regulations in regard to minors' independent decisions to be involved in research. One objection to the lenient stance is that research, such as much epidemiologic research, offers no benefit to the adolescent. [35,47,48] Another criticism is that deception might be required in order to permit the adolescent's participation without parental involvement.[49] A more legalistic argument is that state statutes that allow treatment of mature minors or treatment of minors for specific conditions (such as venereal disease) were clearly not written with research in mind.[48]

By middle or late adolescence, most youth have developed significant decision-making capacity. Because of their budding self-awareness, they desire more personal autonomy. Since we now allow mature minors to make minimal risk treatment decisions, it would seem inconsistent not to afford them the same right when research involves no more than minimal risk. The possibility does exist that epidemiologic research will carry more than minimal risk, but it is unlikely. The major risk presented by such research is the potential for breach of confidentiality, resulting in parents or others finding out about matters that the adolescent preferred to keep private. By taking appropriate measures, this risk can be eliminated. Thus, I recommend that adolescents who are more than fourteen years of age be allowed to assent to minimal-risk epidemiologic research, including AIDS/HIV research, without parental permission; in essence, that they give consent. My recommendation is consistent with what is known about this age group's psychologic capacities, and supports their desires for privacy and self-determination.[17] However, before adolescents can participate in research based solely on their own agreement, the IRB must waive the requirement for parental permission. As a substitute for parental permission, an appropriate mechanism must be put in place to protect the adolescent. For example, a nurse, social worker, or psychologist who is not associated with the research might be used to assist the adolescent in decision making. In addition, the waiver must be consistent with local, state, and federal regulations.

Conclusions

Performing epidemiologic research on children is of great importance to their health and welfare. However, due to their legal incompetence and physical and cognitive vulnerabilities, the question arises as to whether their participation in research is justified, particularly when it does not directly benefit them. Thus, if they are to be research subjects, not only should parental permission and the assent of older children and adolescents be obtained, but the risks of harm should be minimized whenever possible. IRBs are obligated to determine risk levels, but conceptual and practical obstacles sometimes interfere with their ability to characterize minimal risk research. The development of better risk-assessment standards would make epidemiologic research in children more ethically appropriate.

Cultural differences, poverty, and a lack of sophistication about research methods in people of undeveloped countries make the children of these countries vulnerable to exploitation. Investigators from developed nations who conduct epidemiologic research in undeveloped countries must be particularly sensitive to this possibility. The ethical standards for conducting research on children of undeveloped countries should be equivalent to those employed in more advanced nations.

Societal reaction to individuals infected with HIV places them at risk for social stigma and denial of educational and economic opportunities. Thus, detection of the infecion can cause them significant harm. Neonatal HIV infection may occur as a result of intrauterine exposure or in association with the birth process. Not only are the HIV-positive infants affected by the disease, but its detection in them has serious implications for their mothers. Recent advances in technology now permit detection of HIV infection in asymptomatic neonates, who can receive the benefit of treatment and the prevention of PCP. These asymptomatic neonates can be identified by screening all newborns, or by screening the neonates of women known to be HIV positive. Because either method places HIV-infected women at risk for social and economic harms, their consent for neonatal testing should always be sought.

While epidemiologic research usually offers no direct benefit, involving the older adolescent in decisionmaking about the research respects his or her emerging autonomy. Some epidemiologic research touches on sensitive matters that adolescents may not want their parents to know about. To maintain confidentiality in minimal-risk epidemiologic research, it is proposed that parental permission be waived and that mature minors be allowed independent decisionmaking.

ACKNOWLEDGMENTS

I deeply appreciate the helpful comments of Robert Parrott, M.D., and John Sever, M.D. Ph.D., in the preparation of this manuscript.

References

1. Abt, A. *Garrison History of Pediatrics*, ed. I. Abt. Philadelphia: W.B. Saunders, 1965.
2. *The State of the World's Children*. New York: Oxford University Press for UNICEF, 1993.
3. Curran, W. J., Beecher, H. K. "Experimentation in Children: a Reexamination of Legal

and Ethical Principles," *Journal of the American Medical Association* 10 (1969): 77–83.

4. Katz, J. *Experimentation with Human Beings*. New York: Russell Sage Foundation, 1972: 9–65, 633, 1007, 1010.

5. Levine, R. *Ethics and the Regulations of Research*, 2d ed. Baltimore: Urban & Schwarzenberg, 1986: 235–50.

6. *Trials of War Criminals before the Nuremberg Tribunes: United States vs Karl Brandt*, vol. 2. Washington, D.C.: U.S. Government Printing Office, 1979: 181.

7. "World Medical Association Declaration of Helsinki, 1964." In *Research and the Individual: Human Studies*, ed. H. Beecher. Boston: Little, Brown & Co., 1970.

8. National Commission for the Protection of Human Subjects of Biomedical and Behavioral Research. *The Belmont Report: Ethical Principles and Guidelines for the Protection of Human Subjects of Research*. Washington, D.C.: DHEW Pub. No. (OS) 78–0012, App. I, DHEW Pub. No. (OS) 78–0013, App. II, DHEW Pub. No. (OS) 78–0014, 1978.

9. National Commission for the Protection of Human Subjects of Biomedical and Behavioral Research. *Research Involving Children: Report and Recommendations*. Washington, D.C., DHEW Pub. No. (OS) 77–0004 (Appendix), DHEW Pub. No. (OS) 77–0005, 1977.

10. Beecher, H. K. "Ethics and Clinical Research," *New England Journal of Medicine* 274 (1966): 1354–60.

11. National Research Act, Pub. No. 93–348, 1974.

12. Ramsey, P. *The Patient as Person*. New Haven: Yale University Press, 1970.

13. Ramsey, P. "Children as Research Subjects: A Reply," *Hastings Center Report* 7 (1977): 40–42.

14. McCormick, R. "Proxy Consent in the Experimentation Situation," *Perspectives in Biological Medicine* 18 (1974): 2–20.

15. Bartholme, W. "Parents, Children, and the Moral Benefits of Research," *Hastings Center Report* 4 (1976): 44–45.

16. Berenson, G. S., McMahan, C. A., Vorrs, A. W., et al. *Cardiovascular Risk Factors in Children: the Early Natural History of Atherosclerosis and Essential Hypertension*. New York: Oxford University Press, 1980.

17. Leikin, S. "Minors' Assent, Consent, and Dissent to Medical Research," *IRB: A Review of Human Subjects Research* 15 (1993): 1–7.

18. Department of Health & Human Services. "Additional Protections for Children Involved as Subjects in Research." *Federal Register* 48, no. 46 (March 8, 1983): 9814–20.

19. "Proposed Protocol Entitled Myoblast Transfer in Duchenne Muscular Dystrophy: Recommendations." *Federal Register* 56 (Sept. 27, 1991): 49189–190.

20. "Cognitive Function and Hypoglycemia in Children with IDDM," *Federal Register* 58 (July 30, 1993): 40819–820.

21. "Guidelines for the Ethical Conduct of Medical Research Involving Children," *Bulletin of Medical Ethics* (August 1992): 13–22.

22. Australian College of Paediatrics. "Report on the Ethics of Research in Children," *Australian Paediatric Journal* 17 (1981): 162.

23. Medical Research Council of Canada. *Guidelines on Research Involving Human Subjects*. Ottawa: Minister of Supplies and Services, 1987.

24. Papadatos, C. J. "Guidelines for Medical Research in Children," *Infection* 17 (1989): 411–17.

25. Giertz, G. "Ethical Aspects of Paediatric Research," *Acta Paediatrica Scandinavia* 72 (1983): 641–50.
26. *International Ethical Guidelines for Biomedical Research Involving Human Subjects.* Prepared by the Council for International Organizations of Medical Sciences (CIOMS), in cooperation with the World Health Organization (WHO). Geneva, 1993.
27. De Craemer, W. "A Cross-Cultural Perspective on Personhood," *Milbank Memorial Fund Quarterly* 61 (1983): 19–34.
28. *OPRR Reports, Protection of Human Subjects.* Title 45, Part 46, Code of Federal Regulations. Revised June 18, 1991.
29. Lau Y.–L., Yeung, C.–Y. "Parental Perception of the Effect of Venipuncture in Preschool Children in Nontherapeutic Research," *Journal of Paediatric Child Health* 28 (1992): 294–96.
30. Kopelman, L. "When Is the Risk Minimal Enough for Children to be Research Subjects?" In *Children and Health Care*, ed. L. Kopelman and J. Moskop. Boston: Kluwer Academic Publishers, 1989.
31. Janofsky, J. and Starfield, B. "Assessment of Risk in Research on Children," *Journal of Pediatrics* 98 (1981): 842–46.
32. Lascari, A. "Risks of Research in Children," *Journal of Pediatrics* 98 (1981): 759–60.
33. "Ricky Ray, 15, Dies; Known for AIDS Case," *The New York Times* (December 14, 1992): B–10.
34. Jonas, H. "Philosophical Reflections on Experimenting with Human Subjects." In *Contemporary Issues in Bioethics*, ed. T. L. Beauchamp and L. Walters. 3d ed. Belmont CA: Wadsworth, 1989: 432–40.
35. Nolan, K. "AIDS and Pediatric Research," *Evaluation Review* 14 (1990): 465–81.
36. Pizzo, P. "Pediatric AIDS: Problems within Problems," *Journal of Infectious Diseases* 161 (1990): 316–25.
37. "AIDS Spreads Fastest Among Young Women," *The Washington Post* (July 29, 1993): A–1, A–22.
38. "Rising HIV-Related Mortality in Young Americans" (Editorial), *Journal of the American Medical Association* 269 (1993): 3034–35.
39. "AIDS Policy: Two Divisive Issues" (Commentary), *Journal of the American Medical Association* 270 (1993): 494–95.
40. Nolan, K. "Ethical Issues in Caring for Pregnant Women and Newborns at Risk for Human Immunodeficiency Virus Infection," *Seminars in Perinatology* 13 (1989): 55–65.
41. "Testing Newborns for AIDS Virus Raises Issue of Mothers' Privacy," *The New York Times* (August 8, 1993).
42. Working Group on Antiretroviral Therapy: National Pediatric HIV Resources Center. "Antiretroviral Therapy and Medical Management of the Human Immuno-deficiency Virus-Infected Child," *Pediatric Infectious Diseases Journal* 12 (1993): 513–22.
43. Simonds, R. J., Oxtoby, M. J., Caldwell, M. B., Gwinn, M. L., and Rogers, M. F. "*Pneumocystic carinii* Pneumonia among U.S. Children with Perinatally Acquired HIV Infection," *Journal of the American Medical Association* 270 (1993): 470–73.
44. Ackerman, T. F. "Protectionism and the New Research Imperative in Pediatric AIDS," *IRB: A Review of Human Subjects Research* 12 (1990): 1–5.
45. Sigman, G. and Connor, C. "Exploration for Physicians of the Mature Minor Doctrine," *Journal of Pediatrics* 119 (1991): 520–25.

46. Grodin, M. and Alpert, J. J. "Children as Participants in Medical Research," *Pediatric Clinics of North America* 35 (1988): 1389–1401.
47. Veatch, R. M. "Commentary: Beyond Consent to Treatment," *IRB: A Review of Human Subjects Research* 3 (1989): 7–8.
48. Melton, G. B. "Ethical and Legal Issues in Research and Intervention," *Journal of Adolescent Health Care* 10 (1989): 36S–44S.
49. Levine, C. "Teenagers, Research, and Family Involvement," *IRB: A Review of Human Subjects Research* 3 (1981): 8.
50. Grodin, M. A. and Glantz, L. H. *Children as Research Subjects.* New York: Oxford University Press, 1994.

11

The Ethics of Epidemiologic Research with Older Populations

JOANNE M. MCGLOIN
ADRIAN M. OSTFELD

While the elderly as a group have not been identified for special protection under federal research guidelines,[1-5] the researcher of aging populations encounters the stereotypical nursing home patient with multiple impairments as well as the "golden aged" healthy and wealthy retiree, and the grandmother raising AIDS-orphaned grandchildren. Thus, any consideration of ethical issues in studies of this growing population must take into account the heterogeneity of the elderly and the variety of circumstances in which they live. In the discussion that follows, we argue that ageism, a discriminatory attitude toward older people, and paternalism, a condescending attitude toward persons because of real or imagined age-related impairments, should be scrupulously avoided by epidemiologists and other researchers.

The principle of respect for the autonomy of persons requires that the autonomy of all adults be protected. The need for personal autonomy does not retreat with advancing years, and the elderly are as diverse in circumstances and opinion as adults of other ages. Persons with diminished autonomy are entitled to special protections, however.[6] At every stage in life there are subgroups in need of special protection due to mental infirmity, disability, or compromised freedom.

Whereas the principle of nonmaleficence requires us to do no harm, the principle of beneficence requires that benefits be maximized and risks minimized. Thus, analysis of the risk to benefit ratio is part of all research with older subjects. Justice requires the equitable distribution of potential benefits and burdens from research on aging.[52,56] Participation can be an opportunity for expression, a chance for people to speak for themselves and as representatives of their peers.

The tendency of caregivers, institutional review boards (IRBs), and society in general to be overprotective of elderly persons—partly in response to past abuses of some elderly research subjects—may pose obstacles to research concerning the problems of older people.[4,7,8]

As stewards of taxpayer funds, researchers have an obligation to conduct studies of high quality.[9] Rates of participation are one measure of quality. Another aspect, the generalizability of accurate results, depends on representative subject participation. Obtaining desirable participation rates requires the researcher to adapt methods in order to include older persons with varying disabilities, and the tolerance and cooperation of older subjects. Our experience is that older people understand the concept of representation through sampling and that, contrary to the findings of others, older subjects will usually participate in surveys if adequate time is taken to address their concerns.[10]

Our Aging Society

In the past century substantial progress has been made toward the goal of long life for large numbers of people. In 1890, the United States Census found that 2.42 million Americans (4.9% of the population) were age sixty-five or older; the 1990 census enumerated 31.2 million persons over age sixty-five, 12.6% of the total population.[11,12] Growth has been most dramatic in the number of persons age eight-five and older, from 2.24 million in 1980 to 3.08 million in 1990. This represents a 38% increase in one decade alone. While the total population increased by approximately 500% between 1890 and 1990, the number of persons age sixty-five and older grew by 1300%, and the eighty-five-and-older segment by 2800%. These trends are expected to continue. By the year 2040 it is projected that 22% of the population will be sixty-five years of age or older.[13] However, this impressive attainment is a qualified success. The chances of living to age eight-five, seventy-five, or even sixty-five are not equal for all, and long life per se is not synonymous with good health and sustained ability, nor does it ensure an end free of pain, dementia, and isolation.

Research on Aging

Investigations of the predictors of attaining old age, the process of aging, and the common problems among persons of advanced age have a high priority on the national scientific agenda in the United States.[14] The humane and ethical conduct of such human studies raises many questions for the epidemiologic researcher.

The first and most important question is whether the research ought to be undertaken at all.[15] Only if the research question is important, the risk-benefit ratio acceptable, and the current answer to the question unclear should the research be attempted. The second question is whether the value of the research justifies the use of human subjects. The third is whether vulnerable segments of the population, such as those in pain, in institutions, or with compromised decisional capacity, are essential to the conduct of the study.[16] The fourth question is whether the risks of harm to the participants are outweighed by the benefits to society and to those who take part in the research. The impetus for aging research in the United States comes not only from investigators in the field but also from a groundswell of sentiment that ageism is undemocratic and that quality of life among the elderly should be enhanced. Exclusion of today's elderly from epidemiologic research may deprive them and future cohorts of older persons of the benefits of research.[2,17]

In addition to investigations that examine the full range of adult life, the types of research for which elderly populations might be recruited include:

1. *Longevity research*, that is, research aimed at increasing human life span. The personal and social benefits of what has been called "anti-aging research" are unclear.[3] From the perspective of global ecology, it may be hard to justify extending the human life span to the extent that human populations compete with other species for finite resources.[18] Ideally, the phase of life to be extended is healthy adulthood.[19] However, benefits may accrue only to a privileged group and may involve extension of the frailest years, years of compromised quality of life, and years of expensive health care consumption. Public expenditure for research to extend the human life span raises questions of just distribution of resources between first and third world countries and between competing social needs, such as lowering infant mortality rates or AIDS research.

2. *Research to reduce premature mortality.* This type of investigation is aimed at equalizing the chances of reaching an arbitrary point such as sixty-five or eighty-five years of age. One approach would be to study those who are aging "successfully" to learn the secret of their healthy longevity.[18,20] Another method would be to identify disease-prevention and health-promotion strategies to increase the likelihood of survival among groups vulnerable to death in youth or middle age, such as men and minorities.[18,19] The ratio of elderly males to females, which is less than 1 and decreases further with age, highlights this issue.[20] One might argue that priority ought to be given to the health concerns of men and minorities, with the goal of increasing the life expectancies of those groups. However, this approach raises several unanswered questions. Should scientists accept as normative the longer life expectancy of white women, and aim to increase survival rates and life expectancy among males and minority elders? Should older women be deprived of the benefits

of national health research resources because they may age relatively well? Are members of population segments with longer life expectancy simply to be grateful for living so long and not to ask for more in terms of quality of life or morbidity reduction? Should we accept current differences in life expectancies as inherent and limit aging research only to those who survive to old age? A further question is whether success in aging or the presence of diseases of research interest may make certain individuals or segments of the elderly population targets of excessive recruitment and research burden.

3. *Research to reduce morbidity and to improve quality of life.* While not necessarily increasing life span, research aimed at reduction of mortality and improved quality of life includes investigation of the problems of older people living at home or in institutions. In the United States, the problems of advanced age are faced in particular by rapidly growing numbers of white women. Further information is needed about how to treat older patients more effectively and efficaciously at home, and in hospital and long term care settings.[2,7,8] This type of research often can be conducted only with elderly subjects.[5]

The potential value to future generations must warrant the risks and burden to the elderly subject who may not live long enough to benefit directly from the research. In longitudinal aging research and in research with dying persons, for example, it is probable that most benefits from the research will be enjoyed by succeeding generations of older people rather than by the individual research subject.[5] In critically assessing the benefit-to-risk ratio for each study, investigators also have an obligation to consider what benefits might accrue to the individual research subjects. In most nonintervention epidemiologic studies, the benefits are usually limited to recommendations to treat previously unknown problems and to improve control of current chronic illnesses. As the direct benefits to the participants decrease, more than minimal risks become unacceptable. Minimal risks are those that are no greater than risks encountered in daily life or routine testing.[6] Common epidemiologic procedures, such as collection of health history data, observation of events, medical chart review, and routine blood and urine collection are generally considered to be of minimal risk. Examples of higher-risk procedures are exercise stress tests, all-day glucose level monitoring, endurance testing, and invasive procedures.

It is best to avoid collecting information that is potentially damaging to the subject if its confidentiality cannot be protected. For example, research information may be subpoenaed for competency hearings.[21] Self-reports should be distinguished from clinical diagnoses, so that recorded information is not subject to misinterpretation. A further problem is that respondents may be reluctant to report events such as falls if these difficulties could be grounds for discharge or eviction.[22] Confidentiality is a serious responsibility of the investigative staff and one that must be borne even after the study is completed.

The Diversity of Older Persons

The heterogeneity of the elderly has been well documented.[20,23] The majority of older persons are not much different from other adults. There are, however, small but important segments of the elderly population who confront researchers with a special challenge: how to protect these more vulnerable persons from undue risk, while attempting to study all who merit inclusion in the sample and who are able, with or without assistance, to participate voluntarily. The first task is to identify segments of the elderly population whose inclusion in research may be problematic.

Our own experience with the New Haven site of the National Institute on Aging's research initiative, Established Populations for Epidemiologic Studies of the Elderly (EPESE), will be used to illustrate a variety of special situations that arise in epidemiologic research with older persons. We will also use this example to show some of the possible ways of adapting protocols to accommodate various types of vulnerability or disability commonly found among older subjects. Begun as one of three U.S. study sites in 1980, the New Haven EPESE is designed to describe "the health and illness experiences of people as they move through the years beyond age 65."[23] The specific aims of this prospective study are to identify predictors of mortality and morbidity, and to investigate risk factors for chronic disease and for physical and cognitive impairment in the elderly. The overall goal is to disseminate information for prevention of disease and maintenance of functioning and independence for older people.

The study population in New Haven is a stratified cluster sample of 3337 non-institutionalized persons age sixty-five or older who were living in the city in 1982. The sample was stratified by housing type (public housing for the elderly, private housing for the elderly, general community housing). The response rate for the 1982 baseline survey was 82%, with 2812 persons participating. On average, each person interviewed in the baseline survey represents more than five persons in the population sampled. Mechanisms were established to monitor deaths, hospitalizations, and nursing home admissions among respondents. The respondents were 79% white, 19% African-American, and 2% were of "other" racial groups.[23]

Reasons for refusing to participate in the baseline survey included suspicion of research in general, suspicion of the research institution in particular, and being too busy or too ill. The respondents included well elderly with no reported chronic disease or disability (15%); physically disabled persons (7% used walking aids,

2% used wheelchairs, 1% were bed bound); and persons with a wide range of cognitive performance results on the nine-item modified Mental Status Questionnaire (10% had four or more errors; 34% had none).[23,24]

Following the baseline survey, EPESE respondents were contacted annually to monitor change in functional ability as well as incidence of chronic disease and major life events. Follow-up contacts, annually over the eight-year period from 1983 to 1990 and again in 1994, yielded response rates of 90%–97% among survivors.

Sensory Deficits

Two issues need to be addressed in designing surveys for older populations that include persons with sensory deficits. Both have ethical implications. First, there is a need to broaden inclusion criteria as much as possible without compromising the scientific integrity of the study. Second, there is a responsibility to maintain the dignity and reasonable comfort of persons who have given their informed consent to the research.

Sensory deficits among older potential research subjects must be addressed so that they are not excluded from the research in an arbitrary fashion. Such deficits apply to small but important segments of potential elderly research subjects,[10] and are more prevalent among older persons. These problems may be compounded within an individual. The exclusion of persons with hearing or vision deficits limits the generalizability of findings, and may deprive subgroups of the elderly (such as those who are deaf, blind, or nonspeaking) from the benefits of the research. Data must be collected from impaired individuals with care and courtesy, and without distressing the study participants. Sensory deficits may present problems to researchers if a protocol is designed to rely exclusively on verbal or visual cues. However, research methods can be tailored to overcome these challenges with patience, perseverance, and respect for the value of each person's contribution.

In the EPESE baseline survey, 10% of respondents reported being unable to read ordinary newsprint even when wearing glasses or contact lenses.[23] Severe visual impairments by themselves do not require the exclusion of persons from surveys, but such impairments may limit subject participation in postal surveys, in self-administered pencil-and-paper surveys, in cognitive function assessments that require responses to visual cues, and in measures of physical performance that require visual orientation. For example, in asking sensitive questions such as level of income, some protocols offer the respondent a card on which to point to a category rather than requiring a verbal answer. It may be necessary to use materials in Braille to accommodate respondents literate in Braille, or to employ other methods. The ability of the interviewer to read questions in a clear and well-paced fashion is particularly important in such cases. Special care must be taken to avoid breaches in privacy and confidentiality that may result from asking sensitive questions when other persons are close by.

Ten percent of EPESE respondents could not hear a voice at normal sound level even when using a hearing aid.[23] In our experience, several approaches may allow the inclusion of hearing-impaired older persons in epidemiologic research. Some trial and error may be required to identify the method that is most comfortable for the respondent and that the investigator judges to be sufficiently reliable. A questionnaire that is well spaced, clearly laid out, and printed in large type can assist some older persons with visual or hearing impairments to read the questions themselves, and allow respondents who cannot speak to point to responses. This approach is preferable to shouting questions at hearing-impaired older persons, because it does not compromise dignity, privacy, or confidentiality. Employing interviewers trained in sign language is another strategy for including the hearing impaired.

It is important to consider in particular applications whether difficulty in communication can be overcome by such approaches. Problems with speech such as post-stroke aphasia are particularly challenging. A variety of approaches may have to be tried to determine how, or even whether, the intent of the research can be adequately explained to the potential subject. The manner in which the respondent can express his or her assent or refusal to participate may require experimentation and consultation with knowledgeable family members or the physician. For example, simplified answer categories, such as yes/no rather than degrees of agreement, may be required. Visual analogues (for example, a line with a happy face at the top and a sad face at the bottom to gather an assessment of mood) may be useful.[25,26]

Severe arthritis or other disorders that limit flexibility or feeling in the fingers may hamper participation in self-administered pencil-and-paper surveys, as well as in cognitive function tests that require drawing or copying visual images. The sensitive design of instruments with sufficient space for writing may support the dignity of some impaired elderly research subjects.

Cognitive Impairment

A small percentage of the elderly are cognitively impaired.[23] Like physical disability, cognitive impairment can be mild or severe, benign or dangerous. Some cognitively impaired older persons may have good days and bad days, or parts of days in which they function better or worse. Severe cognitive dysfunction is, of course, a serious impediment to voluntary, informed consent. However, the exclusion of all persons who exhibit any cognitive impairment limits the generalizability of results, eliminates the opportunity to examine the association of cognitive impairment with the outcome variables of interest, and may reduce sample size and compromise the value of the study.[10] Cognitive impairment raises two sets of issues for the epidemiologic researcher. First, can the person grant informed consent to participate? Second, can the person provide reliable and valid self-reports of requested information?

A universally accepted set of criteria for competency to consent to research participation has not been established for cognitively impaired adults.[27] Unless there is clear and convincing evidence to the contrary, competency in adults must be assumed no matter how advanced their age.[4] However, as with people of any age who may not be able to concentrate because of fatigue, illness, alcohol, or drugs, it may be necessary to have more than one contact with a potential study subject to determine competency before enrolling the person in the study.

To protect elderly subjects, other authors have argued for two tiers of screening prior to actual study enrollment.[16,28–33] Some authors have also suggested a two step process for obtaining the informed consent of elderly persons: first, giving information about the study, and then, sometimes days later, testing recall of the content and seeking consent.[32,34] However, such screening may deprive older persons of the opportunity to contribute to what may, in fact, be a low-risk protocol. This also increases the length and expense of the study. The exclusion of elderly persons who fail to retain the content of the informed consent procedure over time may be too severe a criterion. Moreover, excessive attention to evaluating cognitive function can be insulting to the potential subject.[2,35] Memory may not be the sole or even a major component of decisional capacity,[7] and excessive screening can be demeaning to the vast majority of older people who have no cognitive dysfunction and who resent the implication that to be old is to be forgetful. Finally, measures of cognitive function are often dependent on educational attainment and language fluency.[20] Low levels of vocabulary and education, as well as advanced age, have been cited as correlates of failure to remember the content of information sheets two to three weeks later.[28,29] Thus, the recent immigrant or uneducated older person may be more likely to be excluded by such screening methods.

Vulnerability Due to Illness

When conducting research with ill persons of all ages, the risk-to-benefit ratio must justify the time and attention required by participation. The importance of the research question must merit personal contact with acutely ill older persons in order to warrant the burden it may impose on them and their care givers. A comparison of older and younger adults who were ill found that both groups were more likely to consent to low-risk rather than high-risk procedures.[36] However, acutely ill persons may feel more dependent on care givers and fail to fully understand their right to refuse consent.

The amount of time needed to complete interviews increases with advancing age and severity of illness. It may be necessary to make multiple but shorter visits, especially if the subject is receiving treatments or needs frequent care by attendants. Interviews are best limited to 45 to 60 minutes to avoid respondent fatigue, although some older persons may be quite willing to be involved for longer periods of time.[10]

Today's elderly were adults in the 1960s when some widely publicized abuses in medical research were brought to light.[37] Some abuses involved nontherapeutic experimentation on aged persons without their consent. Remembering such accounts may cause older adults to resist being used as "guinea pigs," particularly when hospitalized. Reluctance to participate in research must be respected and addressed in a manner that balances compassion for the ill patient with the need to ensure scientific rigor.

Research and care of the ill or disabled should be kept distinct both in the protocol and in the communication with participants. A care provider may endorse the research, but participation must never be a condition for receiving usual care. Usual care should not be used as the "carrot" for research participation, nor must there be any hint that nonparticipation will displease any care providers or institutions.[8]

In times of illness, family members may be especially protective of older persons and attempt to limit the researcher's access to the subject. Unless he or she is legally incompetent, the older patient can give or withhold consent to participate.[4] However, the concerns of family members should not be ignored. In some studies, information is obtained from proxies or caregivers along with patient self-report. Two approaches may be taken if care givers must be approached to obtain access to elderly individuals. The first is simply to listen carefully to the concerns of family members and attempt to adequately answer their questions about the purpose of the research, the use of the data, confidentiality procedures, the time required, and why people who are old and sick are needed as subjects. Respondents should be reassured that participation will not interfere with or influence the elderly person's usual treatment or services. A second approach is to obtain a surrogate interview from the caregiver and, upon its conclusion, to ask if the same questions might be addressed to the elderly subject. This process may reassure the caregiver or proxy respondent that the content of the survey is reasonable.

Among older persons, chronic illness is more prevalent than acute illness, and may contribute to impairment in activities of daily living (ADL) and mobility. If respondents must come to a research center, it is important to minimize travel time, provide convenient parking, and, if necessary, escort service. The research team should maximize ease of access within the medical center for the older study subjects, especially those who are ill.

Social and Economic Factors

The requirements and burdens of research projects vary. These may include filling out forms, sharing personal information over the telephone, allowing a stranger into the home, providing blood samples, urine collection, trips to the medical center, and diagnostic procedures that may be lengthy or anxiety-provoking. In some instances, the subject may feel flattered or be so familiar with these types of procedures that there is no apparent inconvenience. More often, however, participation in a research study is not an everyday occurrence. The experience may also be time-consuming and inconvenient. A trip "downtown," easily accomplished by the researcher with a reserved parking space, may require multiple bus transfers and pose a genuine challenge for a volunteer retiree. The subject's commitment makes him or her a true partner in the research effort. Contributions of time and effort ought to be acknowledged in the informed consent statement.

The varying economic circumstances of older people raise questions about just remuneration for research participation and avoidance of manipulation.[8,38] Many elderly black women, for example, are burdened by extremely low incomes. In 1982, the New Haven EPESE found that more than 60% of black females had incomes of less than $5,000 per year; some had substantially less.[23] Thus, to offer $100 to a subject for devoting a day to blood chemistry monitoring for research may not be enough incentive for some, but it may lead other segments of the elderly population to expose themselves to burdens of the research for a meager return.

Preliminary screening of those who volunteer to be research subjects may eliminate persons motivated by the offer of a stipend who cannot safely endure lengthy procedures such as fasting or stress tests. Such contact also provides the opportunity to fully describe any discomfort involved in testing, and thus aid the potential subject in carefully weighing the risks and benefits of study participation.

Institutionalized Elderly

Until recently, research on the problems of nursing home residents received little attention.[7,8,15] The nursing home was a "black box" and admission an "endpoint." The seriousness and complexity of the issues involved in research on institutionalized populations, underscored by past abuses of nursing home patients, have limited this type of research to low-risk protocols with potential therapeutic benefit for the individual subject.[7] Little attention has been given to resolving the ethical issues inherent in conducting research in long term care (LTC) institution settings.

Consent, competence, confidentiality, and conflict of interest have been identified as four major issues in nursing home research.[8,56] A proper balance of protection and opportunity must be sought for research in this setting.[8] The factors that need to be considered in aging research (institutional review, informed consent, decisional capacity, source of funding, confidentiality, recruitment setting, and research interventions) are the same as those for other human subjects investigation. However, efforts to protect subjects, particularly those who are demented and institutionalized, are not consistently reported in the literature on aging research.[39,40]

The institutionalized elderly may be considered a vulnerable group, not because of their age, but because they reside in a restrictive environment. Their situation is somewhat like that of prisoners; they are at greater risk of manipulation and, perhaps, more fearful of the possible consequences of refusing.[2,8] Consent in this setting may not be truly voluntary, and certainly will often be compromised and clouded by ambivalence.

Nursing home residents are more likely to be female (75%) than male and white (93%) than non-white.[20] Comorbid conditions and other health problems are more common among nursing home residents than among community-living elderly.[41] Almost half of all nursing home residents have some degree of dementia, and impaired cognitive function is more common in this population.[5,20] It is important for the interviewer to actually see and assess institutionalized subjects, as staff evaluations of patients' cognitive ability may not be reliable; this is particularly true in facilities employing personnel from nursing "pools," a practice often associated with high staff turnover and irregular contact between patients and staff. Further, residents referred by staff for research studies may be unsuitable.[8] By insisting on visiting study subjects in nursing homes, we have found some elderly patients to be better able to communicate and participate than staff had assumed.

Many long term care facilities do not have organized ethics committees because institutional review boards are unlikely to be needed and cumbersome to maintain.[7,42] In the EPESE study, larger nonprofit facilities, particularly those with religious affiliations, sometimes had a mechanism to bring discussion of research participation to the board of trustees. More often, however, institutional cooperation was an administrative decision. EPESE investigators approached administrators individually or in groups to explain the purpose of the study. Because the research staff did not burden the clinical staff, and because the subjects' consent to participate in the EPESE study preceded LTC admissions, facilities were generally cooperative.

Confidentiality and privacy are more difficult to maintain in nursing homes than in most private residences.[7,8] It is likely that participation will be observed by staff and other patients. The interviewer may have to shout to be heard. Private space may be limited. Even the highly sensitive issue of a patient's competency may be openly discussed.

Despite the special requirements of research with nursing home residents, one compelling argument for these efforts is that while at any time only 5% of the elderly are institutionalized, the likelihood of an older person spending some time in such facilities is much higher.[20]

Informed Consent

Informed consent can be legally provided by anyone who is psychologically competent, has reached the age of legal competence, and has not been declared incompetent by a court of appropriate jurisdiction. The general presumption of adult competence should not be compromised by lack of intelligence, education, skill, or wisdom.[4] Adults, including the very elderly, are presumed to be of sound mind unless a focused inquiry shows general incapacity.[3,4] The nature of the tasks constituting competence varies with the context.[4] For example, one may no longer be competent to drive but still competent to report a history of driving.

It is the dependent, cognitively impaired, institutionalized person for whom special protections must be devised. Mental infirmity may mean cognitive or emotional impairments or a combination of the two. In some cases the extent of decisional capacity is unclear, because of compromised intellectual, emotional, or judgmental capacity. A patient may be able to consent effectively to participate in an observational study, but not a drug trial.[4] Time of day can also influence respondent understanding, tolerance, and performance. Interviewers may ask care givers what time of day is best for the subject; for marginally cognitively impaired persons, it is usually morning and early afternoon.

Potential risks and burdens to respondents must be presented in a straightforward fashion, and neither minimized nor overstated.[36] The right to refuse participation in any or all parts of the research should be disclosed and protected. Physical contact without consent and with no therapeutic intent could be considered assault.[34,56]

It is also important to use easily understood language, to discuss details with those who wish full information, and to refrain from imposing on those who wish adequate, rather than complete, information.[34] Initial contact materials should include an introductory letter written in large type describing the study, and a more detailed information sheet to be kept by the respondent for future reference. The EPESE letter and information sheet were easy to read, pretested, and simplified prior to the survey. Through pilot testing, we found that a friendly but not overly familiar tone resulted in fewer immediate refusals than a shorter, more formal letter. Attesting to the heterogeneity of the elderly, more inclusive and less presumptuous statements, such as "the many circumstances in which older people live" as opposed to "the problems and needs of the elderly," were better received. It is important to make the data collection process itself pleasant and rewarding for subjects. The risk-benefit ratio may be improved by building in secondary benefits such as altruism, contribution to society, contact with others, a break from routine, and contribution to knowledge.[2,7,8,43]

Use of Proxies

Proxies, or surrogate respondents, are persons other than the study subject who provide information on behalf of the subject and make decisions for the subject. The need for proxies in research studies increases with the age of respondents,[44] and the extent of agreement between self and proxy reports is variable.[9,45] Potential subjects may have been declared incompetent by a court. In such cases, the court-assigned legal guardian or conservator is the most appropriate person to contact about serving as a proxy.[4] More often, persons of varying capabilities are found to be cared for by a variety of informal care givers, most of whom are family members.[46] Whenever a surrogate respondent provides information about a subject, issues such as the right to privacy and the adequacy of informed consent are raised. Since the role of the proxy is often to protect the subject, it may be considered inconsistent to volunteer the subject for any risk that does not carry a therapeutic benefit.[15,35,47] The issue of appropriate surrogate decision making for persons no longer capable of formulating and expressing preference (proxy consent) is a serious contemporary legal dilemma.[46] The constitutional right to privacy has an impact on how much even a legally appointed guardian may disclose about an incompetent person.[4] Further, the choice of possible alternate decision makers is clouded in legal and ethical uncertainty.[4] The proxy may derive some future benefit from the research findings, while the subject remains burdened.[3] For example, nontherapeutic research on Alzheimer's patients is unlikely to benefit the patient, but may provide a later advantage to a proxy, such as a blood relative. It has been argued that such conflicts of interest may be intrinsic to the subject-proxy relationship.[48]

Proxies may be persons who live with respondents (for instance, a spouse, adult child, sibling or other relative, unrelated care giver or other unrelated person), or caregivers or friends who visit regularly.[33] The interviewer must be conscientious about selecting individuals who know the subject and can provide accurate data. In some cases the legal guardian may barely be acquainted with the patient. This is more usual for older people with court-appointed guardians and no families. Sadly, there are severely cognitively impaired people with no social ties and no guardian; their participation is often avoided.[49] In some jurisdictions a shortage of potential guardians limits these appointments to emergency (life or death) situations.

How best to include incapacitated and institutionalized persons, particularly for studies of their quality of life, poses a challenge.[16,50,51] The use of proxies is often problematic in such studies. Many subjective items cannot be asked of a second party. Legally, only a court-appointed guardian can give consent to participate on behalf of an incompetent person and, even then, the best interests of the ward may preclude participation in research with no direct therapeutic benefit to the subject.[4] The right to privacy may also be breached.[52] Unless the subject has positively stated an interest in research participation prior to incompetence, there can be a conflict of interest.[15] In general, modifying protocols to maximize participation by the subjects themselves is preferable to the use of proxies.

Selecting the Collectors of Data

In epidemiologic studies of the elderly, interviewers should be sensitive, intelligent, and able to speak clearly. Other personal characteristics that are advantageous include being pleasant, persistent, and perspicacious. The investigator is advised to seek compassionate persons, unbiased in their approach to each respondent, who can observe without intervening. Role definition and clarity of professional limits are imperative in studies that involve some subjects in distress. The interviewer's function and reason for contacting the elderly research subject are quite narrow. While he or she may make referrals based on specific guidelines, interviewers do not diagnose, treat, or counsel subjects.

Some interviewers recruited to work for the EPESE survey were older persons. The decision to select older staff was in part a response to a high level of awareness in the community of discrimination against older workers, and also a way of allowing federal funds to do "double duty" for the area elderly (producing research findings in the long-term, and helping to support a few older families in the short term).

Bilingual interviewers were also employed. We sought persons who were themselves natives of the countries in which our elderly respondents were born (Puerto Rico, Neapolitan Italy, and Poland), and who were familiar with the dialects spoken in New Haven neighborhoods.

Training of Data Collectors

Training is required even if experienced staff are recruited for a survey of older people.[35] Training provides an opportunity to build awareness of expectations between investigators and field staff. In surveys of older people, bias toward the aged can be addressed during these sessions, as well as how to deal with over-protective relatives, when to use a proxy, the building of trust and rapport, and the importance of clear speech, unbiased probing, tactful handling of digressions, confidentiality, and avoidance of interviewer bias.[9,10] Training also includes the development of listening and communication skills, role playing, and giving non-biasing information.[49]

Protocols for handling unusual occurrences should be part of instruction, along with directives for when to break the protocol.[53,54] For example, extremely ele-vated blood pressure, fainting, falling, shortness of breath, unconsciousness, and references to suicide are urgent conditions of elderly respondents to which the interviewer must respond. Verbal abuse, erratic behavior, and sexual advances are other situations that staff must be prepared to handle.

In the EPESE study, physician investigators and psychiatrists were identified to whom field staff could refer unusual cases. Follow-up training session mod-ules included a psychiatrist's discussion of how to handle respondent anger, sad-ness, and mention of suicide. Interviewers also learned how to identify emer-gency versus non-life-threatening situations, how to respond to unusual events such as medical emergencies, when to call the office, and when to break proto-col and dial 911.

If blood samples were drawn, protocols were followed for informing subjects about abnormal blood values, and for referrals if results had clinical significance. Cut points were established for "borderline" and critically high or low levels of glucose, blood urea nitrogen, and cholesterol. If abnormalities were found, a nurse or physician called the elderly respondent and followed up with a letter urging that a physician repeat the test. A few false positives occurred, which irritated some subjects. However, many more cases in need of treatment were identified, thus providing an important direct benefit to a small number of older subjects.

EPESE interviewer training also included guidance on what types of state-ments to avoid (such as those that are misleading or manipulative). Interviewers were instructed not to promise any direct benefit to the elderly respondents or their families. However, they were allowed to appeal to respondents' altruism and to stress benefits to future generations. They were also told to assure re-spondents that findings would be used responsibly, and would never be given to employers, landlords, or insurance companies.

A further issue is that investigators must ensure the humane and ethical treat-ment of those who collect the data. Interviewer safety is an important concern. If it is not adequately addressed, interviewers can be exposed to serious risks, or participation can be jeopardized if elderly persons live in neighborhoods per-ceived by staff as too dangerous to visit. Risk of disease from exposure to blood and body fluids is another occupational hazard for data collection staff in some studies. Training in universal precautions and hepatitis B immunization may be desirable to protect elderly respondents; flu shots may be offered to interviewers, since persons over age sixty-five are considered to be at increased risk.

Interviewers should be trained to deal effectively with requests for assistance from elderly participants,[55] such as help with unmet health, housing, or human service needs. In the EPESE study, referrals usually consisted of the interviewer giving the respondent telephone numbers for Info-Line (a telephone information and referral service) and the city's Elderly Services Department. Such referrals for nonemergency assistance were made only upon the request of the elderly subjects or their families. A signed release allowing the research staff to contact agencies or physicians on behalf of the respondents, if they were unable to call for themselves, was employed in serious situations. Requests for physician referrals were directed to the principal investigator. Mention of suicidal intent was taken most seriously and promptly brought to the attention of a psychiatrist coinvestigator, who then contacted the respondent directly.

Community Relations

In epidemiologic research, study personnel have an obligation to know the community from which participants come.[22,44] Essential to the design and execution of the study are knowledge of transportation, sources of care, and agencies and facilities with which participants are likely to interact. Such knowledge helps to ensure a more humane protocol for the older participant, and to avoid undue burdens to respondents. In the EPESE study, professional relationships were established with elderly service providers and local aging advocates through presentations and discussions. Both the breadth and limitations of the planned research were presented, as was our willingness to make available aggregate data in forms that did not breach respondent confidentiality. In general, as knowledge in the study accumulates, the judicious presentation of some findings to participants amplifies their knowledge of the risks and benefits of continued participation, and enhances their sense of being active participants rather than passive subjects.

The investigator has a social obligation to use data in a way that provides direct benefit when that can be accomplished without compromising respondents' confidentiality or other rights.[21] For example, the EPESE team has responded to requests for data for local planning efforts and for technical assistance. In one instance, the principal investigator and project director were asked for guidance in developing neighborhood services for elderly residents of a predominantly black census tract. A review of survey data revealed high rates of poor physical function and low income. These were especially striking in black elderly females.[23] Existing services for elderly in the neighborhood and city were then inventoried. Ample numbers of conventional elderly housing units and adult day centers existed, but there was no elderly housing specifically designed for the independent elder with significant ADL limitations. Data provided by EPESE investigators led directly to the establishment of augmented housing for elderly participants in the most needy community. Funding was awarded by the state to build elderly congregate units on a main street in the heart of New Haven's black neighborhood. While research data alone did not make this building a reality, it would not have been built without the involvement of the research team members.

The Funding Source

Topics of aging research and likely benefits to society and subjects ought to be of sufficient importance to warrant the use of limited financial resources and the imposition of burdens on elderly research subjects.

Funding should be adequate to ensure that data are collected and handled in a humane and responsible fashion, without necessitating the hurried or undignified treatment of elderly human subjects. Further, investigators should not pursue research protocols when the funding or time constraints will lead to compromises in the humaneness or quality of the study.

Conclusions

As a segment of the total United States population and in sheer numbers, elderly persons constitute a growing and heterogeneous subgroup. Historically, epidemiologic research has often excluded older persons from study designs, or failed to address the special needs of persons with impairments in order to allow for study participation. Longevity research, research to reduce premature mortality and morbidity, and research to improve quality of life are investigations that require enrollment of elderly persons. While most older people are in good health and able to participate with little or no accommodations, the issues of sensory deficits, cognitive impairment, chronic and acute illness, institutionalization, and other protective living arrangements must be considered in protocol design. These are necessary if a truly representative sample of older persons is to be recruited and if findings are to be generalizable to the broadest possible older population.

Ethical issues related to obtaining informed consent and the use of proxies, while part of most epidemiologic studies, may take on greater significance in studies of older persons.[56,57] Epidemiologic investigators must recruit and train data collectors sensitive to possibly impaired older persons, while avoiding ageism and bias regarding disability. Investigators may benefit from community and professional relations, since "gatekeepers" often belong to this age group.

Funding sources must take account of the extra effort necessary to include the infirm. A heterogeneous range of elderly persons can participate and be retained in longitudinal epidemiologic studies if ethical and standardized methods are honed to the variety of their needs. It is the responsibility of researchers to facilitate their participation in a humane and dignified manner.

References

1. Ostfeld, A. "Older Research Subjects: Not Homogeneous, Not Especially Vulnerable," *IRB: A Review of Human Subjects* 2 (1980): 7–8.
2. Makarushka, J. and McDonald, R. "Informed Consent, Research, and Geriatric Patients: The Responsibility of Institutional Review Committees," *The Gerontologist* 19 (1979): 61–66.
3. Reich, W. "Ethical Issues Related to Research Involving Elderly Subjects," *The Gerontologist* 18 (1978): 326–37.
4. Dubler, N. "Legal Judgments and Informed Consent in Geriatric Research," *Journal of the American Geriatrics Society* 35 (1987): 545–49.
5. Butler, R. "Protection of Elderly Research Subjects," *Clinical Research* 28 (1980): 3–5.
6. The National Commission for the Protection of Human Subjects of Biomedical and Behavioral Research. *The Belmont Report: Ethical Principles and Guidelines for the Protection of Human Subjects of Research.* Washington, D.C.: U.S. Government Printing Office, 1978. DHEW Publication No. (OS) 78–0012.
7. Cassel, C. "Research in Nursing Homes: Ethical Issues," *Journal of the American Geriatrics Society* 33 (1985): 795–99.
8. Cassel, C. "Ethical Issues in the Conduct of Research in Long Term Care," *The Gerontologist* 28 (1988): 90–96.
9. Herzog, A. and Rodger, W. "Age and Response Rates to Interview Sample Surveys," *Journal of Gerontology: Social Sciences* 43 (1988): 200–05.
10. Kelsey, J., O'Brien, L., Grisso, J., and Hoffman, S. "Issues in Carrying Out Epidemiologic Research in the Elderly," *American Journal of Epidemiology* 130 (1989): 857–66.
11. U.S. Dept. of Commerce, Bureau of the Census. *Characteristics of the Population: General Population Statistics: U.S. Summary Part 1, 1980 Census of the Population.* Washington, D.C.: U.S. Government Printing Office, 1982: 26.
12. U.S. Dept. of Commerce, Bureau of the Census, Economics and Statistics Administration. *1990 Census of the Population: General Population Characteristics.* Washington, D.C.: U.S. Government Printing Office, 1992: 19–21.
13. U.S. Bureau of the Census. "Demographic and Socioeconomic Aspects of Aging in the United States," *Current Population Reports.* Series no. 138. Washington, D.C.: U.S. Government Printing Office, 1984: 23.
14. Lonergan, E. and Krevans, J. "Special Report: A National Agenda for Research on Aging," *The New England Journal of Medicine* 324 (1991): 1825–28.
15. Annas, G. and Glantz, L. "Rules for Research in Nursing Homes," *New England Journal of Medicine* 315 (1986): 1157–58.
16. Melnick, V., Dubler, N., Weisbard, A., and Butler, R. "Clinical Research in Senile

Dementia of the Alzheimer Type: Suggested Guidelines Addressing the Ethical and Legal Issues," *Journal of the American Geriatrics Society* 32 (1984): 531–36.

17. Miller, S., Applegate, W., and Perry, C. "Clinical Trials in Elderly Persons," *Journal of the American Geriatrics Society* 33 (1985): 91–92.

18. Cassel, C. "Ethics and the Future of Aging Research: Promises and Problems," *Generations: The Biology of Aging* (fall/winter 1992): 61–65.

19. Butler, R. "Excellence, Efficiency, and Economy Through Aging Research." In *Human Aging Research: Concepts and Techniques*, ed. B. Kent and R. Butler. New York: Raven Press, Ltd., 1988: 1–10.

20. Moritz, D. and Ostfeld, A. "The Epidemiology and Demography of Aging." In *Principles of Gerontology*, ed. R. Andres, E. Bierman, J. Blass, and W. Hazzards. New York: McGraw Hill, 1990: 146–56.

21. Gordis, L. "Ethical and Professional Issues in the Changing Practice of Epidemiology," *Journal of Clinical Epidemiology* 44, suppl. I (1991): 9S–13S.

22. Sorock, G. "Letter to the Editor," *American Journal of Epidemiology* 133 (1991): 317.

23. Cornoni–Huntly, J., Brock, B., Ostfeld, A., Taylor, J., and Wallace, R., eds. *Established Populations for Epidemiologic Studies of the Elderly: Resource Data Book*. U.S. DHHS, National Institute on Aging, 1986.

24. Pfeiffer, E. "A Short Portable Mental Status Questionnaire for the Assessment of Organic Brain Deficit in Elderly Patients," *Journal of the American Geriatrics Society* 23 (1975): 433–41.

25. Aitlen, R. "Measurement of Feelings Using Visual Analogue Scales," *Proceedings Royal Society of Medicine* 62 (1969): 989–96.

26. Stern, R. and Bachman, D. "Depressive Symptoms Following Stroke," *American Journal of Psychiatry* 148 (1991): 351–56.

27. Appelbaum, P. and Roth, L. "Competency to Consent to Research: A Psychiatric Overview," *Archives of General Psychiatry* 39 (1982): 951–58.

28. Taub, H. "Informed Consent, Memory and Age," *The Gerontologist* 20 (1980): 686–90.

29. Taub, H., Baker, M., and Sturr, J. "Informed Consent for Research: Effects of Readability, Patient Age, and Education," *Journal of the American Geriatrics Society* 34 (1986): 601–06.

30. Taub, H. "Comprehension of Informed Consent for Research: Issues and Directions for Future Study," *IRB: A Review of Human Subjects Research* 8 (1986): 7–10.

31. Taub, H. and Baker, M. "A Reevaluation of Informed Consent in the Elderly: A Method of Improving Comprehension Through Direct Testing," *Clinical Research* 32 (1984): 17–21.

32. Miller, R. and Willner, H. "The Two-Part Consent Form: A Suggestion for Promoting Free and Informed Consent," *New England Journal of Medicine* 290 (1974): 964–66.

33. Ratzan, R. " 'Being Old Makes You Different': The Ethics of Research With Elderly Subjects," *Hastings Center Report* 10 (1980): 32–42.

34. Denham, M. "The Ethics of Research in the Elderly," *Age and Aging* 13 (1984): 321–27.

35. U.S. National Institute on Aging. *Protection of Elderly Research Subjects: Summary of a Conference*. Bethesda, MD: U.S. National Institutes of Health, 1977. DHEW Pub. No. (NIH) 79–1801. Conference held at the National Institutes of Health in Bethesda, MD, July 18–19, 1977.

36. Stanley, B., Guido, J., Stanley, M., and Shortell, D. "The Elderly Patient and Informed Consent," *Journal of The American Medical Association* 252 (1984): 1302–06.

37. Beecher, H. "Ethics and Clinical Research," *New England Journal of Medicine* 274 (1966): 1354–60.
38. Lipsitz, L., Pluchino, F., and Wright, S. "Biomedical Research in the Nursing Home: Methodological Issues and Subject Recruitment Results," *Journal of The American Geriatrics Society* 35 (1987): 629–34.
39. Lane, L., Cassel, C., and Bennett, W. "Ethical Aspects of Research Involving Elderly Subjects: Are we doing more than we say?" *The Journal of Clinical Ethics* 1 (1990): 278–86.
40. Sachs, J., Rhymes, J., and Cassel, C. "Research Ethics: Depression and Mortality in Nursing Homes," *Journal of the American Medical Association* 266 (1991): 215–16.
41. Zimmer, A., Calkins, E., Hadley, E., Ostfeld, A., Kaye, J., and Kaye, D. "Conducting Clinical Research in Geriatric Populations," *Annals of Internal Medicine* 103 (1985): 276–83.
42. Libow, L. and Neufield, R. "Research in the Nursing Home: Obstacles and Opportunities." In *Human Aging Research: Concepts and Techniques*, ed. B. Kent and R. Butler. New York: Raven Press, Ltd., 1988: 95–105.
43. Cassel, C. "Informed Consent for Research in Geriatrics: History and Concepts," *Journal of the American Geriatrics Society* 35 (1987): 542–44.
44. Harris, T., Burt, V., and Ezzati, T. "Issues in Carrying out Epidemiologic Research in the Elderly" (Letters), *American Journal of Epidemiology* 133 (1991): 316–18.
45. Magaziner, J., Simonsick, E., Kashner, T., and Hebel, J. "Patient-Proxy Response Comparability on Measures of Patient Health and Functional Status," *Journal of Clinical Epidemiology* 41 (1988): 1065–74.
46. Warren, J., Sobal, J., Tenney, J., Hoopes, J., Damron, D., Levenson, S., DeForge, B., and Muncie, H. "Informed Consent by Proxy," *The New England Journal of Medicine* 315 (1986): 1124–28.
47. Abrams, R., "Dementia Research in the Nursing Home," *Hospital and Community Psychiatry* 39 (1988): 257–59.
48. Cassel, C. "Ethics as an Enabler of Human Aging Research." In *Human Aging Research*, ed. B. Kent and R. Butler. New York: Raven Press, Ltd., 1988: 85–93.
49. Cohen–Mansfield, J., Kerin, P., Pawlson, G., Lipson, S., and Holdridge, K. "Informed Consent for Research in a Nursing Home: Processes and Issues," *The Gerontologist* 28 (1988): 355–59.
50. Lonergan, E., ed. "Research in Biomedical Ethics." In *Extending Life, Enhancing Life*. Washington, DC: Institute of Medicine, National Academy Press, 1991.
51. Melnick, V. "Special Considerations in Geriatric Research: Ethical and Legal Issues," *Drug Information Journal* 19 (1985): 475–82.
52. Coughlin, S. and Beauchamp, T. "Ethics, Scientific Validity and the Design of Epidemiologic Studies," *Epidemiology* 3 (1992): 343–47.
53. Reatig, N. "Ethical Issues in Geriatric Research: Frail Elderly." In *Geriatric Psychiatry: Clinical, Ethical and Legal Issues*, ed. B. Stanley. Washington, DC: American Psychiatric Press, Inc., 1985: 82–89.
54. Yordi, C., Cha, A., Ross, K., and Wong, S. "Research and the Frail Elderly: Ethical and Methodological Issues in Controlled Social Experiments," *The Gerontologist* 22 (1982): 72–77.
55. Strain, L. and Chappell, N. "Problems and Strategies: Ethical Concerns in Survey Research With the Elderly," *The Gerontologist* 22 (1982): 526–31.
56. Wicclair, M. R. *Ethics and the Elderly*. New York: Oxford University Press, 1993.
57. Colsher, P. "Ethical Issues in Conducting Surveys of the Elderly." In *The Epidemiologic Study of the Elderly*, ed. R. Wallace and R. Woolson, New York: Oxford University Press, 1992.

12

Ethics and Epidemiology in the Age of AIDS

CAROL LEVINE

AIDS (acquired immunodeficiency syndrome) now commands an army of specialists and subspecialists in nearly every field of medicine and science, as well as in ethics, law, psychology, sociology, education, economics, journalism, and politics. But in 1981 AIDS was unknown. It was epidemiologists who gave this new disease its name and defined its modes of transmission, and who now monitor its spread, natural history, and the effect of public health and clinical interventions. Each step and misstep in this process has had far-reaching consequences, some of which will be described in this chapter. (More specific accounts of the early years of the epidemic and the role played by epidemiologists have been chronicled elsewhere.[1,2,3])

Epidemiology deals with disease processes and trends in populations. But, as Gerald Oppenheimer points out, "Epidemiology, unlike virology, has a strong social dimension in that it explicitly incorporates perceptions of a population's social relations, behavioral patterns, and experiences into its explanations."[4] When, as in the case of AIDS, those perceptions involve a lethal disease, stigmatized behaviors such as drug use and homosexual sex, and a suspicious and fearful public, the potential for moral problems soars.

After outlining some general considerations relating to ethics and epidemiology, this chapter focuses on three examples, drawn from my own experience, that illustrate the interrelationship of epidemiology and ethics in the case of AIDS. The first describes the conflict in the early years of the epidemic between the need for valid data about a new disease of unknown etiology and subjects' fears of confidentiality breaches. The second concerns the conflict between scientific definitions of the term "disease" and the economic and regulatory uses of these definitions, as well as their impact on individuals. The third pits the epidemiologic value of anonymous serological surveillance techniques against the clinical value of identifying seropositivity in individuals. These three examples are not comprehensive; epidemiology has also played an important role in, for example, cohort studies of HIV-infected persons.

Ethical Issues in Epidemiologic Studies

Although all of the ethical principles that govern research apply to both clinical and noninterventional epidemiologic research, the weight given to one principle or another varies according to the context. Clinical research focuses on the individual as part of a study population. Ethical principles that predominate in clinical research also focus on individuals: respect for autonomous decision making, beneficence (enhancing the welfare of the individual), and nonmaleficence (avoiding harm to individuals). These principles weigh heavily in considerations of the ratio of risks to benefits in medical decision making, informed consent, and privacy and protection of confidentiality.

Epidemiologic studies, on the other hand, focus on populations but may involve identified individuals. The predominant ethical values include the importance of knowledge to be gained and the potential benefit to groups (perhaps future patients or society in general). Questions of justice—in this case, fairness between the selection of subjects who bear the burdens of research and the eventual recipients of any benefits derived from the research—also arise in epidemiologic studies. Some of the ethical problems common in epidemiology are invasion of privacy, violation of confidentiality, conflict of interest, and tension between a researcher's values and those of the communities studied.[5]

Clinical trials and noninterventional epidemiologic research present different types of risks or harms. Risks in clinical trials typically involve adverse physical effects or, less commonly, psychological harm. But, as Alexander Morgan Capron[6] points out:

Epidemiologic research can also involve the risk of harm, but it is typically of a different sort. Since, in most cases, investigators do not physically intervene with the subject and do not even have direct contact of any sort, physical and psychological injuries are unlikely. Yet other sorts of harm may occur. First, if data dealing with sensitive matters— either raw data or final results—can be linked to subjects, they may suffer social harm, such as ostracism or loss of employment. Second, even when individuals cannot be linked to information that is embarrassing (or worse), findings that paint an adverse picture of an entire population may eventuate in harm to that group, either directly or as a result of the adoption of laws or policies that have a negative impact on the welfare of group members.[6]

Furthermore, Capron continues, even when subjects are not physically or psychologically harmed, they may be wronged, for instance, by invasion of privacy without consent or by treating people solely as a means to an end. Such possibilities, he rightly maintains, explain why ethical guidelines are important, even if the risk of direct harm to subjects is negligible.

For these reasons and others, epidemiologic studies are governed by special regulatory requirements, although some types of research are exempt from institutional review board (IRB) oversight. Examples include research involving the collection or study of existing data, records, pathologic specimens, or diagnostic specimens as long as there are no identifiers linking the data to the subjects. IRBs accustomed to reviewing clinical studies may have difficulty in devising appropriate standards for epidemiologic studies.[7]

Confidentiality and the Wary Subject

In 1981 Michael Gottlieb, a Los Angeles physician, reported to the federal Centers for Disease Control and Prevention (CDC) the unexpected occurrence of the rare *Pneumocystis carinii* pneumonia (PCP) in five previously healthy homosexual men he had treated in 1980 and 1981.[4] An editorial note in the *Morbidity and Mortality Weekly Report* (*MMWR*) suggested that some aspect of a "homosexual lifestyle" might be involved.[8] Soon after, a second *MMWR* report described a finding of Kaposi's sarcoma, a cancer rarely seen in the United States, in twenty-six gay men in California and New York City treated in the previous thirty months.[9] Although it is now known that cases of AIDS had been seen as early as 1977, these *MMWR* reports marked the official start of the epidemic.

In mid-1981 the CDC formed a surveillance task force, which contacted state and local health departments to identify suspected cases of what was soon to be called AIDS. (An earlier designation, Gay-Related Immunodeficiency, or GRID, was used until late 1982.[10]) Although the case of a heterosexual woman with AIDS had been reported to the CDC by August 1981, and a New York City investigation of eleven men with PCP included seven drug users, five of them heterosexual, the focus remained on homosexuality as the defining characteristic of the population at risk. By 1983 several investigations were under way involving gay men as subjects. To gather valid data on the sexual, drug-using, and other behavior of gay men, epidemiologists sought to obtain highly detailed and accurate descriptions of these aspects of subjects' lives. The researchers especially focused on the numbers of sex partners—the "promiscuity" theory—and on the use of amyl nitrate ("poppers") during sex. In these interviews the subjects might have revealed information about homosexual behaviors, which are illegal in some states and stigmatized everywhere; about the use of illegally obtained drugs; about criminal activities, such as prostitution; or about illegal entry into the United States. They also might have named other individuals involved in these activities. Many subjects, unwilling to trust government researchers with such potentially damaging information, either refused to cooperate or gave inaccurate or incomplete answers.

While some epidemiologists were sensitive to the subjects' concerns, others failed to see why they should treat information about this disease, or the people who had it, with any special protections. Public health departments were proud of their record of maintaining confidentiality of information about other diseases. Nevertheless, in some instances at least, internal procedures were less than strict. Case folders with identifying names were sometimes left on desks or given to other researchers or agency employees. Local health departments reported cases with identifiers to the CDC. At that time the modes of transmission of this deadly disease were still under investigation. Against a background in which police departments, fire departments, and others were calling for lists of people with AIDS, and against a public barraged by politicians' demands that people with AIDS be isolated, the subjects' concerns were understandable.

At this point ethicists became involved in the issue. Early in 1983, a physician treating gay men and gay men with AIDS involved in epidemiologic research asked the staff of The Hastings Center, then located in Hastings-on-Hudson, New York, to join them in stressing the importance of confidentiality in AIDS research. They specifically sought to bolster their views, which were regarded by some health department officials as self-interested, with the professional and independent standing of ethicists. The center's staff subsequently decided to convene a working group to develop guidelines on this subject. The proposal to the Charles A. Dana Foundation, which funded the project, stated:

There is an inherent tension between the needs of researchers who want access to a maximum of information with a minimum of hindrance and the desires of AIDS patients who want sensitive and identifiable information about themselves given the maximum protection and the most restricted distribution. This tension need not pose an insuperable difficulty. While the legitimate interests of researchers and patients can be accommodated, it will require a serious examination of the contexts in which disclosure takes place, the purposes for which the information may be used, and the people who will have access to it.

The proposal warned that "the future integrity of epidemiological research on AIDS" depended on reaching a mutual understanding.

Given adversarial positions that were hardening, the staff judged that the composition of the working group would be a determining factor in the acceptance of the guidelines. No matter how ethically justifiable or well argued the guidelines were, if they did not have the support of the parties whose interests were at stake, they would have no impact. This was a real-world situation fraught with drama. Many gay men believed that isolation and quarantine in "concentration camps" were distinct possibilities. They were, they believed, facing a hostile, angry, and irrational public. Some researchers and health department officials, for their part, feared a rapidly spreading and uncontrollable epidemic. These perceptions made the issues emotionally explosive.

The working group that was convened included government and academic researchers, epidemiologists, lawyers, privacy specialists, ethicists, physicians, and representatives of gay and AIDS organizations. Most of the "experts" had never talked with the subject representatives of the target population, who were for their part extremely wary of researchers and government officials of any kind. Interestingly, the way epidemiologists had framed the epidemic to that date helped determine the composition of the group. There were no participants representing drug users or women, because these groups or their behaviors had not been formally linked with the disease. There were, however, representatives of the Haitian community, which had been officially termed a "risk group" (a designation later dropped because of protests).[11]

The overall problem addressed in the guidelines was: What procedures and policies will both protect the privacy of research subjects and enable research to proceed expeditiously? The ethical challenge was described as "striking a balance between the principle of respect for the autonomy of persons (which requires that individuals should be treated as autonomous agents who have the right to control their own destinies) and the pursuit of the common good (which requires maximizing possible benefits as well as minimizing possible harms, to society as well as to individuals)."

Despite their different perspectives, members of the working group reached a consensus on all but one of the proposed guidelines. These covered descriptive issues such as what identifiers are necessary, when they are needed, and what precautions should be taken to protect identifiable data; who should and who should not have access to personally identifiable information; the rather severe limitations of current legal protections; steps that should be taken to enhance the legal protections for both research subjects and researchers whose data might be subpoenaed; standards for institutional review boards; and questions of consent.

The single issue on which the working group could not agree was use of the Social Security Number (SSN) as an identifier. The guidelines pointed out that SSNs offer the greatest potential for matching data sets but that they also pose the greatest threat to confidentiality: "Some researchers believe that Social Security numbers are indispensable in longitudinal studies, where it is important to be able to recognize that different sets of data have come from a single person. Those who oppose the use of Social Security numbers stress that these numbers are assigned and held by the federal government. Potential misuse of information by government agencies is one of the strongest fears expressed by subjects in AIDS research."[12]

The SSN question has recurred in the context of the debate over national health reform and increasing concerns about the privacy of data collected under a regional or national system. Most proposals for reform rely on the SSN as a personal identifier. Lawrence O. Gostin and colleagues assert that "perhaps the most critical single decision regarding privacy and security in a reformed health care system is whether to use the Social Security Number . . . as the individual identifier."[13] Pointing out that the SSN currently is not a completely reliable identifier, and that this identifier is used extensively for a variety of non-health-related purposes, Gostin et al. instead recommend a personal health security number, which would have no other purpose and would be essentially as private as a health record itself. Despite the importance of this issue, then and now, it seemed a minor matter in the face of overwhelming consensus on other issues at the time that the confidentiality guidelines were written by the AIDS working group.

The guidelines had no official weight but were cited repeatedly in the course of negotiations over epidemiologic research. The process of their formulation also set some important precedents. At this early stage of the epidemic, ethics was firmly established as integral to public health decision making. Affected communities were involved in recommendations about their interests. Finally, consensus could be achieved on most thorny issues. Even when agreement could not be reached, the dissenting positions could be articulated and clarified.

What Counts as an AIDS Case?

The ethical dimensions of epidemiology come into play well before the design and implementation of specific studies. They are introduced with decisions about what will be studied and how the questions will be framed. While most ethical discussion concerns problems arising in the conduct of studies, there is also an ethical dimension to studies that are never undertaken.

For example, consider the CDC's surveillance case definition of AIDS and the struggle to include medical manifestations of HIV infection that relate specifically to women.[14] Disease classification systems and surveillance definitions are ordinarily tools for epidemiologists and clinicians, not matters for political debate and patient advocacy. It is hard to imagine a protest march complaining about the classification system for colon cancer. But when it comes to AIDS, nothing is ordinary.

The CDC categorizes HIV/AIDS in two ways. The AIDS surveillance case definition sets out the criteria for what counts as a case of AIDS for purposes of public health reporting. Case reporting is the primary, although not the only, surveillance tool in monitoring the incidence and prevalence of disease. The surveillance case definition is intended solely to provide consistent statistical data for public health purposes. The CDC urges clinicians not to rely on this definition alone in diagnosing serious disease caused by HIV infection.

In addition to the official surveillance case definition, the CDC has developed an alternative, comprehensive "classification" system for HIV infection for adults and adolescents. (There is a separate classification system for children.) The classification system covers the broad spectrum of HIV disease, from initial infection, asymptomatic infection, and persistent generalized lymphadenopathy through serious opportunistic infections and cancers. This system combines clinical disease criteria and (since 1993) immunologic markers. The primary purpose is to provide a framework for categorizing HIV-related morbidity and immunosuppression. In the controversy discussed in this section, the surveillance case definition was the primary focus, although the classification system was also involved by virtue of its reliance on the surveillance case definition for criteria for the end stage of AIDS.

The CDC's surveillance case definition of AIDS is used by public health officials, researchers, clinicians, hospital administrators, disability specialists, insurance administrators, health economists, legislators, social workers, psychologists, policy makers, and the media. It has influenced the way the epidemic is perceived, managed, and funded. An AIDS diagnosis triggers a series of benefits and services generally not available to a person with HIV infection.

It is not surprising, then, that the CDC's surveillance case definition of AIDS has transcended epidemiology to become a symbol for the inadequacies of the United States government's response to the HIV epidemic, and a particular symbol for the failure to address adequately the needs of HIV-infected women.

The CDC's surveillance case definition of AIDS has been changed three times (in 1985, 1987, and 1993) since the first version in 1981. The CDC's initial surveillance case definition required the diagnosis of one of eleven opportunistic infections, or of two cancers that were considered "at least moderately predictive of a defect in cell-mediated immunity, occurring in a person with no known cause for diminished resistance to that disease."[15] In 1984, when HIV-1 was discovered, various laboratory tests were developed to measure and confirm the presence of HIV antibodies. Using these tests as diagnostic indicators, the CDC broadened the surveillance case definition of AIDS in 1985 to include additional opportunistic infections or cancers that would be indicative of AIDS in persons with positive HIV antibody test results.[16] The surveillance case definition was further expanded in 1987 to include several severe nonmalignant HIV-associated conditions, including HIV wasting syndrome and neurological manifestations, and to permit "presumptive" diagnoses, such as diagnoses of AIDS based on the presence of one of seven indicator diseases without confirmatory laboratory evidence of HIV.[17]

In 1991 the CDC proposed still another revision of the surveillance case definition and the disease classification system. Under this scheme there would be three categories of HIV disease (asymptomatic, symptomatic, and AIDS). There would also be three categorical levels of $CD4^+$ T-cells per cubic millimeter (mm^3) of blood, which would guide clinicians in recommending therapeutic actions in disease management. Because declining $CD4^+$ T-cell counts have been shown to be reliable indicators of disease progression, individuals with less than 200 $CD4^+$ T-cells per mm^3 would be considered to have AIDS, regardless of their symptoms. No new opportunistic infections or other conditions would be added to the already long list of twenty-three AIDS-defining conditions in the surveillance case definition.[18]

This proposal was greeted with intense and often acrimonious debate. Virtually everyone agreed that the surveillance case definition should be revised, but many disagreed with the CDC's approach. Advocates argued that the "outdated" surveillance case definition artificially lowered the number of cases of AIDS, which was reflected in inadequate federal funding and attention. Officials in states with large numbers of women and drug users with HIV-related illnesses, the groups most likely to fall outside the CDC's 1987 surveillance case definition for AIDS, were concerned that funding formulas based on case reports of CDC-defined AIDS were inequitable. Women's advocates claimed that many women with HIV-related illnesses were improperly diagnosed and treated because the surveillance case definition was developed from data on clinical manifestations in gay men. Moreover, community-based organizations that provide services to individuals, especially women, who are disabled by HIV illness but do not meet the criteria for AIDS found it difficult to obtain various federal, state, and local entitlements and benefits for their clients. A full-page advertisement in *The New York Times* (June 19, 1991), initiated by the AIDS Coalition to Unleash Power (ACT UP) and signed by over 200 individuals and organizations, protested: "Women don't get AIDS. They just die from it."

One group went even further, forcibly handcuffing selected participants (all well-known AIDS advocates, including some physicians) at a meeting at the offices of the American Public Health Association held with CDC officials to discuss the controversy. During the several hours that followed, the group protested the meeting, the attendance by AIDS advocates and the CDC, the proposed revisions and the failure to include conditions specific to women, and the general lack of government action on AIDS.

The CDC claimed that there was insufficient evidence to include specific gynecological conditions. By strict research standards, the evidence was indeed scant, but the studies that would have provided more adequate evidence one way or the other had not been done or had not been started early enough in the course of the epidemic to provide reliable data. The CDC's final revision of the HIV infection classification system and the surveillance case definition for AIDS contained all its original proposals, but it also included one female-specific condition (invasive cervical cancer), as well as pulmonary tuberculosis and recurrent pneumonia.[19] As a result of the expanded surveillance case definition, in 1993 reported AIDS cases increased 111% over cases reported in 1992 (103,500 compared with 49,016),[20] significantly surpassing the 75% rise the CDC had predicted.[21] The number of case reports in the first quarter of 1993 was 178% higher than in the same period of 1992; the rate of increase declined in subsequent reporting periods.

Of cases reported in 1993, 54% were based on conditions added to the definition in that year. Of these, the majority (91%) had only severe HIV-related immunosuppression; 7% had pulmonary tuberculosis; 2%, recurrent pneumonia; and less than 1%, invasive cervical cancer.

The increase in reported cases in 1993 was greater among females (151%) than males (105%). The largest increases were among racial/ethnic minorities, adolescents and young adults, and cases attributed to heterosexual transmission.

The CDC has noted that the increase created by the expanded surveillance case definition will lessen over time. The number of new cases reported during the first half of 1994 (40,079) decreased 65 percent from the number reported during the same period of 1993 (61,743).[22]

The controversy—as acrimonious as any in AIDS history—revealed that surveillance case definitions, disease classification systems, and the CDC's role in both were poorly comprehended. Our understanding of the current state of the epidemic (actually a series of smaller epidemics, which began in different cities at different times and have followed different courses) suffered from the initial, almost single-minded focus on gay men. The controversy also showed how secondary uses of surveillance information can have a far greater impact on individuals than its primary epidemiologic purpose.

HIV Surveillance and the Identification of Infected Newborns

The potential conflict between the values that predominate in epidemiologic studies and those that weigh most heavily in clinical practice has become real in the case of HIV seroprevalence studies conducted in newborns. Under these circumstances the importance of obtaining accurate knowledge about the course of the epidemic, in a way that does not present any risk to individuals, comes into conflict with the importance of identifying and treating individual patients. This is not an instance of one goal being more valuable than the other; it is a case in which one methodology cannot serve both goals equally well.

Discussions about HIV counseling and testing policies for pregnant women and newborns have taken place in the context of a broader debate: Should testing be voluntary with informed consent, mandatory (legally required), or routine (usually interpreted to mean that patients have a right to refuse testing, but health care providers do not have an obligation to inform patients that they are being tested)? With some exceptions (screening of blood donors, military personnel, and immigrants, for example), the debate has been resolved, at least temporarily, in favor of voluntary testing.

All the major organizations and groups that have specifically examined testing policies for pregnant women have concluded that voluntary screening with informed consent is the course most likely to produce the desired effects of education, prevention, and appropriate medical and social service follow-up. The Institute of Medicine in the United States, for example, concluded that "individuals (or their legally recognized representatives) should have the right to consent to or refuse HIV testing (except when such testing is conducted anonymously for epidemiologic purposes)." Opposing mandatory newborn or prenatal screening programs, the Institute of Medicine found "no compelling evidence that women and children should constitute an exception to this principle."[23] Similarly, a working group from the Johns Hopkins University and Georgetown University rejected mandatory screening and recommended a range of voluntary policies.[24]

This consensus is eroding, however, because of new evidence about the benefits of early diagnosis and intervention in pediatric HIV disease, and the results of the AIDS Clinical Trial Group Study 076. This trial showed that transmission from mother to fetus was reduced dramatically (to 8.3% from 25%) in a group of pregnant women treated with zidovudine (AZT).[25] PCP is the most frequent and lethal manifestation of HIV disease in infants. Prophylaxis in adults can prevent or delay PCP; although there are no studies in infants, the U.S. Public Health Service recommends that prophylaxis be initiated in HIV-positive infants with $CD4^+$ T-cell counts lower than 1500 per mm^3.[26] In addition, antiretroviral therapy can begin at an early age and babies can be monitored more closely for other infections. Finally, the risk of HIV transmission from breast milk, while small, can be avoided if an HIV-infected mother does not breast-feed. These benefits, while no panacea, have a significant impact on the ethics of the screening calculus.

Although the potential medical benefits of early diagnosis and prophylactic therapy apply to adults and children, the most vigorous calls for routine or mandatory screening come from pediatricians and primarily stress the benefits to newborns.[27] Nearly all babies born to HIV-infected mothers carry maternal antibodies, but in 3 out of 4 these antibodies disappear by about fifteen months of age. New techniques can more accurately identify truly HIV-infected infants as early as three months of age.[28] Still, screening of newborns for HIV identifies only potentially infected babies. It also may miss some HIV-infected newborns who nonetheless test HIV negative; their mothers may not have developed antibodies by the time they gave birth.

Although HIV testing of newborns cannot definitively identify an infected infant, it almost certainly discloses the mother's HIV status. The irony of this fact is clearly evident in the debates concerning proposals to unblind seroprevalence studies carried out for epidemiologic purposes. Over the past several years, the CDC has developed what it calls a "family" of serological surveys to estimate the prevalence of HIV infection in sentinel areas and groups throughout the country.[29] In June 1989, the New York State Department of Health proposed to "modify its on-going blind newborn HIV antibody testing program to permit voluntary notification of mothers whose infants test positive." Under the proposal, new mothers would have been given the option of learning their baby's test results (and as a consequence, their own HIV status). Several objections were raised to the proposal by community-based health care providers and others. These objections primarily concerned (1) the confusing and psychologically traumatic impact on new mothers of learning about their own HIV infection and the possible infection of their babies at a time when they are physically and emotionally vulnerable; (2) the potential for manipulation or coercion by health care providers, who might not understand or accept a mother's unwillingness to learn the test results at that time; and (3) the lack of health care and support services for women and their children, once identified as seropositive.

Because of these objections, the state Department of Health agreed to postpone the implementation of this proposal in favor of a much more aggressive voluntary program, called the Obstetrical HIV Counseling/Testing/Care Initiative. This program offers voluntary testing, with counseling at twenty-four sites, to women who have given birth without access to prenatal care. Initial results indicate that a growing number of these women are being counseled (64.8% by 1991) and have consented to testing (46.9%), and are being referred for care.[30] Early diagnosis of HIV infection is increasing. In 1991, 45% of children under one year old had been diagnosed with HIV infection prior to their first episode of PCP. In 1992 and 1993, that figure was 60%.[31]

In addition, New York City's Child Welfare Administration (CWA) has revised its policy on HIV testing for infants and children entering foster care. Because newborns in foster care are much more likely to be HIV positive than newborns going home with their mothers, CWA is taking several steps to ensure that they receive appropriate evaluation and follow-up. The administration has expanded the list of risk factors warranting HIV testing and requires a physician's HIV risk assessment for children from birth to the age of two within thirty days of entering foster care. These and other changes are expected to increase the numbers of children identified as HIV positive in the foster care system. The infected children and their foster parents are eligible for special medical and social services.[32]

Despite these two initiatives aimed at increasing the numbers of HIV-infected infants identified at birth, the controversy over newborn testing erupted in the New York State legislature in 1993–94. Nettie Mayersohn, an assemblywoman from Queens, introduced legislation to require the State Department of Health to notify parents if their infant showed positive results on the HIV test that is currently done anonymously. The debate quickly polarized, and raged not only in the legislative halls but also in the media.

To deflect the furor and to table action on the Mayersohn bill, the New York State Assembly's Ad Hoc Task Force on AIDS asked the Governor's AIDS Advisory Council to study the issue. After several months of hearings and debate, in February 1994 a subcommittee convened by the Advisory Council recommended a policy of "mandatory counseling and strongly encouraged voluntary testing for all pregnant and postpartum women," as well as other measures to strengthen counseling and testing and availability of services (p. iii).[31] A group of pediatricians dissented from the report, declaring that this policy was "insufficient to offer the protection which every infant deserves" and that voluntary testing has an "unacceptably high failure rate."[33]

A legislative compromise that would have mandated counseling and encouraged voluntary testing failed on the last day of the session. The New York State Task Force on Life and the Law, another executive branch body, was then asked to restudy the entire issue.

In all the vociferous and voluminous debate, the purpose and importance of blinded seroprevalence studies as an epidemiologic tool were hardly mentioned, and then only to be misunderstood. There are several important objections to unblinding these studies.

Such a policy will compromise the scientific validity of the studies. Blinded surveys test blood samples already collected for other medical purposes and devoid of all personal identifiers. Blinded surveys can generate less biased estimates of HIV prevalence because individuals do not have the opportunity to select whether or not to participate in serological testing. Ethically, blinded surveys do not place any participant at risk of identification, so issues of privacy and confidentiality are not raised.[34] Consequently, study protocols are exempt from IRB review, and individual consent forms and measures to secure the confidentiality of the information obtained are not required. For these reasons, blinded studies are simpler, quicker, and less costly than nonblinded surveys. They have also been remarkably uncontroversial and free of political influence. However, blinded HIV serological surveys on adults or children have been very controversial in England and the Netherlands,[35] and one commentator in the United States has claimed that "surreptitious testing is deceitful" and that "in the quest to eliminate self-selection bias, epidemiologists are ignoring the difference between human subjects and laboratory animals."[36]

The use of blinded surveys is compatible with a parallel system of voluntary counseling and testing in settings where individuals likely to be at risk of HIV infection are treated. One of the purposes of blinded serological surveys is to pinpoint precisely where resources and services are needed, including counseling and testing. But, as the Public Health Service points out, "The surveillance activity, in the case of an HIV prevalence survey, must not be confused with the public health intervention for which the survey may indicate a need."[37] Further, guidelines for unlinked anonymous screening for the public health surveillance of HIV infections, issued by the World Health Organization in June 1989, state: "Voluntary testing (confidential or anonymous) with counselling should be available wherever possible to populations in which UAS [unlinked anonymous screening] is being carried out, so that those individuals who wish to know their HIV-infection status can do so. This is particularly important if the population is estimated to have a moderate to high prevalence of HIV infection. However, such testing should be offered through a separate system."[38]

The debate about newborn screening may shift to screening of pregnant women, if the results of the 076 trial are borne out by further experience. Although it is likely that mandatory screening of pregnant women will be proposed, such a policy would raise serious concerns. As Ronald Bayer puts it, "Mandatory screening of children could become justifiable if therapeutic interventions could substantially extend the lives of infected children, because treatment, regardless of parental objections, would be imperative. By contrast, the mandatory screening of pregnant women is objectionable because mandatory treatment of competent adults is virtually never acceptable."[39] In practical terms, nothing short of incarceration and forced treatment would be feasible if a woman refused the daily regimen of AZT.

As this issue unfolds, it may be appropriate to reevalute the usefulness of the seroprevalence studies that were the initial focus of the debate. Earlier in the epidemic it was important to detect the presence of HIV in various populations and regions, to establish baselines, and to detect trends. For these goals, serological surveys are an appropriate tool. At the current stage in newborn screening, in regions where prevalence levels have been identified and are relatively stable, blinded anonymous serological surveys may only need to be repeated at intervals and not conducted on all newborns. Other surveillance methods can be used to provide additional data. In its draft guidelines on HIV/AIDS surveillance, the World Health Organization states: "While sentinel HIV serosurveillance can be used to monitor the epidemic, it should not be entirely relied upon for estimating the present and future impact of HIV, or for evaluating the impact of a national AIDS programme."[40] In any event, serosurveys should not be used for purposes for which they are not intended. If the clinical benefits of early medical intervention become so compelling that the public health power of the state is used to identify potentially HIV-infected infants, then screening should be done explicitly, without the "cover" of the anonymous blinded serological prevalence studies. In May 1995 the CDC suspended funding of the blinded newborn seroprevalence studies. This move was widely seen as a counter to federal legislation introduced by Rep. Gary Ackerman, who represents Mayersohn's district, to unblind the results of the CDC studies.

Conclusion

While the definitive history of AIDS research is yet to be written, Oppenheimer[10] gives an astute preliminary assessment:

From the beginning of the epidemic, epidemiologists conceptualized HIV infection as a complex social phenomenon, with dimensions that derived from the social relations, behavioral patterns, and past experiences of the population at risk. On the one hand, the epidemiologists' approach may have skewed the choice of models and the hypotheses pursued and may have offered some justification for homophobia. On the other, by defining HIV infection as a multifactorial phenomenon, with both behavioral and microbial determinants, epidemiologists offered the possibility of primary prevention, a traditional epidemiological response to infectious and chronic diseases. Epidemiologists, in effect, established the basis for an effective public health campaign and—through publications, conferences, and the continuous collection of surveillance data—helped make AIDS a concern of policymakers and the public (p. 76).[10]

Ethics, too, will be seen to have played a role in providing a reasoned and principled approach to some of the conflicts that have arisen. But, unfortunately, the end of the epidemic is nowhere in sight, and the ethical issues are likely to become even more pressing and difficult in the future.

References

1. Shilts, R. *And the Band Played On: Politics, People and the AIDS Epidemic.* New York: St. Martin's Press, 1987.
2. Fee, E. and Fox, D. M. *AIDS: The Making of a Chronic Disease.* Berkeley, CA: University of California Press, 1992.
3. Bayer, R. *Private Acts, Social Consequences: AIDS and the Politics of Public Health.* New York: The Free Press, 1989.
4. Oppenheimer, G. M. "In the Eye of the Storm: The Epidemiological Construction of AIDS." In *AIDS: The Burdens of History,* ed. E. Fee and D. M. Fox. Berkeley: University of California Press, 1988: 267.
5. Last, J. M. "Epidemiology and Ethics," *Law, Medicine & Health Care* 19 (1991): 166–74.
6. Capron, A. M. "Protection of Research Subjects: Do Special Rules Apply to Epidemiology?" *Law, Medicine & Health Care* 19 (1991): 185.
7. Cann, C. I.   and Rothman, K. J. "IRBs and Epidemiological Research: How Inappropriate Restrictions Hamper Studies," *IRB* 6 (1984): 5–7.
8. Centers for Disease Control. "*Pneumocystis* Pneumonia—Los Angeles," *Morbidity and Mortality Weekly Report* 30 (1981): 250–252.
9. Centers for Disease Control. "Kaposi's Sarcoma and *Pneumocystis* Pneumonia Among Homosexual Men—New York City and California," *Morbidity and Mortality Weekly Report* 30 (1981): 305–307.
10. Oppenheimer, G. M. "Causes, Cases, and Cohorts: The Role of Epidemiology in the Historical Construction of AIDS," in *AIDS: The Making of a Chronic Disease,* ed. E. Fee and D. M. Fox. Berkeley, CA: University of California Press, 1992: 62, 76.
11. Farmer, P. *AIDS and Accusation: Haiti and the Geography of Blame.* Berkeley, CA: University of California Press, 1992.
12. Bayer, R., Levine, C., and Murray, T. H. "Guidelines for Confidentiality in Research on AIDS," *IRB: A Review of Human Subjects Research* 6 (November/December 1984): 1–7.

13. Gostin, L. O., Turek–Brezina, J., Powers, M., Kozloff, R., Faden, R., and Steinauer, D. D. "Privacy and Security of Personal Information in a New Health Care System," *Journal of the American Medical Association* 270 (1993): 2488.

14. Levine, C. and Stein, G. L. "What's in a Name? The Policy Implication of the CDC Definition of AIDS," *Law, Medicine and Health Care* 19 (1991): 278–90.

15. Centers for Disease Control. "Update on Acquired Immune Deficiency Syndrome (AIDS)—United States," *Morbidity and Mortality Weekly Report* 31 (1982): 507–14.

16. Centers for Disease Control. "Revision of Case Definition of Acquired Immunodeficiency Syndrome for National Reporting—United States," *Morbidity and Mortality Weekly Report* 34 (1985): 373–75.

17. Centers for Disease Control. "Revision of the CDC Surveillance Case Definition for Acquired Immunodeficiency Syndrome," *Morbidity and Mortality Weekly Report* 36 (Suppl.): 1S–15S.

18. Centers for Disease Control. "1992 Revised Classification System for HIV Infection and Expanded Case Definition for Adolescents and Adults," Draft, November 15, 1991.

19. Centers for Disease Control. "1993 Revised Classification System for HIV Infection and Expanded Surveillance Case Definition for AIDS Among Adolescents and Adults," *Morbidity and Mortality Weekly Report* 41, no. RR–17 (1992): 1–5.

20. Centers for Disease Control and Prevention. "Update: Impact of the Expanded AIDS Surveillance Case Definition for Adolescents and Adults on Case Reporting—United States, 1993," *Morbidity and Mortality Weekly Report* 43 (1994): 160–61, 167–70.

21. Centers for Disease Control and Prevention. "Impact of the Expanded AIDS Surveillance Case Definition on AIDS Case Reporting—United States, First Quarter, 1993," *Morbidity and Mortality Weekly Report* 42 (1993): 308–10.

22. From data cited in the Centers for Disease Control and Prevention. *HIV/AIDS Surveillance Report* 5(1) (1993); 5(2) (1993); and 6(1) (1994).

23. Institute of Medicine. *HIV Screening of Pregnant Women and Newborns.* Washington: Institute of Medicine, 1991: 2–3.

24. Faden, R., Geller, G., and Powers, M. *AIDS, Women and the Next Generation.* New York: Oxford University Press, 1992: 333–34.

25. Hauger, S. M., Nicholas, S. W., and Caspe, W. B. *Guidelines for the Care of Children and Adolescents with HIV Infection (Report of the New York State Department of Health AIDS Institute Criteria Committee for the Care of HIV-Infected Children).* St. Louis: Mosby-Year Book, Inc., 1991 (Suppl. to *Journal of Pediatrics* 119 [1, Part 2]: July 1991).

26. Centers for Disease Control. "Guidelines for Prophylaxis Against *Pneumocystis* carinii Pneumonia for Children Infected with Human Immunodeficiency Virus," *Morbidity and Mortality Weekly Report* 40 (1991): RR–2.

27. Angell, M. "A Dual Approach to the AIDS Epidemic," *New England Journal of Medicine* 324 (1991): 1500.

28. Quinn, T. C., Kline, R. H., Halsey, N., Hutton, N., Ruff, A., Butz, A., Boulos, R., and Modlin, J. F. "Early Diagnosis of Perinatal HIV Infection by Detection of Viral-specific IgA Antibodies," *Journal of the American Medical Association* 266 (1991): 3439–42.

29. Pappaioanou, M., Dondero, Jr., T. J., Peterson, L. R., Onorato, I. M., Sanchez, C. D., and Curran, J. W. "The Family of HIV Seroprevalence Surveys: Objectives,

Methods, and Uses of Sentinel Surveillance for HIV in the United States," *Public Health Reports* 105 (1990): 113–19.

30. New York State Department of Health, AIDS Institute. *Women and Children with HIV Infection in New York State: 1990–92 AIDS Institute Program Review*. Albany, NY: New York State Department of Health, 1992.

31. New York State AIDS Advisory Council. *Report of the Subcommittee on Newborn HIV Screening of the New York State AIDS Advisory Council*. Albany, NY: February 10, 1994: 17, iii.

32. New York City, Human Resources Administration, Child Welfare Administration. *Draft Bulletin: HIV Testing of Children in Foster Care*, April 23, 1993.

33. Dissenting Comments on the January 31, 1994 Report of the Subcommittee on Newborn Screening to the AIDS Advisory Council, February 4, 1994.

34. Bayer, R., Levine, C., and Wolf, S. M. "HIV Antibody Screening: An Ethical Framework for Evaluating Proposed Programs," *Journal of the American Medical Association* 256 (1986): 1768–74.

35. Bayer, R., Lumey, L. H., and Wan, L. "The American and Dutch Responses to Unlinked Anonymous HIV Seroprevalence Studies: An International Comparison," *AIDS* 4 (1992): 4283–90.

36. Isaacman, S. I. "HIV Surveillance Testing: Taking Advantage of the Disadvantaged" (Letter), *American Journal of Public Health* 83 (1993): 597.

37. Dondero, T. J., Pappaioanou, M., and Curran, J. W. "Monitoring the Levels and Trends of HIV Infection: The Public Health Service's HIV Surveillance Program," *Public Health Reports* 103 (1988): 213–20.

38. Global Programme on AIDS, World Health Organization. *Unlinked Anonymous Screening for the Public Health Surveillance of HIV Infections: Proposed International Guidelines*. Geneva, Switzerland: WHO, June 1989.

39. Bayer, R. "Ethical Challenges Posed by Zidovudine Treatment to Reduce Vertical Transmission of HIV," *New England Journal of Medicine* 331 (1994): 1224.

40. World Health Organization. *Guidelines for HIV/AIDS Surveillance and AIDS Case Definitions in Adults*. Geneva, Switzerland: WHO, May 25–27, 1992: 15.

V

THE REGULATORY CONTEXT AND PROFESSIONAL EDUCATION

13

The Institutional Review Board*

ROBERT J. LEVINE

The Declaration of Helsinki[1] establishes as the international standard for biomedical research involving human subjects the requirement that "each experimental procedure involving human subjects should be clearly formulated in an experimental protocol which should be transmitted for consideration, comment and guidance to a specially appointed committee independent of the investigator and sponsor." (Article I.2.) In most of the world such committees are called *research ethics committees*. In the United States, federal law assigns to these committees the name *institutional review board* (IRB) and the authority and responsibility for approving or disapproving proposals to conduct research involving human subjects (ref. 2, p. 323ff., and ref. 3.). In Canada, *research ethics boards* have similar authority to approve or disapprove research proposals, not merely to offer "consideration, comment and guidance."[4] (p. 48)

The Council for International Organizations of Medical Sciences (CIOMS), in collaboration with the World Health Organization (WHO), has formulated the *International Ethical Guidelines for Biomedical Research Involving Human Subjects*. These guidelines assign to research ethics committees the authority and responsibility for review and approval of research proposals before they may be initiated.[5] In their 1991 *International Guidelines for Ethical Review of Epidemiological Studies*, CIOMS and WHO extend the requirement for committee review and approval to research in the field of epidemiology.[6]

History

The Nuremberg Code (1949) and the original Declaration of Helsinki (1964) made no mention of committee review. These documents placed on the investi-

*Some passages in this chapter are adapted from *Ethics and Regulation of Clinical Research*.[2]

gator all responsibility for safeguarding the rights and welfare of research subjects. The first mention of committee review in an international document was in the Tokyo revision of the Declaration of Helsinki (1975). The first international document to require review *and approval* by an independent committee was the *Proposed International Guidelines for Biomedical Research Involving Human Subjects*, promulgated by CIOMS in collaboration with WHO in 1982.[7] This document states that its purpose is to indicate how the ethical principles embodied in the Declaration of Helsinki can be effectively applied, particularly in developing countries (p. 1).[7] Nevertheless, it goes beyond Helsinki in that it requires committee approval.

In the United States, the first federal document requiring committee review was issued November 17, 1953. Titled Group Consideration for Clinical Research Procedures Deviating from Accepted Medical Practice or Involving Unusual Hazard, its guidelines applied only to research conducted at the newly opened Clinical Center at the National Institutes of Health (NIH).[8] Little is known about peer review at other institutions during the 1950s other than that it existed, at least in some medical schools. In 1961 and again in 1962, questionnaires were sent to American university departments of medicine. Approximately one-third of those responding reported that they had review committees, and one-quarter either had or were developing procedural documents.[9]

On February 8, 1966, the Surgeon General of the United States Public Health Service (PHS) issued the first federal policy statement requiring research institutions to establish the committees that subsequently became known as IRBs.[9] The policy obligated recipients of PHS grants in support of research involving human subjects to specify that "the grantee institution will provide prior review of the judgment of the principal investigator or program director by a committee of his institutional associates. This review shall assure an independent determination: (1) Of the rights and welfare of the . . . individuals involved, (2) Of the appropriateness of the methods used to secure informed consent, and (3) Of the risks and potential medical benefits of the investigation."

The evolution of the federal government's charges to review committees and of its recognition of the need for diversity in their composition was reflected in several revisions of its policy between 1966 and 1969 (ref. 2, pp 322–325, and ref. 10); these will be discussed later in this chapter.

Purpose

The purpose of the IRB is to ensure that research involving human subjects is designed to conform to relevant ethical standards. Originally, the IRB's primary focus was on safeguarding the rights and welfare of individual research subjects, concentrating on the plans for informed consent and the assessment of risks and anticipated benefits. In 1978, the National Commission for the Protection of Human Subjects of Biomedical and Behavioral Research (National Commission) added a requirement that the IRB ensure equitableness in the selection of research subjects (p. 67ff.).[2] The National Commission was concerned primarily with protecting vulnerable subjects from involvement in unjustifiably risky research and from bearing a disproportionately large share of the burdens of research. Subsequently, as participation in some types of research became widely perceived as a benefit, IRBs also assumed responsibility for ensuring disadvantaged persons equitable access to such benefits.[11,12]

The authority and responsibility of the IRB is limited to review and approval of research involving human subjects. The IRB's domain is customarily identified by defining *research* and distinguishing it from other seemingly similar activities that lie outside its province. The following definitions are compatible with those found in United States federal regulations.

The term *research* refers to a class of activities designed to develop or contribute to generalizable knowledge. Generalizable knowledge consists of theories, principles, or general relationships (or the accumulation of data on which they may be based) that can be corroborated by accepted scientific observation and inference. The *practice* of medicine or behavioral therapy refers to a class of activities designed solely to enhance the well-being of an individual patient or client. The purpose of medical or behavioral practice is to provide diagnosis, preventive treatment, or therapy.[2]

While the IRB has neither the responsibility nor the authority to review activities that conform to the definition of *practice*, it often is properly called upon to review research designed to evaluate the safety and efficacy of various *practices*, including diagnostic, therapeutic, and preventive modalities. Similarly, the activities of some epidemiologists may be difficult to classify as either research, program evaluation, or surveillance. The latter two categories, which refer to the practices of epidemiologists, need not ordinarily be reviewed by an IRB (pp. 3–10; 145–146).[2]

According to CIOMS/WHO *International Guidelines for Ethical Review of Epidemiological Studies* (pp. 22–23):[6]

It may at times be difficult to decide whether a particular proposal is for an epidemiological study or for evaluation of a programme on the part of a health-care institution or department. The defining attribute of research is that it is designed to produce new, generalizable knowledge as distinct from knowledge pertaining only to a particular individual or programme.

For instance, a governmental or hospital department may want to examine patients' records to determine the safety and efficacy of a facility, unit or procedure. If the examination is for research purposes, the proposal should be submitted to [an IRB]. However, if it is for the purpose of programme evaluation . . . the proposal may not need to be submitted to ethical review; on the contrary, it could be considered poor practice and unethical not to undertake this type of quality assurance. . . .

If it is not clear whether a proposal involves epidemiological study or routine practice, it should be submitted to the [IRB] responsible for epidemiological protocols for its opinion on whether the proposal falls within its mandate.

A source of continuing controversy is whether the IRB has an obligation to approve, disapprove, or require revision of the scientific design of research protocols for any reasons other than ethical flaws (pp. 20–25).[2] Those who argue that IRBs do or should have such an obligation point out that each of the leading international codes for research involving human subjects establishes an ethical requirement for good scientific design. As noted in the CIOMS/WHO *international ethical guidelines* for example, "scientifically unsound research on human subjects is *ipso facto* unethical." Moreover, the argument goes, the IRB's obligation to determine that risks to subjects are reasonable in relation to anticipated benefits necessarily relies on a prior determination that the scientific design is adequate, for if it is not, there will be no benefits and any risk must be considered unreasonable.

Opponents to assigning such an obligation to the IRB, while conceding these two points, argue that the IRB is not designed to make expert judgments about the scientific merits of research proposals. Such judgments require evaluation of two different features of the protocol—value and validity.[10,13] Evaluation of the value entails an appraisal of what the Nuremberg Code calls "the humanitarian importance of the problem to be solved" (Principle 6). Some commentators, myself included, believe that the properly constructed IRB has the capacity and authority to make reasonably reliable assessments of scientific value in this sense. Others, however, point with concern to the numerical dominance on most IRBs by scientists and health professionals, and suggest that such persons value things differently than does the majority of the population. Almost certainly, for example, health professionals and scientists typically place a higher value on the pursuit of knowledge for its own sake than do persons outside the health professions or academia.

Most IRBs do not have the competence to provide more than a superficial assessment of the validity of the scientific methods or the results. In the majority of cases, scientists in the institution who are most qualified to evaluate the scientific validity of a research plan are the investigators who have proposed the research; federal regulations require that they be excluded from the IRB's discussion of their protocol, even if they are IRB members. In general, responsibility for assessment of scientific validity is and ought to be delegated to committees designed to have such competence—for example, scientific review committees either within the institution or at funding agencies such as the National Institutes of Health (pp. 21–23).[2]

According to the CIOMS/WHO *international ethical guidelines*:

Committees competent to review and approve scientific aspects of clinical trials must be multidisciplinary, much like those specified earlier for assessment of safety. In many cases such committees operate most effectively at the national level. A national scientific review committee offers several advantages over local committees. First, consolidating the necessary expertise in one group allows members to deepen their knowledge in the field, thereby improving the quality and utility of the review. Second, a national committee's awareness of all proposals for research in the country facilitates the performance of another essential function, the selection of those protocols most likely to achieve the nation's health research objectives.

If an ethical review committee considers a research proposal scientifically sound, or verifies that a competent expert body has found it so, it will then consider whether any known or possible risks to the subjects are justified by the expected benefits (and whether the methods of carrying out the research will minimize harm and maximize benefit) and, if so, whether the procedures proposed for obtaining informed consent are satisfactory and those proposed for selection of subjects are equitable. (p. 38)[5]

Membership

The Surgeon General's 1966 memo called for prior review by "a committee of [the investigator's] associates," commonly called *peer review*. As of 1968, 73% of committees were limited in membership to immediate peer groups of scientists and physicians (p. 443).[9]

On May 1, 1969, PHS guidelines were revised to indicate that a committee constituted exclusively of biomedical scientists would be inadequate to perform the functions by then expected of such a committee: "The membership should possess . . . competencies necessary in the judgment as to the acceptability of the research in terms of institutional regulations, relevant law, standards of professional practice and community acceptance."

Regulations of the U.S. Department of Health and Human Services (HHS), first promulgated in 1974 and since revised several times, reflect the spirit of the 1969 PHS policy. The HHS regulations require IRBs to have at least one nonscientist (such as a lawyer, ethicist, member of the clergy) and at least one member who is not otherwise affiliated with the institution (commonly but incorrectly called a "community representative"). Persons having conflicting interests are to be excluded; this concern is also reflected in the Declaration of Helsinki's requirement of a "committee independent of the investigator and sponsor." Gender diversity is also required.

According to Robert Veatch, the IRB is an intermediate entity between two models of the review committee:[10] The "interdisciplinary professional review model," made up of diverse professionals such as doctors, lawyers, scientists, and clergy, brings professional expertise to the review process, while the "jury model . . . reflects the common sense of the reasonable person." In the jury model, "expertise relevant to the case at hand is not only not necessary, it often disqualifies one from serving on the jury." Veatch concedes that in order to perform all of its functions, the IRB requires both professional and jury skills. However, he argues that the presence of professionals makes it more difficult for the IRB to be responsive to the information needs of the reasonable person or to be adept at anticipating community acceptance.

John Robertson[14] would correct the "structural bias" of professional domination by introducing a "subject surrogate," an expert advocate for the subjects' interests. According to federal regulations (Section 46.107a)*: "If an IRB regularly reviews research that involves a vulnerable category of subjects, . . . consideration shall be given to the inclusion of one or more individuals who are knowledgeable about and experienced in working with these subjects."[15] For research involving prisoners, for example, regulations require that at least one member of the IRB be either a prisoner or a prisoner representative. There is unresolved controversy over whether persons with AIDS should be appointed to membership on all IRBs that review research in the field of HIV infection.[16]

If representatives of the various populations of prospective research subjects were to be added to the IRB, the committee would become much too large to be an effective deliberative body. In the typical university hospital, it would be necessary to include patients with cancer, heart disease, diabetes, stroke, and hypertension, to name just a few categories of diseases having a far greater incidence and prevalence than HIV infection. Moreover, if it were decided to include a person with HIV infection as a committee member, should this person be a gay white male, a user of illicit intravenous drugs or a heterosexual sex partner of one, a male or female sex worker, a person with hemophilia, or a representative of any of the other subsets of the population with HIV infection? Members of each of these subsets may have vastly different perspectives on matters relevant to the design and conduct of research. IRBs must have access to accurate information about the various populations of prospective research subjects in their institutions. Gaining such access must be accomplished without crippling the IRB's ability to take effective action; this may be facilitated through the use of consultants or such means as community consultation (ref. 2, pp. 90–91, and ref. 16), surrogate consultation (pp. 227–228),[2] establishment of advisory committees,[16] and other means beyond the scope of this chapter.

---

* Federal regulations are cited in this chapter in the following form: Section 46.107a.[15] "15" is the reference in this paper to the "final common rule" promulgated in 1991 that is applicable to all federal departments. The proper form of citation of these regulations without reference to any specific federal department is "__107a." I consistently use the form "46.107a" because I assume that most readers are primarily concerned with the regulations of the Department of Health and Human Services, Part 46. The corresponding citation for regulations of the Food and Drug Administration, for example, would be 56.107a, or for the Environmental Protection Agency, 26.107a. Although this is called the "final common rule" there are some variations across departments.

Locale

In the United States the first IRBs were established in the institutions in which research was conducted. The 1966 Surgeon General's policy statement required a committee of "institutional associates." In 1971, the FDA promulgated regulations that required committee review only when regulated research was conducted in institutions—hence the name, institutional review committee (IRC). Regulations proposed in 1973 by the Department of Health, Education and Welfare, forerunner of the Department of Health and Human Services, also reflected a local setting in their term, organizational review board (ORB). In 1974, the National Research Act established a statutory requirement for review by a committee, to which it assigned the name institutional review board (IRB), a compromise between the two names then in use.

IRBs are required to comply with federal regulations when reviewing activities involving FDA-regulated "test articles" such as investigational drugs and devices, and when reviewing research supported by federal funds.[3] Moreover, all institutions that receive federal research grants and contracts are required to file "statements of assurance" of compliance with federal regulations. In these assurances virtually all institutions voluntarily promise to apply the principles of federal regulations to all research they conduct regardless of the source of funding.

These similarities notwithstanding, each IRB has a decidedly local character. They have various names, such as Human Investigation Committee or Committee for the Protection of Human Subjects. Each is appointed by its own institution and each lends its own interpretation to the requirements of federal regulations. For example, at one university medical students are forbidden to serve as research subjects, whereas at another, involvement of medical students as research subjects is sometimes required as a condition of approval of a study (pp. 80–82).[2]

The National Commission recommended that IRBs be "located in institutions where research ... is conducted. Compared to the possible alternatives of a regional or national review ... local committees have the advantage of greater familiarity with the actual conditions (pp. 1–2)."[18] The National Commission envisioned the local IRB as an ally of the investigator in safeguarding the rights and welfare of research subjects, as well as a contributor to the education of both the research community and the public.

FDA's change in regulations in 1981 to require IRB review of all regulated research regardless of where it was done created a problem for the numerous physicians who were conducting investigations in their private offices, many of whom had no ready access to IRBs. In response, private corporations developed non-institutional review boards (NRBs).[18] There are reasons to question the validity of NRB review—for example, they do not, in the words of the National Commission, "have the advantage of familiarity with" local conditions. Nevertheless, many of them appear to be performing satisfactorily.

In 1986, FDA began to waive the requirement for local IRB review for some protocols designed to evaluate investigational new drugs or to make them available for therapeutic purposes, particularly drugs intended for the treatment of patients with HIV infection.[19,20] In such cases IRBs were offered the option of accepting review by a national committee as fulfillment of the regulatory requirement for IRB review. Such practices have caused some commentators to question the strength of the government's commitment to the principle of local review.

The purpose of waiving the requirement for local IRB review was to reduce the delays that are inevitable when several IRBs examine a protocol that is to be conducted at multiple sites. It has been recognized for many years that investigators who conduct studies involving a number of institutions—for example, multi-institutional clinical trials and survey research—may encounter formidable bureaucratic problems. Apparently, each IRB interprets the regulations differently and imposes requirements for revision of protocols that may be inconsistent. A dramatic example of the problems presented to investigators by such behavior was published by Kavanagh et al.[21] Their proposal to conduct survey and interview research on genetic counseling services in 51 institutions was reviewed by IRBs in each of these institutions. Securing final authorization to proceed with the research took over a year and involved 384 distinct communications between IRBs and the investigators. Of the 51 institutions, 11 decided that IRB review was not required, 28 approved the protocol as submitted, and 12 approved the protocol after requesting one or more modifications. Rothman calculates that the investigator-hours required to secure all the necessary IRB approvals to initiate a large-scale epidemiologic survey may approximate 3% of an epidemiologist's active professional career.[22]

Section 46.114 of the federal regulations, as revised in 1981, was designed to reduce the bureaucratic burdens of IRB approval for research involving multiple institutions. In contrast to the 1974 regulations it replaced, the revision permitted "reliance upon the review of another qualified IRB, or other similar arrangements aimed at avoidance of duplication of effort (Section 46.114)."[23] The 1991 revision of the regulations added to Section 46.114 that such arrangements require the "approval of the [federal] department or agency head" (Section 46.114).[15] The effect of the latter revision may be to increase the bureaucratic burden, particularly if it is interpreted to require approval of the head of the federal agency or department in advance each time an investigator intends to employ an arrangement designed to avoid duplication of effort.

Internationally, there is much less concern about the location of the ethical review committees. The CIOMS/WHO *International Ethical Guidelines for Biomedical Research Involving Human Subjects* require IRB approval for all research involving human subjects and recognize the validity of review at a regional or, "in a highly centralized administration," a national level (p. 40).[5]

Moreover, in their commentary on "multicentre research," the guidelines state: "In some such studies, scientific and ethical review may be facilitated by agreement among institutions to accept the results of review by a single review committee (p. 41)."[5] In many European countries, research ethics committees are regional.[24]

Several commentators have expressed concern that in the United States the local institution has too much power in the protection of human research subjects. Robertson, for example, alerts us to "the danger . . . that research institutions will use [IRBs] to protect themselves and researchers rather than subjects."[14] Others point to the dominance of investigators in IRB membership, the regulatory requirement for "legally effective informed consent," and close associations between IRBs and risk-management offices in many institutions as evidence that IRBs are being used in the manner Robertson suggests.

Given the legal climate of the United States, it is definitely in the interest of the institution to safeguard the rights and welfare of research subjects. In my view, the IRB should be highly attentive to the interests of institutions and investigators, as well as those of research subjects. Moreover, it is part of the IRB's function to educate investigators and institutional officials on the good reasons for ensuring that their interests are not at odds with those of research subjects. Obtaining legally and ethically valid informed consent is not only responsive to the subject's rights, it also affords the institution and the investigators protection against litigation. In addition, ensuring the equitable selection of subjects and the reasonable balance of risks and benefits respects the rights of research subjects, and also fosters good relations between the institution and the community. What institution wants to see a story in the local newspaper that compares its research activities with the Tuskegee Syphilis Experiment? When IRBs are functioning at their best, they harmonize the interests of the institution, the investigators, and the subjects to the extent that there is little or no conflict.

Multinational Research

Epidemiologists often conduct research in countries other than their own. Of particular concern are research protocols designed by investigators and sponsors in technologically developed countries and then carried out in developing (or underdeveloped) countries or communities. What if there are differences in ethical values between the two cultures? In such cases, whose ethical standards should be followed? How are review committees in the external sponsoring country to know what kinds of information are considered private in the host country or what kinds of material compensations would be considered undue inducements? There is an extensive body of literature on the differing perceptions that exist in various cultures of the world on issues such as the nature of personhood, gift exchange traditions, the nature and causation of disease, medical ethics, and other matters pertinent to assessing the ethical propriety of proposals to conduct research involving human subjects. Interested readers may find their way into this literature by consulting Ohnuki-Tierney,[25] De Craemer,[26] Hall,[27] Christakis,[28,29] Barry,[30] and Levine.[31]

At the root of debates over the legitimacy of differing ethical perspectives and standards across cultures is the age-old tension between ethical universalism and ethical pluralism. Universalists hold that ethical standards are or ought to be the same in all places and in all times. Variations across cultures indicate that some societies are behind others in the degree of "moral progress" they have attained.[32] Those who most closely approximate the universalist position in arguing for uniform standards for the conduct of research involving human subjects are IJsselmuiden and Faden[33] and Angell.[34] Ethical pluralists, by contrast, contend that since ethics are constructed in the course of debates held in particular societies, they will necessarily reflect the histories and traditions of the particular cultures. Pluralists regard variations across cultures in ethical standards as both inevitable and legitimate. Among the leading proponents of ethical pluralism in the development of guidelines for research involving human subjects is Christakis.[28,29]

I have argued that there should be a compromise between the two extremes.[31] Some ethical principles seem to be universally valid. For example, there is a universal proscription against inflicting injury on a person without justification. But what counts as justification in various societies differs substantially. The principle of respect for persons, when stated at a sufficient level of abstraction (that is, enjoining people to treat persons as ends and not merely as means), is universally applicable. However, when this principle is elaborated to require that all persons are to be treated as self-determining, it loses its relevance to some cultures in which individual self-determination is less highly valued than it is in the United States.

American universalists would argue that persons in such cultures must be educated; they must be taught to value self-determination as much as we do. Some might add that they must learn to value and protect the right to be self-determining or else they will remain vulnerable to exploitation by those who have decisionmaking authority. Pluralists counter this argument by pointing out that the society seems functional as it is; if we impose on it our ethical standards, it may have a destructive effect on the culture; we should show respect for a society by allowing it to be self-determining.

In the specific context of research involving human subjects, there are some research and development activities that must be carried out in order to be responsive to the urgent health needs of persons who live in societies in which self-determination is not merely not highly valued, it is considered antisocial. There are, for example, certain tropical diseases that exist only or primarily in such societies. It seems inappropriate to say to persons in these cultures that we will conduct research addressed to your health problems but only if you allow us to replace your ethical standards with our own. In my view, human subjects research in such populations that undergoes appropriate committee review but uses consent procedures that may fall short of the requirements of Western civilization is responsive to the universally applicable requirement to refrain from using persons merely as means to the ends of others.

The CIOMS/WHO *international ethical guidelines* reflect what I consider a satisfactory compromise position, holding that some ethical standards are universal while recognizing the legitimacy of some degree of ethical pluralism. These guidelines set forth procedures to be followed when research is initiated and financed in one country (the external sponsoring country) and carried out by investigators from the external sponsoring country in another country (the host country) involving as subjects residents of the host country:

Special responsibilities may be assigned to review committees in the two countries when a sponsor or investigator in a developed country proposes to carry out research in a developing country. . . .

Committees in the external sponsoring country . . . have a special responsibility to determine that the scientific methods are sound and suitable for the aims of the research, whether the drugs, vaccines or devices to be studied meet adequate standards of safety, whether there is sound justification for conducting the research in the host country rather than in the country of the external sponsoring agency, and that the proposed research does not in principle violate the ethical standards of the external sponsoring country. . . .

Committees in the host country have the special responsibility to determine whether the goals of the research are responsive to the health needs and priorities of the host country. Moreover, because of their better understanding of the culture in which the research is proposed to be carried out, they have special responsibility for assuring the equitable selection of subjects and the acceptability of plans to obtain informed consent, to respect privacy, to maintain confidentiality, and to offer benefits that will not be considered excessive inducements to consent.

In short, ethical review in the external sponsoring country may be limited to ensuring compliance with broadly stated ethical standards, on the understanding that ethical review committees in the host country will have greater competence in reviewing the detailed plans for compliance in view of their better understanding of the cultural and moral values of the population in which the research is to be conducted. (p. 44)[5]

Further, the following passage from the CIOMS guidelines is of interest in considering the ethical propriety of proposals in different cultures:

The ability to judge the ethical acceptability of various aspects of a research proposal requires a thorough understanding of a community's customs and traditions. The ethical review committee must have as either members or consultants persons with such understanding, so that the committee may evaluate proposed means of obtaining informed consent and otherwise respecting the rights of prospective subjects. Such persons should be able, for example, to identify appropriate members of the community to serve as intermediaries between investigators and subjects, to decide whether material benefits or inducements may be regarded as appropriate in the light of a community's gift-exchange traditions, and to provide safeguards for data and personal information that subjects consider to be private or sensitive. (p. 27)[5]

Criticisms of IRBs

Before 1962, as William Curran put it, "a general skepticism toward the development of ethical guidelines, codes, or sets of procedures concerning the conduct of research" prevailed in the medical research community.[9] In the 1970s several biomedical scientists were harshly critical of the IRB system, claiming that it tended to stifle creativity and impede progress (pp. 345–348).[2] Survey research sponsored by the National Commission, however, showed that only 25% of biomedical researchers agreed with the statement that: "The review . . . is an unwarranted intrusion on the investigator's autonomy—at least to some extent (p. 75)."[17] Behavioral and social scientists were considerably less accepting of review, claiming that their research activities were not as likely as those of the biomedical scientist to harm subjects. Some argued that since all they do is talk with subjects, review was an unconstitutional constraint on their freedom of speech.[2] As a consequence of such arguments, several classes of research involving human subjects are exempt from coverage by federal regulations. Among those commonly employed by epidemiologists are, as stated in Section 46.101b:

Research involving the use of . . . survey procedures, interview procedures or observation of public behavior unless: (i) Information obtained is recorded in such a manner that human subjects can be identified directly or through identifiers linked to the subjects; and (ii) any disclosure of the human subjects' responses outside the research could reasonably place the subjects at risk of criminal or civil liability or be damaging to the subjects' financial standing, employability, or reputation.

Research involving the collection or study of existing data, documents, records, pathological specimens, or diagnostic specimens, if these sources are publicly available or if the information is recorded by the investigator in such a manner that the subjects cannot be identified, directly or through identifiers linked to the subjects.[15]

Although these activities are exempt from coverage by federal regulations, the investigators who engage in such activities are not exempt from relevant ethical obligations. One may not, for example, conduct survey research without first securing the informed consent of the respondents. Moreover, many institutions require IRB review of some or all of the research activities exempted by the regulations. And finally, these exemptions are not recognized by the international codes of research ethics.

In many institutions, review of research protocols in the categories exempted by the federal regulations is conducted by use of an expedited review procedure, which is described in Section 46.110b.[15] Expedited review entails review by "the IRB chairperson or by one or more experienced reviewers designated by the chairperson from among members of the IRB." Apart from review of exempt categories of research, use of expedited review procedures is limited by the regulations to: (1) a list published in the *Federal Register* of "categories of research" (actually a list of specific procedures such as venipuncture) when they present no more than minimal risk; and (2) "minor changes in previously approved research during the period . . . for which approval is authorized."

According to Williams, IRBs do an inadequate job of ensuring that risks will be reasonable in relation to anticipated benefits.[35] He argues that this defect is inevitable for three reasons: (1) Federal regulations on this standard are written in vague language, in contrast to the more clear direction provided for protecting subjects' rights. Moreover, since the regulations permit consideration of the long-range effects of applying knowledge as benefits but not as risks, they create a bias in favor of approval. (2) The membership of the committee, dominated as it is by professionals, is likely to place a higher value than laypersons would on the benefit of developing new knowledge. (3) Groups confronted with choices involving risks may be either more or less cautious, or "risk aversive," than the average of individuals within the group; this is known as the "risky shift" or "group polarization phenomenon." Williams[35] and Veatch[10] believe that in the context of IRBs, the groups are likely to be more tolerant of higher levels of risk than they would be as individuals.

Several commentators have proposed that IRBs could enhance their effectiveness by sending members to the sites of the actual conduct of research to verify compliance with protocol requirements[14] or to supervise consent negotiations.[36] Others respond that while such activities should be done when there are reasons to suspect problems in specific protocols, routine monitoring activities might be detrimental to the successful functioning of the committee by eroding its support within the institution (p. 341ff).[2]

Evaluation of IRBs

Critics of the IRB system claim that little or no objective evidence exists that IRB review prevents the conduct of inadequate research. For example, a national survey of IRBs revealed that the rate of rejection of protocols is less than 1 in 1000 (p. I-216).[17] Supporters of the system respond that the actual rejection rate is much higher if one includes protocols withdrawn because investigators refuse to modify them as required by IRBs. Moreover, rejection rates may be a poor indicator of the IRB's quality; protocols may be improved in anticipation of the IRB's requirements, and investigators may decide not to submit proposals they think might be rejected.

It is difficult to evaluate the IRB's performance objectively, and satisfactory subjective evaluations can be made only by experienced IRB members and administrators (p. 358–359).[2] Jerry Mashaw concludes in his excellent theoretical analysis of IRBs that "If [the IRB] is to do its core job well, we must live with its inevitable incompetence at other tasks. Moreover, we must also live with the rather vague regulatory standards and with the continuing inability of the federal funding agencies to know for sure whether [IRBs] are functioning effectively. If we would have wise judges and paternalistic [skilled in protecting subjects' rights and welfare interests] professionals, we can neither specifically direct nor objectively evaluate their behavior" (p. 22).[37]

Conclusion

Institutional Review Boards originated in isolated American institutions in the 1950s, became legally mandated in the United States in the 1970s, and in the 1990s became required by international ethical guidelines. They are the most important social control mechanism to assure the ethical conduct of research involving human subjects, by contributing to the education of researchers in matters related to research ethics in general, as well as by guiding researchers to comply with ethical and legal expectations as they carry out specific research projects. In the 1940s through the 1960s, great reliance was placed on investigators to safeguard the rights and welfare of research subjects, and on informed consent to authorize the involvement of any particular individual as a research subject. Subsequently, there has been a partial shift in these responsibilities; the IRB is now relied on to help decide whether the relation of risks to benefits is such that individuals should be invited to enroll as subjects, and what kinds of individuals or groups should be considered eligible to receive such invitations.

There are some limits to the IRB's capability to assure the ethical conduct of research involving human subjects. For example, although it is generally agreed that the ethical justification of such research requires that it be scientifically sound, the IRB is usually not competent to render authoritative judgments about scientific merit. In such cases, the IRB has the responsibility to assure that scientific validity has been evaluated and approved by some competent agency.

It is widely agreed that IRBs are most effective when located in the institutions where the research is to be carried out. Nevertheless, there are many cases in which research is conducted in institutions far removed from the IRB that has reviewed and approved it, apparently without serious repercussions. The greatest challenge to the principle of local review is presented when research is designed in an external sponsoring country to be carried out by investigators from that country in a host country. For such contingencies, the CIOMS/WHO *International Ethical Guidelines for Biomedical Research Involving Human*

Subjects specify divisions of responsibility and authority for ethical review committees in each of the two countries.

When IRBs were introduced for the review of biomedical research, there were many angry and resentful criticisms from biomedical researchers about unnecessary and unwarranted stifling of creativity and obstruction of progress. Subsequently, when the scope of IRB authority was extended to include social and behavioral research, researchers in those fields protested that this was an unconstitutional restraint on their freedom of speech. Although some criticisms remain, they are now focused on details of the IRB's performance and how it might be improved, rather than on the legitimacy of the entire concept of IRB review.

Finally, it is difficult, and perhaps impossible, to evaluate the IRB's performance objectively, and satisfactory subjective evaluations can be made only by experienced IRB members and administrators. This is an inevitable consequence of the fact that adequate performance of the IRB's essential tasks necessarily entails the exercise of professional judgment, rather than conformity to a regulatory algorithm.

References

1. World Medical Association. *Declaration of Helsinki* (as amended by the 41st World Medical Assembly, Hong Kong, September, 1989). Reprinted as Annex I in Council for International Organizations of Medical Sciences. *International Ethical Guidelines for Biomedical Research Involving Human Subjects*. Geneva: Council for International Organizations of Medical Sciences, 1993.
2. Levine, R. J. *Ethics and Regulation of Clinical Research*. 2d ed. Baltimore: Urban & Schwarzenberg, 1986.
3. Robertson, J. A. "The Law of Institutional Review Boards," *UCLA Law Review* 26 (1979): 484–549.
4. Medical Research Council of Canada. *Guidelines on Research Involving Human Subjects*. Ottawa: Medical Research Council of Canada, 1987: 48.
5. Council for International Organizations of Medical Sciences. *International Ethical Guidelines for Biomedical Research Involving Human Subjects*. Geneva: Council for International Organizations of Medical Sciences, 1993.
6. Council for International Organizations of Medical Sciences. *International Guidelines for Ethical Review of Epidemiological Studies*. Geneva: Council for International Organizations of Medical Sciences, 1991: 22–23.
7. Council for International Organizations of Medical Sciences. *Proposed International Guidelines for Biomedical Research Involving Human Subjects*. Geneva: Council for International Organizations of Medical Sciences, 1982: 1.
8. Lipsett, M. B., Fletcher, J. C., and Secundy, M. "Research Review at NIH," *Hastings Center Report* 9, no. 1 (1979): 18–21.
9. Curran, W. J. "Government Regulation of the Use of Human Subjects in Medical Research: The Approaches of two Federal Agencies," In *Experimentation with Human Subjects*, ed. P. A. Freund. New York: Braziller, 1970: 402–454.

10. Veatch, R. M. "Human Experimentation Committees: Professional or Representative?" *Hastings Center Report* 5, no. 5 (October 1975): 31–40.
11. Levine, C. "Has AIDS Changed the Ethics of Human Subjects Research?" *Law, Medicine & Health Care* 16 (1988): 167–73.
12. Levine, R. J. "The Impact of HIV Infection on Society's Perception of Clinical Trials," *Kennedy Institute of Ethics Journal* 4, no. 2 (1994): 93–98.
13. Freedman, B. "Scientific Value and Validity as Ethical Requirements for Research: A Proposed Explication," *IRB: A Review of Human Subjects Research* 9, no. 6 (1987): 7–10.
14. Robertson, J. A. "Ten Ways to Improve IRBs," *Hastings Center Report* 9, no. 1 (1979): 29–33.
15. Federal Policy for the Protection of Human Subjects; Notices and Rules. *Federal Register* 56, no. 117: 28001–28032, Tuesday, June 18, 1991.
16. Levine, C., Dubler, N. N., and Levine, R. J. "Building a New Consensus: Ethical Principles and Policies for Clinical Research on HIV/AIDS," *IRB: A Review of Human Subjects Research* 13, nos. 1 & 2 (1991): 1–17.
17. The National Commission for the Protection of Human Subjects of Biomedical and Behavioral Research. *Institutional Review Boards: Report and Recommendations.* Washington, 1978, DHEW Publication No. (OS) 78–0008.
18. Herman, S. S. "A Noninstitutional Review Board Comes of Age," *IRB: A Review of Human Subjects Research* 11, no. 2 (1989): 1–6.
19. Food and Drug Administration. *Waiver of Institutional Review Board Review of Certain Clinical Studies of Azidothymidine (AZT) Unsigned memorandum,* September 30, 1986.
20. Department of Health and Human Services: Expanded Availability of Investigational New Drugs Through a Parallel Track Mechanism for People with AIDS and other HIV-related Disease. *Federal Register* 57, no. 73 (April 15, 1992): 13244–259.
21. Kavanagh, C., Matthews, D., Sorenson, J. R., and Swazey, J. P. "We shall overcome: Multi-institutional Review of a Genetic Counseling Study," *IRB: A Review of Human Subjects Research* 1, no. 2 (April, 1979): 1–3, 12.
22. Rothman, K. J. "The Rise and Fall of Epidemiology, 1950–2000 A.D.," *New England Journal of Medicine* 304 (1981): 600–02.
23. Department of Health and Human Services: Final Regulations Amending Basic HHS Policy for the Protection of Human Subjects. *Federal Register* 46, no. 16 (January 26, 1981): 8366–92.
24. McNeill, P. M. "Research Ethics Committees in Australia, Europe, and North America," *IRB: A Review of Human Subjects Research* 11, no. 3 (1989): 4–7.
25. Ohnuki-Tierney, E. *Illness and Culture in Contemporary Japan: An Anthropological View.* New York: Cambridge University Press, 1984.
26. De Craemer, W. "A Cross-cultural Perspective on Personhood," *Milbank Memorial Fund Quarterly* 61 (winter 1983): 19–34.
27. Hall, A. J. "Public Health Trials in West Africa: Logistics and Ethics," *IRB: A Review of Human Subjects Research* 11, no. 5 (Sept./Oct. 1989): 8–10.
28. Christakis, N. A. "Ethics are Local: Engaging Cross-cultural Variation in the Ethics of Clinical Research," *Social Science and Medicine* 35 (1992): 1079–91.
29. Christakis, N. A. "The Ethical Design of an AIDS Vaccine Trial in Africa," *Hastings Center Report* 18, no. 3 (June/July, 1988): 31–37.
30. Barry, M. "Ethical Considerations of Human Investigation in Developing Countries: The AIDS Dilemma," *New England Journal of Medicine* 319 (1988): 1083–86.

31. Levine, R. J. "Informed Consent: Some Challenges to the Universal Validity of the Western Model," *Law, Medicine & Health Care* 19 (1991): 207–13.
32. Macklin, R. "Universality of the Nuremberg Code," In *The Nazi Doctors and the Nuremberg Code: Human Rights and Human Experimentation*, ed., G. J. Annas and M. A. Grodin. New York: Oxford University Press, 1992: 240–57.
33. IJsselmuiden, C. B. and Faden, R. R. "Research and Informed Consent in Africa— Another Look," *New England Journal of Medicine* 326 (1992): 830–34.
34. Angell, M. "Ethical Imperialism? Ethics in International Collaborative Clinical Research," *New England Journal of Medicine* 319 (1988): 1081–83.
35. Williams, P. C. "Success in Spite of Failure: Why IRBs Falter in Reviewing Risks and Benefits," *IRB: A Review of Human Subjects Research* 6, no. 3 (1984): 1–4.
36. Robertson, J. A. "Taking Consent Seriously: IRB Intervention in the Consent Process," *IRB: A Review of Human Subjects Research* 4, no. 5 (1982): 1–5.
37. Mashaw, J.L. "Thinking about Institutional Review Boards," In The President's Commission for the Study of Ethical Problems in Medicine and Biomedical and Behavioral Research. *Whistleblowing in Biomedical Research: Policies and Procedures for Responding to Reports of Misconduct*, pp. 3–22, Washington, 1982.

14

Scientific Misconduct in Epidemiologic Research

COLIN L. SOSKOLNE
DOROTHY K. MACFARLANE

Many people believe that those following a career in any of the health sciences are virtuous, can be trusted to protect the public interest, and possess a scrupulous desire to pursue truth.[1,2] This belief, however, does not always accurately reflect reality. The theft of intellectual property, the creation or fabrication of data, and even the falsification of data to better support one's desired belief or agenda are known to occur in science. Such practices fall under the general rubric of scientific misconduct and are contrary to science, whose fundamental value is the pursuit of truth in the public interest.

Recent surveys have attempted to establish an estimate of the prevalence or incidence of scientific misconduct. Because of poor response rates in these surveys, estimates have been difficult to ascertain.[3–5] Nonetheless, it is apparent that misconduct has occurred in the past[6–10] and continues into the present across science[11–15] and in epidemiology in particular.[16,17]

Scientific misconduct is the term that has been adopted as the North American designation for failures to maintain honesty and integrity in science, whereas the Danes prefer the term *scientific dishonesty*.[18,19] The definition of scientific misconduct has been modified in the recent past (as discussed below under "Evolution of the Definition of Scientific Misconduct"). Interpretations of scientific misconduct tend to focus on ensuring that the scientific pursuit of truth is not intentionally compromised. A further facet of scientific misconduct relates to the public nature of science; because science is often publicly funded, there is an implicit social trust in the integrity of the scientific enterprise, especially that science can and will protect the common interest. The latter provides substantial motivation for science to be both publicly accountable and self-regulating.[7,15,20]

Besides disregard for the pursuit of truth and protection of the public interest, there is a further dimension to scientific misconduct. It relates to the various aspects of interpersonal behavior not only among scientists, but also between scientists and the various constituency groups with which they work.

The theft of intellectual property (plagiarism) falls within the scope of scientific misconduct among peers, although such theft tends to be difficult to prove and therefore can be controversial. A related concern is the accurate attribution of both intellectual contribution and effort, as drawn from relationships between colleagues, mentors and students, and employers and employees.

Another form of misconduct among peers involves conflicting interests that can derive from personal self-interest[17] or manifest as professional jealousies when one's self-interest is allowed to interfere with objectivity[21]. Shamoo[17] has admirably addressed the issue of conflicting interests using as an example research in the pharmaceutical industry, where concern for profitability can cloud safety concerns at the drug testing stage. Professional jealousy can be illustrated when one considers that epidemiologists have a reputation for being their own worst enemies, or for "eating their young." They are trained to be critical of research study proposals/papers, and it is therefore relatively easy for them to exercise power within the peer review system by evaluating the work of others without objectivity. It is also possible that a lack of objectivity in critiquing the work of perceived competitors could stem from an epidemiologist reviewer's wish to maintain or enhance professional standing.[15,22]

Two moral foundations on which good collegial relationships rest are those of integrity and mutual trust, which, when eroded, severely damage interactions between colleagues. In addition, the work intended to serve the public interest itself could be harmed.[15] Overzealousness also may drive misconduct. This can happen when the excitement the researcher feels over his or her work leads to behaviors that are, at best, lacking in objectivity or, at worst, irrationally biased. In these circumstances, the objectivity of the scientist is lost.

Constituencies with which epidemiologists work include government departments and agencies, universities, labor unions, industry, the media, private foundations, statutory granting agencies, nongovernmental organizations, and activist groups. Each of these groups has its own agenda and hence promotes its own interests. Good conduct on the part of epidemiologists includes adequate disclosure or openness in dealing with various constituencies. An ethical dilemma that can arise in attempts to be open relates to the timing of public disclosure of study findings. Release of information prior to its verification (as opposed to its replication or corroboration), perhaps because of pressure from interested groups, could be morally inappropriate. Such issues often are addressed both in ethics guidelines[23–27] and in standards of practice.[15,28,29] The scientific ethic requires that a policy of openness guides scientists. Hence, all scientists have an obligation to submit their methods and results to peer review and publication in a responsible and timely manner.

"Whistle-blowing" has become a concern for fear of job loss or at least some type of retaliation, especially if those accused are in positions of authority over the person making the allegations of scientific misconduct or malpractice.[30-32] Nevertheless, whistle-blowing has received some justification in many recent codes of ethics and ethics guidelines.

Justice is often a consideration in the reporting of misconduct. Guidelines for the handling of allegations of misconduct have been difficult to manage, and the issue of due process has become preeminent in investigations of this nature. Because allegations do not always prove to be true, the reputation of the accused should be protected unless guilt is established. The principle "innocent until proven guilty" applies. Hence the process for investigating charges of misconduct has had to be developed and administered with care and respect for due process.[33-36]

The saying, "He who pays the piper calls the tune" has particular relevance to epidemiology. There are instances in which reputable consultants have been accused of being "in the pocket" of the interest group that has retained their services, causing potential harm to the work they have critiqued and to the public interest when science is derailed in the process.[20,37-39] Guidelines used to socialize students could be applied in minimizing instances of misconduct, not only among epidemiologists employed in the public sector, but also among those working or self-employed in the private sector.

Concern about misconduct in science is established, with a growing body of literature on the subject. In particular, a thoughtful overview of the issue—dealing with definitional questions, prevalence issues, likely determinants, and suggestions to reduce the incidence of fraud— has recently appeared[7]; the reader is encouraged to refer to these other perspectives.

Two Recent Investigations of Scientific Misconduct

First Case Study: Actual Misconduct

In 1993, a high-profile case of scientific misconduct was reported by the United States' Office of Research Integrity (ORI).[40,41] It concerned the effectiveness of alternative surgical procedures for female breast cancer. This impropriety was not exposed in the media until some nine months later, concurrent with demands for a return of funds that had been provided to the institution of the guilty scientist.[42-46]

The physician-scientist, Roger Poisson, was found to have inappropriately manipulated (falsified) data associated with a series of major multicenter breast cancer clinical trials. His case has provided an example of direct relevance to epidemiologists. Much public consternation was aroused by the delay in disclosure that data falsification had occurred in a study upon which many women had made life dependent decisions.[47–49] The scientific question addressed by the study was whether lumpectomy was as effective as radical mastectomy in terms of survival in the treatment of breast cancer.

The misconduct in this example appears to have been based in the fact that Poisson had, among other things, revised records concerning the eligibility criteria for participation in the study. Poisson reportedly claimed that he had conducted himself in the patient's best interests.[42,50] However, there appears to have been a persistent disregard for the relevant scientific methods.

Second Case Study: Alleged Misconduct

In 1992, there was a highly publicized environmental epidemiology case in which scientific misconduct had been alleged. This case involved the methods of analysis used by H. L. Needleman[51–55] in his pioneering work in the late 1970s on neurobehavioral effects of environmental lead exposure in children. Despite a reanalysis of the data several years earlier in response to concerns about the appropriateness of the analytical methods used,[56] accusations of scientific misconduct resurfaced. Ultimately, this case of alleged scientific misconduct was dismissed and Needleman's name was cleared. However, errors in the questioned papers were identified and corrections to the literature recommended by the investigative bodies. Some have claimed that self-interest was the motive for the allegations, giving rise to concerns about conflicting interests on the part of the lead industry.

The case raised substantial consternation among both professionals and the public and, clearly, the considerable effort expended on the part of the accused and the sizeable teams required to investigate the allegations were costly.

The potential of scientific misconduct to damage the entire scientific enterprise is evidenced in a very real way by the first case study. Public confidence in the manner in which science is both conducted and managed was clearly eroded.

Because science must be concerned with issues of self-regulation (see below), not only is it paramount for investigations of misconduct to be visible, but also to take reasonable steps to protect the accused's confidentiality. Even if a person charged with misconduct is proven innocent, or if the charges are dismissed, his or her name could remain tarnished from the experience.

The amount of money and resources directed to investigating misconduct are substantial. Each time a scientist is implicated in wrongdoing, the whole scientific enterprise is harmed through the erosion of public support and diminished public confidence.[57,58] Yet, science must be accountable to the public in whose interest science is conducted and through whose purse it is generally funded.

Accountability and Professional Self-Regulation

Society, through government, relegates some control of the professions to the professional bodies themselves.[20] Therefore, to ensure the highest possible standards of professional practice, it is incumbent on the professions to remain vigilant concerning possible malpractice or misconduct among their memberships. Epidemiologists have only recently begun, however, to formally consider this responsibility.[20]

The new professional endeavor has been encouraged partly by pressure on institutions, as a prerequisite to seeking National Institutes of Health (NIH) funding support, to demonstrate their compliance with NIH guidelines. These guidelines require the existence of formally established programs and mechanisms within each institution that address issues of professional responsibility and accountability. For example, to qualify for NIH funding ethics training must be offered in graduate programs supported by the NIH,[59] and procedures must be promulgated for investigating allegations of misconduct.[60-63] Despite these requirements, problems of implementation persist.[64]

Issues surrounding scientific misconduct were addressed at a symposium on "Ethics and Law in Environmental Epidemiology," held in conjunction with the International Society for Environmental Epidemiology (ISEE) annual meeting in Cuernavaca, Mexico, in 1992. The symposium was organized in response to highly publicized cases (including that of Needleman) of alleged epidemiologic misconduct, and to cases recently judged as misconduct by the former Office of Scientific Integrity (OSI). The symposium proceedings[18,21,33-36] provide a useful basis for education and further development and refinement of ethics guidelines. Insight is offered through discussion of process issues in the two countries (United States and Denmark) known to have formally addressed these matters, and also through extensive commentary on specific case studies from these countries. In addition, the proceedings document situations presented by the international symposium participants, discussed in depth by the symposium panelists.

Activities such as symposia and workshops provide a basis for professional education and are essential for ensuring grass-roots participation in professional guideline development. The ISEE ethics and law symposium was designed to involve epidemiologists at the grass-roots and thereby to extend the ethics guidelines in the hope of preventing future acts of misconduct. Despite the several draft guidelines that have been published,[23-28] each of which to some extent does address the need for integrity in science, the absence of grass-roots involvement in their development reduces the likelihood of adherence to them.

Misconduct Extended to Consensus Building

Epidemiology provides the bridge from animal to human studies and hence has the potential to influence not only medical care, but also national health and social policies. The extent of epidemiology's impact on society is therefore substantial. Out of concern for the effect that fraud, deception, or delusion could have on policy, Feinstein[65] drew attention to these problems as they relate to the milieu of consensus conferences, where judgements can be influenced by political and nonscientific forces. Instead of consensus conferences, Feinstein urged the exclusive use of "unequivocally valid scientific methods, evidence, and interpretations" when seeking scientific truths.

The Office of Research Integrity (ORI)

Background

The Office of Research Integrity (ORI) in the United States (which replaced the Office of Scientific Integrity, OSI) evolved within the United States Department of Health and Human Services (HHS) in response to several highly publicized scientific misconduct cases of the late 1970s, and to Congressional questions about related actions taken by the National Institutes of Health (NIH). In July 1986, NIH issued written guidance on this issue.[66] Misconduct was defined as "(a) serious deviation, such as fabrication, falsification or plagiarism, from accepted practices in carrying out research or in reporting the results of research; or (b) material failure to comply with Federal requirements affecting specific aspects of the conduct of research—e.g., the protection of human subjects and the welfare of laboratory animals." The definition specifically excluded "certain types of possibly inappropriate practices that should be of concern to scientists everywhere, but do not necessarily call for Federal action. These include, for example, co-authorship practices, recognition of collaborators and multiple publication."

The *NIH Guide* noted further that the United States Public Health Service (PHS) was developing a regulation to implement the Health Research Extension Act of 1985 (PL 99–158). The *Guide* stated that institutions that accept PHS funds have an obligation to: (a) develop their own policies and procedures for dealing with possible misconduct; and (b) inform PHS of the initiation of a formal investigation of possible misconduct. The proposed rules were published in September 1988.[67]

Evolution of the Definition of Scientific Misconduct

Scientific misconduct was defined, in 1989, as "fabrication, falsification, plagiarism or other practices that seriously deviate from those commonly accepted within the scientific community for proposing, conducting, or reporting research. It does not include honest error or honest differences in interpretation or judgment of data."[60,68] The preamble to the regulation describes the reasons for the changes in the definition of misconduct. The second clause, regarding material failure to comply with other requirements for the conduct of research, was already covered by existing regulations and another office that dealt with human subject and animal protection (Office for Protection from Research Risks). Deception was specifically omitted, since it was recognized that deception is an acceptable and necessary component of some types of research. A sentence was added to exclude "honest error or honest differences in interpretations or judgments of data." The phrase "other practices that seriously deviate" was retained, despite considerable disagreement from those who contended that it might be interpreted to include innovative research approaches.

Some of the comments on the proposed rule recommended that the scientific misconduct definition be expanded to include duplicate publication and intellectual piracy. Why these were not added is not addressed in the preamble.

Establishment of the Offices of Scientific Integrity and Scientific Integrity Review

In March 1989, the PHS established two offices to "improve its methods for protecting against scientific misconduct."[69] The Office of Scientific Integrity was placed in the Office of the Director, NIH, as a focal point for the PHS. Its charge was to promote high standards for research through a prevention and education program, oversee scientific misconduct investigations at awardee institutions, investigate allegations of misconduct when necessary, and make recommendations to the Assistant Secretary for Health regarding misconduct allegations.

A second office, the Office of Scientific Integrity Review, was established in the Office of the Assistant Secretary for Health. It was to be responsible for "overseeing the PHS scientific misconduct activities and ensuring that these activities are carried out in an independent and neutral manner."

This structure continued until June 1992, when the two offices were consolidated, placed directly under the authority of the Assistant Secretary for Health, and renamed the Office of Research Integrity (ORI).[70] In addition, the existing regulations were supplemented by a notice published on November 6, 1992,[71] which provided for an interim procedure for an individual to seek a hearing on ORI findings of scientific misconduct and the proposed PHS administrative action. The hearing would be conducted by a Research Integrity Adjudications Panel under the direction of the HHS Departmental Appeal Board. The NIH Revitalization Act (PL 103-43), signed June 10, 1993, made ORI an "independent entity reporting to the Secretary."

Authority

The authority of the ORI to make findings of scientific misconduct and propose PHS administrative actions is founded in statute and regulation. The purpose of the ORI is to protect the research mission of the PHS. Therefore, the administrative actions proposed are geared to safeguard research and the funds available to support research. They include debarment from eligibility to receive research funding, prohibition from service on PHS advisory boards, or oversight of research applications submitted by the individual found to have engaged in scientific misconduct. Also authorized are remedial actions designed to rectify the scientific literature, such as correction or retraction of published research. Since June 1993, ORI has published in the *Federal Register* a summary of each case in which a misconduct finding was made, including the administrative actions imposed.[41]

Procedures

The role of ORI is defined and limited by statute and by the published PHS regulations. Questions raised about the due process protection afforded the respondent led to addition of a hearing process, available as an option to any individual found by ORI to have committed scientific misconduct.[33,61,72–74] The hearing process is an evaluation of the facts of the case by an independent panel appointed by the HHS Departmental Appeals Board. For the most part, the board consists of lawyers trained to conduct hearings of this type, although a scientist will be invited to join the panel when either party requests it. Hearing results are binding on HHS except when debarment is recommended. This recommendation must be separately approved by the department's debarment official.

The Definition of Scientific Misconduct

The interpretation of the definition of *scientific misconduct* has been a subject of debate since the original NIH guidelines were published in 1986. The most frequently questioned clause of the current definition regards "other practices that seriously deviate from those commonly accepted within the scientific community." Objections have ranged from a concern that innovative research methods might be considered misconduct to a fear that the vagueness of the phrase makes it impossible to interpret and accurately apply to new cases with new facts.

Whether authorship disputes, credit given to collaborators, and duplicate publication are appropriately handled as scientific misconduct issues also have come into question. Although these practices are not explicitly excluded from the 1989 definition, as they were from the 1986 version, it is noted that they also are not specifically included as had been suggested by some comments received following publication of the proposed rule. In general, these behaviors are viewed as serious matters that deserve the attention of scientists and ethicists, but they are not considered to constitute scientific misconduct that requires federal action. That is, scientific misconduct pertaining to the public interest per se is deemed to warrant federal action, while matters of misconduct pertaining to colleagues are best handled and resolved within the profession.

An additional problem has been in determining whether fabrication, falsification, and plagiarism always represent research misconduct, or whether there are "acceptable" minor transgressions that do not rise to the level of misconduct. In general, ORI has found that when the intention to fabricate, falsify, or plagiarize exists, these three types of behaviors always constitute misconduct. However, certain types of plagiarism may not always involve an intent to deceive or to take credit for someone else's unique contributions, as, for example, in a verbatim repetition of a description of a standard method used in a scientific experiment.

Fabrication, usually of data or results, appears to present the most clear-cut form of misconduct. It is difficult to imagine a condition under which the fabrication of data, methods, or results would be acceptable behavior. In contrast, falsification presents intermediary problems. It is difficult in some cases to distinguish between honest error and falsification. The Departmental Appeals Board has ruled that the exclusion of honest error from the definition places a burden on ORI personnel to prove that the false data or statements could not have occurred by error, that is, that the falsification was intentional.

Further refinements of the definition of scientific misconduct will be necessary to resolve these issues of interpretation. It is important that the definition not be so strict (sensitive) that scientists are at risk because of sloppiness or unintentional lapses. Further, definition must not be so specific that serious yet unforeseen circumstances are excluded, which would require frequent updating to cover every act that might constitute scientific misconduct. The standards that are applied in the investigation of scientific misconduct are identical across all areas of science, including epidemiologic research.

ORI Record

The case load of the ORI has remained remarkably constant since it opened as OSI in 1989. Statistics show that the office began 1991 with 69 cases and ended 1992 with 71 active cases. During the same two-year period, 57 cases were opened and 55 cases closed. During 1993, 35 cases were opened and 28 closed. It should be noted that a substantial number of complaints brought to ORI's attention did not proceed to ORI cases because the alleged actions did not meet the definition of scientific misconduct, the research was not related to PHS funding or a PHS application, or the allegation was not substantial enough to pursue. Of 314 allegations or queries made during 1991 and 1992, only 36 proceeded to a formal inquiry or investigation. Fifty were determined to represent types of misconduct handled by other offices, and were referred to the proper authorities (such as Office for Protection from Research Risks, Food and Drug Administration, and offices responsible for financial reviews of grants, contracts and cooperative agreements). The remaining allegations were judged either to not be within the jurisdiction of the ORI or any other federal office, or were considered not substantial enough to pursue.

From June 1992 until July 1993 ORI made findings of misconduct in 22 cases. In 13 of these cases, the findings and proposed administrative actions were accepted by the respondent. Nine respondents requested hearings. Two of the 9 were resolved without a full hearing and resulted in acceptance of the terms proposed by ORI. Two findings of misconduct were upheld, 2 were overturned, and 1 was settled. In 2 cases, the ORI withdrew prosecution. During 1993 and the first half of 1994, ORI negotiated voluntary settlements with 6 individuals found to have engaged in scientific misconduct. In most of these cases, the respondents agreed to voluntarily exclude themselves from applying for or receiving PHS research funding for periods ranging from 2 to 5 years.

Conclusions and Recommendations

Guidelines relating to scientific integrity and honesty are not an end in themselves, but rather a means to the end of ensuring the pursuit of truth and the maintenance of proper ethics. The end is believed to be most attainable through interested stakeholders and colleagues engaging in an open discussion of issues and concerns. Such discussion might serve to prevent instances of misconduct.

The notion of prevention is central to epidemiology. Hence, application of epidemiologic methods to elucidate the determinants of misconduct would seem a natural area of interest for epidemiological pursuit; at least the idea ought to enjoy the support of epidemiologists. In practice, however, such support requires incentives. Perhaps, as an initial step, the policy makers within the granting agencies could request proposals to stimulate research in scientific misconduct among epidemiologists.

Institutions and professional organizations could assist in preventing misconduct by the top-down example of good conduct[75] and by establishing confidential avenues for discussing even suspicions of misconduct. In the absence of such a model, disincentives prevail in the form of ignorance and a lack of protection for so-called whistle-blowers.

A distinction is drawn between scientific misconduct on the one hand and acts of unprofessional conduct, such as medical malpractice, on the other. The existence of guidelines is relatively recent for epidemiologists. Now that various draft guidelines are in place, there is a bench mark against which standards of conduct can begin to be assessed. Such assessment does lead to the specter of enforcement, which presents difficult and sensitive problems to the profession. Volunteer officers elected to run the professional subspecialty organizations of epidemiologists have not traditionally seen their role as one of policing the profession.

Even in the absence of formal guideline enforcement mechanisms and procedures, the age-old deterrent of peer pressure can be applied. Epidemiologists should call colleagues on perceived wrongdoing and remain vigilant about ensuring that minimum acceptable standards of conduct in the profession are maintained. When misconduct of any degree is detected, the penalties range from censure through professional ostracism and even criminal charges. Clearly, not all forms of misconduct should be responded to with equal force. There also may be a need for the scientific community to offer rehabilitation to those found guilty of misconduct; it may be in the public interest to retain their expertise instead of dismissing them from the practice of their science completely. After all, the potential for misconduct and dishonesty exists in all people. Consider the enthusiastic researcher who goes beyond the data in her interpretation, or the one who fails to do a thorough analysis because the findings obtained by one approach satisfy his own bias. Consider the discussion with a colleague over lunch, and later incorporating that colleague's ideas in a grant application without involving her in the process. Surely, most epidemiologists can relate to these scenarios. Yet it is these very scenarios that can lead one to misconduct.

Integration of ethics into training programs, adequately supported by case-study material, is an essential component for the prevention of scientific misconduct and dishonesty. It is also important for the general socialization of students aspiring to enter the field of epidemiology. This process includes sensitizing students to prevailing professional norms and values. However, there remains a need to evaluate the impact of such programs, which have been required only since 1990.[59]

Various epidemiological organizations have begun integrating ethics into their professional activities by, for example, providing a forum at their respective annual scientific meetings for the discussion of ethical issues and concerns. These ought to be promoted as ongoing activities, in recognition that ethics require the application of values and principles to issues that generate problems and tensions among thoughtful people engaged in professional pursuits.

Because values are subject to change over time, any appeals to ethical principles may need to be periodically reevaluated. Fora at scientific meetings not only provide the opportunity for a fuller discussion of concerns and issues and can generate ideas for resolutions; they also could provide reasonable justification to revise existing ethics guidelines and standards of conduct. Further, they could provide the case-study material so useful for the curriculum of ethics training programs.

One method by which ethics could be reinforced at the training level is through the establishment of an incentive program in which students discuss their particular approach to an ethical problem and, where applicable, its resolution. The incentive program could be an annual competition for students with a prize for the best paper selected, to be awarded at the profession's annual scientific meeting.

In order for each profession to be self-regulating, it must establish an infrastructure whose purpose is to promote ethical conduct in the public interest among its members. Existing committees include the American College of Epidemiology's Ethics and Standards of Practice Committee, the International Society for Environmental Epidemiology's Standing Committee on Ethics and Philosophy, and the International Society for Pharmacoepidemiology's Ethics/Public Policy Committee. The American College of Epidemiology committee includes representatives from the major epidemiologic subspecialties.

Some argue that the mandate of ethics committees should be broadened to include resources for mediation in disputes, for counseling that could prevent the need for misconduct charges, and for the power to intervene in circumstances of sufficient public interest. Further, some suggest that the professions need to have some leverage in debarring a member from practice in the event of proven misconduct. The ORI goes part of the way in denying PHS research funding in cases of serious scientific misconduct. This perspective needs to be weighed against the benefits to be derived through voluntary rehabilitation.

Scientific misconduct can have an extremely negative impact on the public's perception of the scientific enterprise. This, in turn, can impact on public resources that are made available for science. In addition, scientific misconduct can impede the pursuit of truth, leading scientific inquiry down wasteful paths. Ultimately, the public in general, and the disenfranchised and impoverished in particular, will bear a disproportionately greater burden of illness if epidemiology loses funding or reputation. In view of these serious consequences, the professions must consider their direct role in minimizing the likelihood of scientific misconduct. Indeed, any type of misconduct, whether poor peer relations, malpractice, or scientific wrongdoing, that damages the fabric that nurtures science warrants the serious attention of the professions. Implementation is encouraged of mechanisms described in this chapter that will serve to prevent such problems. Another mechanism, not addressed here, is the proposition that formal auditing of research be undertaken[8,10,15,17] by appropriate public interest agencies to deter scientific dishonesty. The longer the profession waits to act on these matters, the greater the likelihood that government could intervene and that public support for the profession could be eroded.

References

1. Pellegrino, E. D. "Character and the Ethical Conduct of Research," *Accountability in Research* 2 (1992): 1–11.
2. Pellegrino, E. D., Veatch, R. M. and Langan, J. P., eds. *Ethics, Trust, and the*

Professions: Philosophical and Cultural Aspects. Washington, D.C.: Georgetown University Press, 1991.

3. Goldberg, L. A. and Greenberg, M. R. "Ethical Issues for Industrial Hygienists: Survey Results and Suggestions," *American Industrial Hygiene Association Journal* 54 (1993): 127–34.

4. Greenberg, M. R. and Martell, J. "Ethical Dilemmas and Solutions for Risk Assessment Scientists," *Journal of Exposure Analysis and Environmental Epidemiology* 2 (1992): 381–89.

5. Frankel, M. S., ed. "In the Societies," *Professional Ethics Report. Newsletter of the American Association for the Advancement of Science* 1 (winter 1992): 2–3.

6. Broad, W. and Wade, N. *Betrayers of the Truth: Fraud and Deceit in the Halls of Science.* New York: Simon & Schuster, 1982.

7. Lowy, F. H. and Meslin, E. M. "Fraud in Medical Research." In *Textbook of Ethics in Pediatric Research,* ed. G. Koren. Ch. 24. Malabar, Florida: Kreiger Publishing Company, 1993: 293–307.

8. Shamoo, A. and Annau, Z. "Ensuring Scientific Integrity" (Letter), *Nature* 327 (June 18, 1987): 550.

9. Dawson, N.J. "Ensuring Scientific Integrity" (Letter), *Nature* 327 (June 18, 1987): 550.

10. Shamoo, A. E. and Annau, Z. "Data Audit—Historical Perspective." In *Principles of Research Data Audit,* ed. A.E. Shamoo. Ch. 1. New York: Gordon & Breach, 1989: 1–11.

11. Teich, A. H. and Frankel, M. S. *Good Science and Responsible Scientists: Meeting the Challenge of Fraud and Misconduct in Science.* Directorate for Science and Policy Programs, American Association for the Advancement of Science (AAAS Publication Number 92–13S) (1992).

12. American Association for the Advancement of Science, American Bar Association, National Conference of Lawyers and Scientists, and the Office of Scientific Integrity Review, Public Health Service, U.S. Department of Health and Human Services. *Misconduct in Science: Recurring Issues, Fresh Perspectives.* Conference Executive Summary. (November 15–16, 1991). Cambridge, Massachusetts.

13. The Associated Press. "Misconduct is Common—Scientists," *The Edmonton Journal* (November 13, 1993): A14.

14. Swazey, J. P., Anderson, M. S., and Seashore, L. K. "Encounters with Ethical Problems in Graduate Education: Highlights From National Surveys of Doctoral Students and Faculty," *Professional Ethics Report. Publication of the American Association for the Advancement of Science, Scientific Freedom, Responsibility and Law Program* VI(4) (fall 1993): 1–7.

15. Glick, J. L. and Shamoo, A. E. "A Call for the Development of 'Good Research Practices' (GRP) Guidelines," *Accountability in Research* 2 (1993): 231–35.

16. Bernier, R., ed. "NIH Actions Against Breast Cancer Researcher Raise Issues for Epidemiologists," *The New Epidemiology Monitor* 15 (1994): 1–2.

17. Shamoo, A. E. "Policies and Quality Assurance in the Pharmaceutical Industry," *Accountability in Research* 1 (1991): 273–84.

18. Grandjean, P. and Andersen, D. "Scientific Dishonesty: A Danish Proposal for Evaluation and Prevention," *Journal of Exposure Analysis and Environmental Epidemiology* 3 (Suppl. 1) (1993): 265–70.

19. Andersen, D., Attrup, L., Axelsen, N., and Riis, P. *Scientific Dishonesty & Good Scientific Practice.* The Danish Medical Research Council, 1992.

20. Soskolne, C. L. "Epidemiology: Questions of Science, Ethics, Morality, and Law," *American Journal of Epidemiology* 129 (1989): 1–18.
21. Soskolne, C. L. "Introduction to Misconduct in Science and Scientific Duties," *Journal of Exposure Analysis and Environmental Epidemiology* 3 (Suppl. 1) (1993): 245–51.
22. McCutchen, C. W. "Peer Review: Treacherous Servant, Disastrous Master," *Technology Review* (October 1991): 28–40.
23. Beauchamp, T. L., Cook, R. R., Fayerweather, W. E., Raabe, G. K., Thar, W. E., Cowles, S. R. and Spivey, G. H. "Ethical Guidelines for Epidemiologists," *Journal of Clinical Epidemiology* 44 (Suppl. 1) (1991): 151S–169S.
24. Russel, E. and Westrin, C-G. "Ethical Issues in Epidemiological Research: Guidelines Containing the Minimum Common Standards of Practice Recommended for Use by Project Leaders and Participants in the Operation of Future Concerted Actions." In Commission of the European Communities. *Medicine and Health: COMAC Epidemiology*, ed. Hallen and Vuylsteek. Luxembourg, 1992, pp. 19–22.
25. IEA Workshop on Ethics, Health Policy and Epidemiology. "Proposed Ethics Guidelines for Epidemiologists," ed. J. Last. *American Public Health Association (Epidemiology Section) Newsletter* (winter 1990): 4–6.
26. *Council for International Organizations of Medical Sciences International Guidelines for Ethical Review of Epidemiological Studies.* Geneva: CIOMS, 1991: 31.
27. *Council for International Organizations of Medical Sciences International Ethical Guidelines for Biomedical Research Involving Human Subjects.* Geneva: CIOMS, 1993: 63.
28. The Chemical Manufacturers Association's Epidemiology Task Group. "Guidelines for Good Epidemiology Practices for Occupational and Environmental Epidemiologic Research," *Journal of Occupational Medicine* 33 (12) (1991): 1221–29.
29. Office of the Assistant Secretary for Health, Public Health Service. *Guidelines for the Conduct of Research Within the Public Health Service.* U.S. Department of Health and Human Services, January 1, 1992, p. 18.
30. Weiss, T. "Too Many Scientists Who 'Blow the Whistle' End up Losing Their Jobs and Careers," *Chronicle of Higher Education* (June 1991): A36.
31. Westman, D. P. *Whistleblowing: The Law of Retaliatory Discharge.* Bureau of National Affairs, 1991.
32. Glazer, M. *The Whistleblowers: Exposing Corruption in Government and Industry.* New York: Basic Books (1989).
33. Price, A. R. "The United States Government Scientific Misconduct Regulations and the Handling of Issues Related to Research Integrity," *Journal of Exposure Analysis and Environmental Epidemiology* 3 (Suppl. 1) (1993): 253–64.
34. Sharphorn, D. H. "Integrity in Science: Administrative, Civil and Criminal Law in the U.S.A.," *Journal of Exposure Analysis and Environmental Epidemiology* 3 (Suppl. 1) (1993): 271–81.
35. Dale, M. L. "Integrity in Science: Misconduct Investigations in a U.S. University," *Journal of Exposure Analysis and Environmental Epidemiology* 3 (Suppl. 1) (1993): 283–95.
36. Soskolne, C. L., ed. "Questions from the Delegates and Answers by the Panelists Concerning 'Ethics and Law in Environmental Epidemiology,'" *Journal of Exposure Analysis and Environmental Epidemiology* 3 (Suppl. 1) (1993): 297–319.

37. "Tobacco Company Suppressed Addiction Study, Scientists Say," *The Edmonton Journal* (April 29, 1994): B12.
38. Soskolne, C. L. "Epidemiological Research, Interest Groups, and the Review Process," *Journal of Public Health Policy* 6 (1985): 173–184.
39. Soskolne, C. L. "Ethical Decision-Making in Epidemiology: The Case-Study Approach," *Journal of Clinical Epidemiology* 44 (Suppl. 1) (1991): 125S–130S.
40. Office of Research Integrity (ORI). "Case Summary: Fabricated and Falsified Clinical Trial Data," *ORI Newsletter* 1 (2) (April 1993): 2.
41. Office of Research Integrity (ORI). "Findings of Scientific Misconduct," *Federal Register* 58 (117) (June 21 Notices 1993): 33831.
42. "Downfall of a Breast Cancer Pioneer," *The Edmonton Journal* (April 10, 1994): C6.
43. "Second Hospital Investigated for False Data," *The Edmonton Journal* (March 30, 1994): A3.
44. The Associated Press. "Breast Cancer Research Data Falsified—Report," *The Edmonton Journal* (March 13, 1994): A4.
45. Adolph, C. "Cancer Patients Never Told Their Files Had Been Falsified." *The Edmonton Journal* (March 15, 1994): A3.
46. Anonymous. "Data Examined," *The Edmonton Journal* (March 16, 1994): A3.
47. "Decisions Based on False Data Still the Right Choice—Agency," *The Edmonton Journal* (April 14, 1994): D14.
48. The Canadian Press. "Fear, Anger Follow Revelation of False Data on Breast Cancer," *The Edmonton Journal* (March 14, 1994): A3.
49. Editorial. "When Science Turns to Fraud," *The Edmonton Journal* (March 18, 1994): A14.
50. Anonymous. "Cancer Patients Reassured: Conclusions of Study Still Valid Despite Some False Data," *The Globe and Mail* (March 15, 1994).
51. Shapiro I. M. "Speaking Out: Petition for a Colleague," *Almanac* (March 17, 1992): 3.
52. Begley, S. "Lead, Lies and Data Tape," *Newsweek* (March 16, 1992): 62.
53. Wohleber, C. "OSI Asks for Internal Inquiry. Needleman Challenged Again on Landmark 1979 Study of Low-Lead Exposure's Effects," *University Times* (January 9, 1992): 4.
54. Twedt, S. "Pitt Expert on Toxic Lead Has Research Challenged," *The Pittsburgh Press* (December 29, 1991): A1.
55. Spice, B. "Pitt to Review Charges Against Lead Researcher," *Pittsburgh Post-Gazette* (December 30, 1991): 4.
56. Needleman, H. L., Geiger, S. K. and Frank, R. "Lead and IQ Scores: A Reanalysis," *Science* 227 (1985): 701–04.
57. Committee on Government Operations Together with Dissenting and Additional Views. *Are Scientific Misconduct and Conflicts of Interest Hazardous to our Health?* Nineteenth Report. 101st Congress, 2d Session. Union Calendar No. 430, House Report 101–688, U.S. Government Printing Office, Washington, 1990, p. 74.
58. Francis, J. R. "The Credibility and Legitimation of Science: A Loss of Faith in the Scientific Narrative," *Accountability in Research* 1 (1989): 5–22.
59. *NIH Guide to Grants and Contracts* 18 (45) (December 1989).
60. *Federal Register* 54 (151), August 8 Rules and Regulations (1989): 32446–32451. DHHS-PHS 42 CFR Part 50. Responsibilities of awardee and applicant institutions for dealing with and reporting misconduct in science.

61. Mishkin, B. "PHS Rules on Scientific Integrity: Major Progress and Some Remaining Questions," *Professional Ethics Report. Newsletter of the American Association for the Advancement of Science* V (1) (1992): 5–6.

62. Medical Research Council of Canada, Natural Sciences and Engineering Research Council of Canada, Social Sciences and Humanities Research Council of Canada. *Integrity in Research and Scholarship: A Tri-Council Policy Statement.* (1994) Cat. No. CR22–29/1994; ISBN no. 0–662–60220–X.

63. Tosteson, D. C. *Faculty Policies on Integrity in Science.* Faculty of Medicine, Harvard University, 1992, p. 27.

64. Office of Research Integrity (ORI). "Research Ethics Training Supported in Principle, But not in Practice," *ORI Newsletter* 1 (2) (April 1993): 4–8.

65. Feinstein, A. R. "Fraud, Distortion, Delusion, and Consensus: The Problems of Human and Natural Deception in Epidemiologic Science," *The American Journal of Medicine* 84 (1988): 475–78.

66. *NIH Guide for Grants and Contracts Policies and Procedures for Dealing with Possible Scientific Misconduct* (July 1986).

67. *Federal Register* 53:181, (September 18, 1988), p. 36344.

68. Mishkin, B. "Report From the Trenches: Scientific Misconduct Definitions and Rules Revisited," *Professional Ethics Report. Publication of the American Association for the Advancement of Science, Scientific Freedom,* Responsibility and Law Program VI (2) (spring 1993): 4–5.

69. *Federal Register* 54:50, March 16 (1989), p. 11000.

70. Office of Research Integrity (ORI). "PHS Reorganizes Effort to Handle Research Misconduct," *ORI Newsletter* 1 (1) (January 1993): 1, 5.

71. *Federal Register* 57:216, November 6 (1992), p. 29809.

72. Barnes, D. M. "Focus on Fraud Shifts From the Conduct of Science to the Conduct of Investigations," *The Journal of NIH Research* 3 (1991): 35–37.

73. Hallum, J. W. and Hadley, S. W. "Scientific Misconduct: The Evolution of Method," *Professional Ethics Report. Newsletter of the American Association for the Advancement of Science* III (3) (summer 1990): 4–5.

74. "Opportunity for a Hearing on Office of Research Integrity Scientific Misconduct Findings." *Federal Register* 57(216) (November 6 Notices 1992): 53125–53126.

75. Hall, W. D. *Making the Right Decision: Ethics for Managers.* New York, NY: John Wiley & Sons, 1993: 248.

15

Toward an Ethics Curriculum in Epidemiology

KENNETH W. GOODMAN
RONALD J. PRINEAS

Additions to established university curricula are often viewed as avoidable entanglements. The schedule is full, the students busy, and the faculty stretched thin. Further, when specialized topics are considered, there is the additional problem of finding qualified faculty. Nevertheless, progress and problems in science and other disciplines inevitably force revisions and additions to existing curricula. We argue here that developments in epidemiology and ethics have attained such importance that they merit (1) development of course materials, (2) training of appropriate faculty members, and (3) inclusion of new courses in epidemiology, public health and other curricula. In addition, preliminary efforts to include ethics and epidemiology sessions in professional conferences should be expanded, and short courses, perhaps on special topics or problems, should be developed for students, practitioners, and university faculty.

There are a number of reasons for broadening the emphasis on ethics and epidemiology. First, epidemiology is a basic discipline whose security and rigor are essential for the development of an enlightened health policy. Because sloppy research or ethical shortcomings weaken scientific conclusions—or public confidence in them—there is a need to instruct students and practitioners in professional practice standards and in the ethical foundations of scientific inquiry. If flawed science is used as a basis for public health policy, it can have adverse health and economic consequences. To the extent that incompetent science can lead to wasted public resources or, worse, to poorer public health, it can be characterized as a misappropriation of public funds or a threat to public health.

Ethics-in-epidemiology courses need to be developed and linked in some way to courses on research design and analysis and health policy. Research issues are already a central part of epidemiology courses offered in North American universities and colleges; pedagogical links between epidemiology and health policy are less common. Coherent attempts to wed ethics with such hybrids are essential.

A second motivation for expanded bioethics education is that further development of appropriate curricula will stimulate research in bioethics and epidemiologic science. Serious and sustained attention to ethical issues in epidemiology is comparatively recent. This inchoate subfield is rich with opportunities to identify and analyze new issues, clarify existing problems, and contribute to decision making procedures for practitioners, policy makers, public officials, students, and others. Scientific research that could be stimulated by curricular development includes work on topics in which uncertainty or methodological controversy raise ethical issues (such as study design and meta-analysis). Several other avenues for research will be apparent in the discussion later of core components of an ethics-in-epidemiology course.

Third, a commitment to epidemiology, public health, or even science itself can lack focus and rigor and is weakened in the absence of a clear understanding of the values that shape inquiry and of the conflicts engendered by competing values. Expanded educational horizons offer opportunities to improve such understanding.

That scientific wrongdoing is blameworthy is neither controversial nor of special philosophical interest. Of greater interest is the fact that there are many ethical issues and conflicts that are more difficult to analyze and about which reasonable people disagree. There is a need, therefore, to provide a conceptual or analytical framework for critical decision making. Ethical problems and issues arise in a wide variety of circumstances, and it is not feasible to review or anticipate all possible situations. Nonetheless, introducing an analytical framework for ethical thinking can provide students with some of the tools necessary for evaluating different and even novel kinds of problems. Such thinking also prepares students to meet future problems of scientific misconduct.

A fourth reason for broadened attention to ethics is that idealistic graduate students may be put off by unethical behavior of others and dissuaded from research careers. Anecdotes are legion of would-be scholars ceasing to work in a particular field because of personal disillusionment due to unethical behavior of others (including mentors) in the field. Formal course work in ethics might help prevent this loss to scholarship by reassuring students about the profession's core values, and providing them with a yardstick for measuring and recognizing unethical practice.

There is nothing unique to epidemiology in these considerations. Concern about integrity is important in all areas of human inquiry. That epidemiology may be said to lag behind some areas of basic science, clinical research, and health policy in attention to ethics should be seen as providing an additional reason for development of a more fully fledged ethics component.

Finally, the rise of bioethics as a distinct field in the past twenty or twenty-five years has seen the emergence of a wide and rich variety of conceptual tools and unprecedented attention to ethical issues in medicine, scientific research, and health policy. Many of these issues are at the core of clinical practice and involve problems arising at the end of life, in obtaining valid consent, when protecting confidentiality, in assessing competence, when allocating resources, and the like. But bioethics and its curricula have also encompassed issues at the periphery of most medical and nursing practice. These include some areas of transplant medicine, such as xenographic transplants; questions that arise with rare diseases or disorders, including a growth of interest in problems in the medical subspecialties; and puzzles presented when patients have strange or false beliefs about the world or causation. Ethics in epidemiology and public health deserve at least as much attention as these rarely encountered components of what we may call "boutique ethics."

We are not suggesting that rare topics are not worthwhile targets for sustained conceptual analysis and policy debate. There is almost always much to be learned from such analyses and debate—and often much that can be applied in more familiar domains. Rather, we are arguing that the intersection of ethics and epidemiology is a fundamentally important domain on its own. The point can be made from another direction. Many bioethicists are competent to discuss ethical issues and problems in clinical medicine, nursing, surgery, critical care, and so forth. They are also well acquainted with ethical issues related to HIV and AIDS, resource allocation, human subjects research, and the like. However, few bioethicists have evidenced familiarity with issues in epidemiologic ethics and the growing literature in this area.

Some empirical evidence indicates support among epidemiologists in academia for broadened ethics curricula. A survey of faculty at U.S. schools of public health suggested that 86% of respondents thought ethics should be included in the curriculum; 66% said they had already included discussion of ethical issues in other courses.[1]

The upshot is that ethical issues in epidemiology should at least be offered—and, ideally, *featured*—in the epidemiology and public health curricula, and perhaps also in medical school curricula, graduate science curricula, nursing school curricula, and in appropriate courses in philosophy and the humanities. Links should be forged between and among these disciplines.

Core Components of a Course in Ethics and Epidemiology

We will now lay out some of the components of a course in ethics and epidemiology. Most of what follows will be intuitively obvious, and we will try to provide motivations for the rest.

Epidemiologists and moral philosophers have for some time recognized that epidemiology raises a number of interesting and important ethical issues. Some of these issues will be familiar to those who have an acquaintance with or background in bioethics and research ethics: informed consent, confidentiality, risk-benefit assessment, patient-subject rights, conflict of interest, allocation of resources, and so forth. Nevertheless, epidemiology often offers—or, rather, demands—a broader set of problems under these headings. For instance, what are a researcher's obligations in terms of informed consent in cultures in which family or village leaders are by custom expected to provide "consent by proxy" for kin or community (questions addressed by Tom Beauchamp in Chapter 2 and Robert Levine in Chapter 13)? Such cultural differences in ethical norms pose an ensemble of interesting challenges for epidemiologists.

Many ethical issues of concern to epidemiologists are rarely addressed in general bioethics. These include, to name just a few, the notion of "ethical imperialism,"[2,3] the danger of social and ethnic stigma arising from epidemiological findings,[4] and the tensions surrounding decisions whether, to what extent, and by which means to reveal public health risks to study communities.[5,6]

Fortunately, there is a rapidly accreting literature that focuses on these and other issues. In addition to this volume, a number of other collections have been prepared, and supplementary readings and topics might be drawn from them.[7-9]

A course in ethics and epidemiology should have the following immediate goals (as distinguished from the overarching goals surveyed earlier):

- To help students identify ethical issues, problems, and conflicts in epidemiology and public health.
- To examine the ways in which ethical issues in epidemiology are either like or unlike ethical issues in other health sciences.
- To provide a decision making procedure for approaching ethical issues, problems, and conflicts.
- To make plain the connections between sound science and (ethically and socially) responsible science.

The course should cover several specific topics, depending on available faculty resources. The topics itemized below are drawn from a graduate course, apparently one of the first of its kind, offered in 1994 in the Department of Epidemiology and Public Health at the University of Miami School of Medicine, and from a course offered in 1995 at Tulane University Medical Center's School of Public Health and Tropical Medicine.[10] The former was based in part on a review of some key texts in epidemiological ethics prepared for the American College of Epidemiology's Ethics and Standards of Practice Committee.[11]

Moral Foundations

It is here that students may be introduced to core concepts in moral philosophy and bioethics. Tom Beauchamp's review in Chapter 2 provides a useful survey of key issues in moral philosophy, with particular attention to epidemiological contexts. In general, students should be exposed to utilitarianism, a philosophy that right actions are those that produce the best possible social consequences, and Kantianism, a philosophy that demands that we respect persons as autonomous agents and never use them as means to another end. The long-standing conflict between these two theories is a rich source of moral debate and insight—though they are by no means the only important types of theory in moral philosophy.

Students should also be exposed to major current approaches to bioethics, another source of illuminating disagreement among philosophers. Depending on available time, student background, and faculty familiarity and intrepidness, students would profitably be exposed to a number of approaches to ethical decision making. (Selecting appropriate texts can be a challenge, and in the references immediately below the standard volumes are followed by more accessible articles.) The approaches emphasize: principles such as respect for autonomy, nonmaleficence (do no harm), beneficence (contribute to welfare), and justice;[12,13] moral rules and moral ideals supported by all rational and impartial persons;[14,15] casuistry, or case-based reasoning;[16,17] and some account of rights that emphasizes human rights.

At least as important is a review of relativism and universalism. Universalists argue that there are knowable truths that are independent of culture, era, and nationality, and that these different beliefs can be objectively assessed. The universalists are prepared to say that some cultures just have it wrong and that their activities violate human rights. Relativists deny this and identify morality as a more or less local phenomenon that cannot be separated from history, culture, nationality, or the like. They reject the possibility of finding a morally neutral vantage point from which to judge the correctness of other cultures' beliefs. *Cultural* relativism—the uncontroversial fact that different cultures embody different customs and values—is the source of a number of difficult and important problems in epidemiological ethics. These include varying stances toward, for example, informed consent (Marjorie Shultz, Chapter 5), acceptable risk (Steven Coughlin, Chapter 7), and confidentiality (Ellen Gold, Chapter 6). Research in cultures different from one's own provides a rich and ready source of examples. Students should be challenged to grapple with the differences between cultural relativism and moral relativism, and urged to identify and take a stand on the kinds of public health values that are often promoted as universal but sometimes disdained by local communities.

Duties, Responsibilities, and Practice Standards

Broadly shared values can and have been transmitted between generations of scientists. The universalist will say these are the best values, or the true ones; the relativist, simply *our* values. In either case, it is appropriate to share such values with students. This is the place to evaluate the relation between science and ethics, and to show that poorly wrought or sloppy science is not only an inefficient way to learn about the world, but is also wrong. It squanders resources, potentially puts people at risk, and wastes colleagues' time. These are *moral*—not merely *economic* or *efficiency*—considerations. We should affirm science's commitment to objective inquiry and not to special interests, mentors' responsibilities for students, and the open and unfettered enterprise of inquiry. Here too is an opportunity to raise several of the touchstone principles of scientific scholarship: the need to give credit where credit is due; the obligation not to fabricate or falsify data; the requirement to respect the scientific corpus and not bloat or pollute it with unnecessary or spurious publications; and the need to maintain coherent records and to share data. These topics are visited below, under the heading Communication, Publication, Intellectual Property, and Education.

The current fascination with ethical dilemmas creates the mistaken impression that ethics is chatty and impotent. It masks the fact that in case after case of scientific misconduct, what is wanted is not a clearer sense of right and wrong, but just the nerve or mettle to do right.

Valid Consent and Refusal

One of the most difficult problems facing epidemiologists is that of valid consent for subjects to participate in research (discussed by Tom Beauchamp in Chapter 2 and Marjorie Shultz in Chapter 5). This course component might address the following points and issues:

• Minimal criteria for valid consent (sufficient information, absence of undue coercion, and competence).
• The nature and context of valid refusal (informed refusal to participate).
• Embedded criteria addressing questions such as the competence requirement in psychological, psychiatric, drug use, and similar studies; the level of detail that is minimally required for informing potential subjects about risks; and whether monetary and other inducements constitute coercion or manipulation.
• Special problems that attach to informed consent forms and their readability, and the relation of readability to the criterion of "adequate information."
• Circumstances, if any, under which informed consent is not necessary.

- The role, function, and constitution of institutional review boards and other forms of supervisory review.
- The potential need for community consent.

Instructors should also familiarize students with historical milestones and documents that chart the evolution of relevant principles and requirements.

Privacy and Confidentiality

People expect that details about their personal lives will not be made public, and that they have a right not to have intruders gain inappropriate access to such information. As data-gathering and storage techniques progress, however, these presumptions are increasingly under strain (see Chapter 5, by Marjorie Shultz, and Chapter 6, by Ellen Gold). The following points and issues should be reviewed:

- Privacy and the degree to which it must be protected, and circumstances under which privacy may be violated.
- Right of epidemiologists to use data bases for purposes not originally foreseen, to advance science and inform policy.
- Confidentiality and minimal criteria for keeping linked records from inappropriate publication or other disclosure.
- Standards for data-base security and access, addressing criteria for legitimate requests for access.
- The relatively free use of unlinked information (where data and a person's identity are decoupled); the relation of this to contexts in which valid consent is presumed unnecessary.
- The need for explicit and rigorous justifications for use or maintenance of linked records.

The wedding of biology, genetics, and epidemiology also raises a number of important, but so far inadequately articulated, issues. Use of computers and networks to store and retrieve genetic information is a recent and growing phenomenon; it is reasonable to be concerned about the use of information retrieval techniques to identify genetic patterns or regularities or to acquire genetic information about individuals or groups.[18]

Risks, Harms, and Wrongs

The distinction among risks, harms, and wrongs (as well as potential benefits) is an important one (addressed by Steven Coughlin in Chapter 7). Epidemiologists should be given standards for evaluating the following:

- The notion of "acceptable risk."
- What constitutes a harm, and how this may vary by culture, community, or even individual.
- What constitutes a wrong, and how wronging differs from harming.
- The need to eliminate or minimize risks, harms, and wrongs, and steps for accomplishing this.
- Success in crafting ethically optimized studies, or those that maximize and justly distribute benefits and minimize risks.
- What constitutes a risk, harm, or wrong to a group or community, including the problem of research-related stigma.
- Relationship among risks, harms, and wrongs and their inclusion in informed consent documents and processes.
- The need for and role of truth telling by observers and experimenters; whether and in what contexts deception can be permitted.
- Use of placebos in clinical trials.[19]
- Role of disease prevention and issues in mass screening.
- Problems and issues that arise in studies involving special or vulnerable populations, including children, the elderly, indigenous peoples, and mental patients.

Sponsorship and Conflict of Interest

The question of professional allegiance finds its most difficult context in the arena of research sponsorship. The following topics should be addressed:

- Criteria for identifying appropriate and inappropriate sponsorship.
- Obligations, and limits to obligations, to sponsors and employers.
- What constitutes a conflict of interest.
- The extent to which the *appearance* of a conflict of interest should be avoided.
- Contexts in which potential or real conflicts should be revealed to subjects and others.

Communication, Publication, Intellectual Property, and Education

Unpublished research cannot easily advance the primary goal of improving public health. But publication of scientific results is sometimes problematic. The following considerations should be evaluated:

- Duties to communicate and problems in communicating study results to subjects, communities, sponsors, and others.
- Difficulties in accurate and balanced communication of risks, harms, and wrongs.

- Obligation to publish study results; effects of publication; responsibilities to colleagues and science.
- Issues in data management.
- Issues in publication and authorship, including overpublication and redundant publication.
- "Ownership" of results, as by a corporate sponsor; nature of intellectual property in epidemiology.
- Role of popular news media in communicating public health information.

Advocacy and Intercultural Conflict

While the primary epidemiological goal of improving public health is obvious, less clear is the appropriate stance researchers should take in attempts to use their findings. That is:

- In what contexts, if any, should epidemiologists become advocates for a particular health policy?[20]
- How should epidemiologists as advocates address issues of cultural difference? What if sincere health policy advocacy conflicts with values prevalent in a study community?
- Should the results of meta-analyses be relied on in formulating health policy?
- To what extent is it realistic and proper to demand of researchers a measure of sympathy and respect for values and customs that, for instance, they find objectionable? Contrarily, is it appropriate to use study results to advocate change in values, customs, or programs?

Integrating Ethics into the Epidemiology Curriculum

The course outlined above is but one component in a complete, institutional commitment to ethics in epidemiology. While it would be a happy development if all training programs in epidemiology and public health offered a course in ethics, it would leave unrealized an ensemble of curricular opportunities. Also, to offer a discrete ethics course and nothing else on the topic sends the tacit message that ethics can be dealt with autonomously or in isolation. An integration of bioethics will, in addition to a special course or courses, feature prominent discussion of bioethics in research methods, biostatistics, and other staples of the curriculum. It might include visiting speakers who give presentations on ethics, or special seminar, workshop, or journal club series that focus on ethical, policy, and social issues. Sessions for discussing current events might be both instructional and popular.

A commitment to bioethics will also realize the opportunity to teach and use faculty from other schools or departments—for example, exciting mixes of epidemiologists, statisticians, philosophers, lawyers, and public-policy experts. Journalists can help clarify some of the problems that arise in reporting risks. Computer scientists can be helpful in identifying issues in data-base security. Physicians and nurses can examine local public health problems that are culturally mediated. Links to course offerings in philosophy departments (such as philosophy of science, ethics, bioethics) and law schools could be especially useful for students with advanced interests.

In a much more ambitious program, an epidemiology ethics "track" or subspecialization could be contemplated. Consider the following sequence:

- Introduction to Bioethics (philosophy department)
- Introduction to Ethics in Epidemiology and Public Health (EPH)
- Ethical Theory (philosophy)
- Philosophy of Science (philosophy)
- Advanced Epidemiologic Ethics (EPH)
- Special Topics (various departments; an example would be a course on International Health Policy and Ethics [or Human Rights] in an international studies program)
- "Internship" on an institutional review board

Each of these components is already available or could be developed without undue administrative hardship at many universities. The real challenge will be to develop the introductory and advanced ethics and epidemiology courses.

Opportunity flows in more than one direction. Epidemiologists with some background in bioethics may be valuable to colleagues in other departments. Further, in addition to academic, institution-based graduate courses, as outlined above, there are other opportunities for developing curricula and promulgating practice and research in ethics in epidemiology. They can be considered under two headings: post-graduate short courses and workshops at epidemiologic society scientific meetings.

Post-Graduate Courses

Requirements for teaching ethics in epidemiology are currently embodied only in National Institutes of Health rules for support of research training programs. The requirements are for ethics training, without detailed specification of duration, format, or content. We believe that these requirements are often inadequately met by brief, infrequent, and poorly structured institutional lectures.

Because of the dearth of graduate course offerings, there is a continuing need for the development of formal, short courses in ethics in epidemiology for post-doctoral epidemiologists. The first such courses were offered in 1995 as part of well-known summer programs in Boston by the New England Epidemiology Institute and Tufts University, and in Ann Arbor by the University of Michigan School of Public Health.

Excellent models for the structure of intensive programs also exist in national and international courses in cardiovascular disease epidemiology supported by the National Heart, Lung and Blood Institute and the American Heart Association. The U.S. course is now in its eighteenth year and takes place in one location (Lake Tahoe, Nevada) for one week in August of each year. Here, selected faculty and students (limited to approximately thirty) meet in retreat surroundings, learning and living together for the duration of the course. Morning lectures are followed by article analysis seminars. In addition, separate discussion sessions are dedicated to research design or student-selected research problems.

Short courses have several distinct advantages over other presentations. First, students and faculty have maximum opportunity for learning from one another. Second, a bonding between students occurs, establishing a network of investigators, and resulting in the formation of new collaborative studies and national and international academic, institutional-based graduate courses. Third, students are immediately engaged by professional group discussion of problems and investigative areas with which they are directly involved.

Such courses require a dedicated core faculty and consulting researchers and thinkers in the field to examine progress and cutting-edge research and education.

Epidemiologic Society Workshops

In recent years, meetings of the American College of Epidemiology and the Society for Epidemiologic Research have featured brief (two-to-three-hour) seminars presented by faculty recruited by the American College of Epidemiology's Ethics and Standards of Practice Committee (ACE ESOPC). These seminars are an outgrowth of discussions of the ACE ESOPC, which was appointed by the ACE Board of Directors in 1990, and their primary focus has been the discussion of selected case histories by seminar faculty. The ACE ESOPC is collecting case histories for use in future ethics workshops and courses.

As formal graduate and post-graduate courses of ethics in epidemiology multiply, epidemiologic society involvement in ethics teaching and research could develop in a number of ways. These could include separate sessions for presentation of ethics research (including student papers), and debates of ethical issues that have not found universal consensus or resolution. Invited lecturers might also address ethical issues affecting health policy.

Such development requires ongoing support for ethics and standards-of-practice committees in their respective epidemiologic societies, and perhaps an interchange between and among societies.

Conclusions and Recommendations

There is a need to address ethical issues in a more complete and rigorous manner in epidemiology and public health curricula, and at the post-graduate and professional levels. There is a concomitant need for high-quality course materials, and for their evolution. Appropriate faculty members must be found or trained for these purposes. Such course development will improve the quality of public health research, stimulate research in science and ethics, clarify the values that guide epidemiologic inquiry, reduce attrition of idealistic students discouraged by unethical mentors, and raise epidemiology and public health ethics to a pedagogic level commensurate with their importance.

We are advocating nothing less than a change in the "standard of care" in epidemiology education. That is, the arguments here are not intended to support mere curricular niceties, but as *requirements* for training programs in epidemiology and public health. A failure to include some measure of bioethics training in the curriculum is itself both educationally and ethically blameworthy. Put differently, there has evolved an ethical obligation to address ethical issues.

Institutions, professional societies, industry, and government should devote appropriate financial resources and personnel to realizing these goals. Surely ethics in epidemiology and public health should enjoy a role that reflects their importance, their potential contributions, and their role in science and society.

Appendix
The Role of Moral Philosophy in Bioethics Training

It will be useful to address briefly a foundational problem that arises whenever bioethics is taught outside a philosophy department or to a group of people not formally trained in philosophy. If bioethics and other kinds of professional ethics are instances of applied philosophy, it is reasonable to require that students (construed broadly) acquire the relevant background in philosophical ethics. To reject this training altogether is comparable to contending that one might learn medicine and omit physiology, learn law and omit torts, or learn epidemiologic research methods and forgo biostatistics.

On the other hand, we have suggested, at least tacitly, that bioethics is a domain with which any epidemiology student, practitioner, or researcher ought to be familiar. It is preposterous to demand that nonphilosophers become philosophers for the sake of learning ethics in their discipline. Too many nonphilosophers have made outstanding contributions to bioethics for that to be required. The problem may be cast as follows: How is it possible to reconcile the need for instruction in professional ethics with the limited background in moral philosophy brought to bear by most students? It seems we risk either trivializing philosophy or daunting students.

This problem is related to the main goals of teaching medical, nursing, legal, and business ethics to college and graduate students. In the first section of this chapter we identified several goals that constitute reasons for expanding instruction in ethics and epidemiology. Three theses run through these, and they are paralleled in discussions about the main goals for teaching ethics to medical students.[21,22,23,24] Ethics instruction seeks either (1) to create moral practitioners; (2) to give practitioners tools for ethical decision making; or (3) to improve outcomes. The first goal may be unattainable if the objective is to form or reform *character*. However, the second and third goals are realistic, and we now have considerable experience in how to achieve them in professional ethics.

For our purposes, the following seems a reasonable and practical objective: Professional training in ethics in epidemiology, medicine, nursing, etc., must be at least leavened with philosophical instruction in basic categories and methods. But the nature of this goal should be made completely clear to students. These are exciting times in bioethics, with a variety of competing approaches, methods, and systems on the table. Students should learn of them, if not master them. They should understand that more than one moral philosophy may be helpful to them in their thinking. Administratively, this underscores the value of including a person well-trained in moral philosophy in any serious attempt to introduce ethics into epidemiology curricula. Otherwise, valid concerns will inevitably arise about the blind leading the blind.

References

1. Rossignol, A. M. and Goodmonson, S. "Are Ethical Topics in Epidemiology Included in the Graduate Epidemiology Curricula?" Washington, D.C.: Presentation to American Public Health Association annual meeting, 1994.
2. Angell, M. "Ethical Imperialism? Ethics in International Collaborative Research," *New England Journal of Medicine* 319 (1988): 1081–83.
3. Levine, R. J. "Informed Consent: Some Challenges to the Universal Validity of the Western Model," Z. Bankowski, J. H. Bryant, and J. M. Last, eds. *Ethics and Epidemiology: International Guidelines*. Geneva: Council for International Organizations of Medical Sciences (CIOMS), 1991: 47–58.
4. Gostin, L. "Ethical Principles for the Conduct of Human Subject Research: Population-Based Research and Ethics," *Law, Medicine and Health Care* 19 (1991): 175–183.
5. Sandman, P. M. "Emerging Communication Responsibilities of Epidemiologists," W. E. Fayerweather, J. Higginson, and T. L. Beauchamp, eds., Industrial Epidemiology Forum's Conference on Ethics in Epidemiology. *Journal of Clinical Epidemiology* 44 (Suppl. I) (1991): 41S–50S.
6. Higginson, J. and Chu, P. "Ethical Considerations and Responsibilities in

Communicating Health Risk Information," *Journal of Clinical Epidemiology* 44 (Suppl. I) (1991): 51S–56S.

7. Fayerweather, W. E., Higginson, J., and Beauchamp, T. L., eds. Industrial Epidemiology Forum's Conference on Ethics in Epidemiology, *Journal of Clinical Epidemiology* 44 (Suppl. I) (1991).

8. Bankowski, Z., Bryant, J. H., and Last, J. M., eds. *Ethics and Epidemiology: International Guidelines*. Geneva: Council for International Organizations of Medical Sciences (CIOMS), 1991.

9. Coughlin, S. S., ed. *Annotated Readings on Ethics in Epidemiology and Clinical Research*. Newton, MA: Epidemiology Resources, Inc., 1995.

10. Coughlin, S. S. "Ethics, Epidemiology and Public Health Research." New Orleans: Tulane University, School of Public Health and Tropical Medicine, draft syllabus, 1994.

11. Goodman, K. W. "Review and Analysis of Key Documents on Ethics and Epidemiology." Miami: University of Miami Forum for Bioethics and Philosophy manuscript, 1993, revised 1994.

12. Beauchamp, T. L. and Childress, J. F. *Principles of Biomedical Ethics*. 4th ed. New York: Oxford University Press, 1994.

13. Beauchamp, T. L. "The Four-principles Approach." In *Principles of Health Care Ethics*, ed. R. Gillon. London: John Wiley & Sons, 1994: 3–12.

14. Gert, B. *Morality: A New Justification of the Moral Rules*. New York: Oxford University Press, 1989.

15. Clouser, K. D. and Gert, B. "A Critique of Principlism," *Journal of Medicine and Philosophy* 15 (1990): 219–36.

16. Jonsen, A. R. and Toulmin, S. E. *The Abuse of Casuistry*. Berkeley: University of California Press, 1988.

17. Jonsen, A. R. "Casuistry as Methodology in Clinical Ethics," *Theoretical Medicine* 12 (1991): 295–307.

18. Goodman, K. W. "Ethics, Genomics and Information Retrieval," *Computers in Biology and Medicine*, in press.

19. Rothman, K. J. and Michels, K. B. "The Continuing Unethical Use of Placebo Controls," *New England Journal of Medicine* 331 (1994): 394–98.

20. Weed, D. L. "Science, Ethics Guidelines, and Advocacy in Epidemiology," *Annals of Epidemiology* 4 (1994): 166–171.

21. Culver, C. M., Clouser, K. D., Gert, B., et al. "Basic Curricular Goals in Medical Ethics," *The New England Journal of Medicine* 312 (1985): 253–56.

22. Pellegrino, E. D., Siegler, M., and Singer, P. A. "Teaching Clinical Ethics," *The Journal of Clinical Ethics* 1 (1990): 175–180.

23. Hafferty, F. W., and Franks, R. "The Hidden Curriculum, Ethics Teaching, and the Structure of Medical Education," *Academic Medicine* 69 (1994): 861–71.

24. Reiser, S. J. "The Ethics of Learning and Teaching Medicine," *Academic Medicine* 69 (1994): 872–76.

Index